Contents

Foreword

Being with persons who are dying has been one of the gifts in my work as a nurse. These experiences have greatly influenced my understanding of death and loss and my ability to be with individuals and families throughout this process. Helping nursing students become aware of their personal experiences with grief and loss has been the focus of a course I taught on *Death, Loss, Transition and Change* in my university life as a professor of nursing.

My teaching and practice as a nurse and psychotherapist have been greatly influenced by the work of Carl R Rogers and the person-centered approach developed by him. When I discovered his writings in my doctoral studies they gave voice to my own life experiences both personally and professionally. Soon thereafter, I had the opportunity to meet Carl which opened up a whole new chapter in my life as I became part of the network of people influenced by his work.

I have read Richard Bryant-Jefferies' book from both of these perspectives as well as my personal experiences in the deaths of loved ones. I believe the dialogues will be helpful to therapists in understanding the processes of grief and loss and the person-centered approach to counseling in response to them.

In *Counselling for Death and Dying: person-centered dialogues* Richard presents the experiences of two client-therapist relationships and the accompanying sessions the therapists have with supervision. The format for the dialogues is very useful and will be helpful for the therapist-reader who is seeking to understand both the person-centered framework and the issues that arise in bereavement counseling.

The dialogues are presented including the thoughts and feelings which come into the therapist's awareness. The information presented makes clear the therapist's responses in the person-centered framework. The path the therapist takes in maintaining his sensitivity to the client's process is easily followed. The thoughts of the therapist make clear the choices the therapist considers at various points in the process. In addition, the explanation of what is happening in the dialogue is interpreted by the author by material presented in boxes. This material is informative to the reader without disrupting the flow of the dialogue.

In the dialogues the inner life of the clients, Billy and Barbara, become real as they struggle to express their feelings of loss – Billy in the loss of his father and the meanings it held for him and Barbara in facing a diagnosis of cancer and impending death. Both of them explore their issues of loss, including the impact of their situations with family members.

For the therapists (and readers) the dialogues create rumblings in our own feelings of what it is like to lose loved ones, of what it might be like to face ones' own death. These stirred emotions are the focus for the supervision explorations presented.

What is most striking about the dialogues is the realness of the feelings present in this all too human experience as lived by the clients. What is most beautiful is the relationship of acceptance shared in being in this most intimate place together as client and therapist. The healing that occurs is understandable in the strength of their connectedness.

Perhaps the essence of the person-centered approach presented can be understood in the following discussion of empathy by the author:

> Therapeutic empathy is a genuine heartfelt response to a sensed presence within the client that is conveyed through the texture and tone of the therapeutic relationship into awareness of the therapist. It impacts on the therapist's awareness as a result of their being openly present and available to the client and to themselves. It is a level of relatedness that takes place beneath the words. Whether it is psychological depth or a matter of the degree of physical contact, is a matter for further reflection. But in these special moments there is a mutual reaching out and connecting. And in these moments it seems a healing energy becomes present, made possible by the presence of the therapeutic conditions (pp. 111–12)

Nowhere in the dialogues does one see evidence of stages of grief. Each person is unique in the feelings and meanings explored in their journeys through grief and loss.

Grace H. Chickadonz PhD, RN
Center for Human Encouragement
Rochester, NY
Professor Emeritus
Syracuse University, NY
June 2006

Foreword

I first started working with people facing life-threatening and life-shortening ill-nesses in the late seventies and early eighties. This was in the early days of what became known as Acquired Immune Deficiency Syndrome (AIDS) and the Human Immunodeficiency Virus (HIV). In those years being told you had AIDS, and even HIV, was seen as a confirmed diagnosis of very early death. My first training in counselling/therapy was in the psychodynamic approach. With this, and armed with an in-depth knowledge of the stage theories of loss and bereave-ment (for example, Elizabeth Kübler-Ross and Colin Murray Parkes), I was stunned to find that counselling/therapy didn't 'work'. I couldn't get people through the stages (which to be fair was never the intention of Kübler-Ross and Parkes in the first place) and I couldn't see how I could help. It was about the same time I came across the work of Carl Rogers. Here was a theorist and practitioner who articulated something that I was becoming vaguely aware of – that simply entering into a relationship with people (in my case those facing life-shortening conditions) truly, deeply, with love and without fear was what 'worked', was what helped. Perhaps I should be clear what I mean by it 'worked'. People found the fortitude and courage to deal with their prognosis in a way that was most healthy for them. For some that meant moving in and out of the stages of grief we know (in theory) so well. For others, it meant moving in and out of some stages and not experiencing others. For yet other people, it meant facing death and bereavement in a completely different way. If you look carefully at the rela-tionships written of in this book, you will find evidence of the stages of loss and bereavement. You will also find evidence of how people move towards their own solutions in their own ways, ways that don't fit with traditional theories of loss and bereavement.

I'm not really sure why death and dying has received so little attention in person-centred writings. Perhaps it is because, unlike other issues practitioners face, it is guaranteed that we will all be faced with death and dying. Does this feel too much to deal with? Is it too much of a challenge to our congruence? It seems to me that for us to practise effectively in our work as counsellors/thera-pists it is imperative that we address this issue. The dynamic of loss generally is, I believe, an important motif in all our work as counsellors/therapists. People come to us because they are no longer happy (they have lost their happiness) or some-thing is not quite right (they have lost their ease). Whilst the issues raised in this book may seem specific to death and dying, they are present in most, if not all, of our work. The questions of how we respond remain the same; they are simply more challenging.

Richard has a deep understanding of the approach both in theory and practice and has brought this understanding to this greatly neglected area in person-centred literature. When he first embarked on this series of Person-Centred Dialogues, I have to admit to being a bit doubtful. I was doubtful as to whether such an endeavour, that of bringing to life the therapeutic process, could be achieved without either caricaturing the person-centred counselling/therapy or denigrating the experience of those who come to counselling and/or therapy. The worst case scenario was, of course, that both my fears would be confirmed. The profundity and emotional texture of each counselling experience, unique to client and therapist alike, is extremely difficult to convey to another person. It is not unlike trying to explain the dream I had last night. I can give a general feel, a general outline of what happened, but am not able to fully communicate the subtle moods, colours and landscapes of the dream. Just like in the telling of my dream, I am trying to describe happenings in one state of consciousness (the therapeutic meeting) whilst in another state of consciousness (outside the therapeutic meeting). Whilst this is typical for all orientations in counselling/therapy, it is particularly true of person-centred counselling/therapy. Person-centred practitioners only have themselves to offer to a client; no specific interventions, no techniques that can be more easily described, no treatment plans, no speculation as to the motives of the client – only themselves. How could such a process be translated into black and white print on a flat page? With the publication of *Time Limited Therapy in Primary Care* my fears were allayed. Richard has the talent as a writer to honour the client, the counsellor/therapist, the supervisor and the process in all its intricacies. As each book in the series has been written, this talent and skill has developed and so we come to the last in the series, *Counselling for Death and Dying*.

I was asked if I would like to write a foreword to this book six months after my partner had died and two or three weeks after my mother had died. I wasn't sure that I was up to it, both in terms of my own process (for example not being able to string coherent sentences together, never mind write them!) and in terms of being able to read a book of this nature. I'm glad I accepted. Richard has produced a book that, to my mind, captures the pain, the joy, the challenge of being with someone bereaved and someone facing death. It also captures the pain and hurt and confusion of being that person who is bereaved or facing death. The dialogues in this book, between client and therapist, therapist and supervisor, also capture what it is to be a person-centred counsellor/therapist and how we might fully enter the world of another person who is in pain. That he has managed to capture all these aspects is a testament to his writing talent, his commitment to the person-centred approach, and his deep dedication to the person-hood of those people we call clients.

Sheila Haugh
Senior Lecturer
Convenor, British Association for the Person-Centred Approach
June 2006

Preface

Counselling for Death and Dying: person-centred dialogues has been written with the aim of demonstrating the counsellor's application of the person-centred approach (PCA) in working with this client group which is becoming an increasing feature of our society. This theoretical approach to counselling has, at its heart, the power of the relational experience. It is this experience that I believe to be at the very heart of effective therapy, contributing to the possibility of releasing the client to realise greater potential for authentic living. The approach is widely used by counsellors working in the UK today: in a membership survey by the British Association for Counselling and Psychotherapy in 2001, 35.6% of those responding claimed to work to the person-centred approach, while 25.4% identified themselves as psychodynamic practitioners. However, whatever the approach, it seems to me that the relationship is the key factor in contributing to a successful outcome – though this must remain a very subjective concept, for who, other than the client, can really define what experience or change is to be taken as a measure of a successful outcome?

The success of the preceding volumes in the *Living Therapy* series, and the continued appreciative comments received from readers and by independent reviewers, is encouragement enough to once again extend this style into exploring the application of the person-centred approach to counselling and psychotherapy to another challenging area of human experience – working with the bereaved, or those who are facing the imminent prospect of their own death or that of a loved one. Again and again people remark on how readable these books are, how much they bring the therapeutic process alive. In particular, students of counselling and psychotherapy have remarked on how accessible the text is. Trainers and others experienced in the field have indicated to me the timeliness of a series that focuses the application of the person-centred approach to working therapeutically with clients who have particular issues. And counsellors and therapists from other approaches have also indicated the value of the style of these books, offering an opportunity to reflect on how, from their theoretical perspective, they would respond to the clients and the issues I present.

However, this, the seventeenth English language title, is planned to be the last one in the *Living Therapy* series. People often ask me what motivates me to write them. My answer is simply the hope that through these books I can make a difference, a positive difference, to people and to their lives. I firmly believe that while human relationships can and do damage people, they are also the most marvellous source of healing. And for me, the principles and values of the person-centred approach, as described in this volume and the preceding ones, set the standard. Whatever the approach to therapy, the relationship between client and therapist is crucial and, from the person-centred approach, key. I don't think we fully understand or appreciate the power of human relationship. I don't believe we understand the mechanisms through which relationship impacts on consciousness. For me this *is* the next frontier in understanding human beings.

Throughout the series I have wanted the style of writing to draw people into the narrative and make them feel engaged with the characters and the therapeutic process. I have wanted this series to be what I would term 'an experiential read'. I was heartened that in my last title, *Counselling Young Binge Drinkers* (Bryant-Jefferies, 2006), Peter Wilson wrote in his Foreword of how:

> too often in case presentations, the emphasis is on the client's disturbance and with due reference to theory. Less attention is paid to the emotional texture of what it is that is happening between the participants involved. What is it that goes through the heads of psychotherapists and counsellors as they practise and what is on the minds of those in receipt of such practice? What is the experience on either side of the table as it were and what is developing beyond the realms of established technique and strategy?

I like the notion of 'emotional texture' and the idea of 'something developing beyond the realms of established technique and strategy'. I hope that I have managed to convey some insight and some answers to his questions not only in this volume, but throughout the series.

As with the other volumes of the *Living Therapy* series, *Counselling for Death and Dying: person-centred dialogues* is composed of fictitious dialogues between fictitious clients and their counsellors, and between the counsellors and their supervisors. Within the dialogues are woven the reflective thoughts and feelings of the clients, the counsellors and the supervisors, along with boxed comments on the process and references to person-centred theory. I do not seek to provide all the answers, or a technical manual expounding on the right way to work with people facing death or the consequences of a person's death. Rather, I want to convey something of the process of working with representative material that can arise so that the reader may be stimulated into processing their own reactions, reflecting on the relevance and effectiveness of the therapeutic responses, and to thereby gain insight into themselves and their practice. Often it will simply lead to more questions, which I hope will prove stimulating to readers and encourage them to think through their own theoretical, philosophical and ethical positions and their boundary of competence.

Counselling for Death and Dying: person-centred dialogues is intended as much for experienced counsellors as it is for trainees. It provides real insight into what can occur during counselling sessions. I hope it will raise awareness of, and inform, not only person-centred practice within this context, but also contribute to other theoretical approaches within the world of counselling, psychotherapy and the various branches of psychology. Reflections on the therapeutic process and points for discussion are included to stimulate further thought and debate. This volume also contains material to inform the training process of counsellors and others who seek to work with those affected by death, dying and bereavement.

I hope this book will demonstrate the value, relevance and effectiveness of this approach, providing as it does a very human response to what is the one inevitable experience that we all have to face at some time in our lives – the death of a loved one, and thoughts and feelings with regard to our own deaths. I hope that in this volume I am able to address a range of themes that leave you, the reader, with much to reflect on and to take into your professional work, whether it is counselling or some other discipline, and whatever the setting.

Richard Bryant-Jefferies
June 2006

About the author

Richard Bryant-Jefferies qualified as a person-centred counsellor/therapist in 1994 and remains passionate about the application and effectiveness of this approach. Between early 1995 and mid-2003 Richard worked at a community drug and alcohol service in Surrey as an alcohol counsellor. Since 2003 he has worked for the Central and North West London Mental Health NHS Trust. While his permanent role has been to manage substance misuse services within the Royal Borough of Kensington and Chelsea in London, he is currently working to promote equality and diversity issues across the Trust. He has experience of offering both counselling and supervision in NHS, GP and private settings, and has provided training through 'alcohol awareness and response' workshops. He also offers workshops based on the use of written dialogues as a contribution to continuing professional development and within training programmes. See www.bryant-jefferies.freeserve.co.uk

Richard had his first book on a counselling theme, *Counselling the Person Beyond the Alcohol Problem*, published in 2001 (Jessica Kingsley Publishers). It provides theoretical yet practical insights into the application of the person-centred approach within the context of the 'cycle of change' model that has been widely adopted to describe the process of change in the field of addiction. Since then he has been writing for the *Living Therapy* series, producing an ongoing series of person-centred dialogues: *Problem Drinking*; *Time Limited Therapy in Primary Care*; *Counselling a Survivor of Child Sexual Abuse*; *Counselling a Recovering Drug User*; *Counselling Young People*; *Counselling for Progressive Disability*; *Relationship Counselling: sons and their mothers*; *Responding to a Serious Mental Health Problem*; *Person-Centred Counselling Supervision: personal and professional*; *Counselling Victims of Warfare*; *Workplace Counselling in the NHS*; *Counselling for Problem Gambling*; *Counselling for Eating Disorders in Men*; *Counselling for Eating Disorders in Women*; *Counselling for Obesity*; and *Counselling Young Binge Drinkers*. The aim of the series is to bring the reader a direct experience of the counselling process, an exposure to the thoughts and feelings of both client and counsellor as they encounter each other on the therapeutic journey, and an insight into the value and importance of supervision.

In 2006, Pen Press will publish what Richard has entitled *A Little Book of Therapy*. This little book offers a series of statements that clients might make during periods of stress, self-doubt or uncertainty, and affirmations to help reframe their perspective and offer opportunity for the reader to engage with the inner resources for change that people have within them.

Richard has written his first novel, *Dying to Live*, a story of traumatic loss, alcohol use and the therapeutic process. He is currently seeking a publisher. He has also adapted *Counselling a Survivor of Child Sexual Abuse* as a stage or radio play, and plans to do the same to other books in the series if the first is successful. He is currently seeking an opportunity for it to be recorded or staged.

Bringing the experience of the therapeutic process, from the standpoint and application of the person-centred approach, to a wider audience is an important motivation for Richard. He is convinced that the principles and attitudinal values of this approach and the emphasis it places on the therapeutic relationship are key to helping people create greater authenticity both in themselves and in their lives, leading to a fuller and more satisfying human experience. By writing fictional accounts to try and bring the therapeutic process alive, to help readers engage with the characters within the narrative – client, counsellor and supervisor – he hopes to take the reader on a journey into the counselling room. Whether we think of it as pulling back the curtains or opening a door, it is about enabling people to access what can and does occur within the therapeutic process.

Acknowledgements

With this book being the last in the *Living Therapy* series I feel caught between wanting to acknowledge those directly involved in my writing of this current title, and those involved over recent years in my writing the whole series.

I would like to thank Sheila Haugh from the UK for her foreword to *Counselling for Death and Dying*, and acknowledge her courage in agreeing to write for this book. Sheila was one my trainers in person-centred counselling and psychotherapy in the early 1990s and she agreed to write her foreword having only recently lost her partner and then her mother. I know that what she has written is an expression of her own experience of living through the process of being with loved ones facing death and coming to terms with her own sense of loss.

I would also like to thank Grace Chickadonz from the USA who has both a nursing and psychotherapy background, for her foreword, particularly given her experience of training nurses in Death, Loss, Transition and Change. She too has had her own deeply personal experiences of death of close relatives.

I also wish to thank the Cancer Information Nurses at Cancer Research UK* for their help in providing me with extremely pertinent information to ensure that the scenario in Part 2 is clinically realistic.

Insofar as the *Living Therapy* series is concerned, I wish to thank everyone at Radcliffe Publishing who have been involved in all aspects of producing this series: editorial, sales, promotion and marketing. So many people have contributed to making the series possible. In particular Maggie Pettifer for her encouragement, editorial input and for putting me in touch with Radcliffe Publishing in the first place! Thank you all.

I also wish to acknowledge once again my partner, Movena Lucas, for her continued support and input throughout this creative process, for the many discussions we have had about themes and content, and for her continued support for the project from beginning to end. Coming into my life when you did, you have been the major catalyst in triggering this particular creative process. Thank you, Movena.

I would like to thank once again all the foreword writers from around the world, and all those friends and colleagues who have fed back constructive

---

* Cancer Research UK, PO Box 123, London WC2A 3PX. Tel: 020 7061 8355. http://www.cancerresearchuk.org; cancer.info@cancer.org.uk. Also their website for patient information: http://www.cancerhelp.org.uk

comment to me that has contributed to the content of each volume and to the series development.

And finally, I wish to acknowledge my clients and supervisees from over the years who have opened my heart and mind to the diversity of human experience, the issues, the challenges, the hopes, the pain, the struggles and the achievements that people face. I have learned that becoming a person-centred counsellor offers an opportunity for self-learning and development. You step on to a conveyer belt of learning. I hope this series has given something back. Yes, the books may be written for counsellors and therapists to read, but in the final analysis they have been written to have constructive effect on clients, on the people who are struggling with issues, or trying to make sense of their lives. I hope that the reading of these books will make a difference and encourage therapists, of all persuasions, approaches and indeed all helping professionals to more deeply understand the living application of the person-centred, and to acknowledge that relationship truly lies at the heart of therapeutic effectiveness.

Introduction

It seems a strange question to ask, but what do we mean by death and dying? We know what these terms mean in relation to the actual physical process. But what of the psychological process? What happens for a person emotionally, psychologically and spiritually when confronted by the reality of the death of a loved one, or the impending death of someone close to them, or their own death?

It seems to me that this is a very personal experience and that there is a danger in suggesting that people have to pass through sequential stages of experiencing when 'adjusting' (if that is the best term) to a life-threatening diagnosis or the loss of a loved one. From a person-centred perspective there is a need to honour the uniqueness of each person in finding their own way to come to terms with what can be one of the most profound, challenging and painful aspects of being alive. In the book *Reflective Helping in HIV and AIDS* (Anderson and Wilkie, 1992), which focuses specifically on working with people with HIV, Anderson suggests a 'need to avoid using particular descriptive theories in a prescriptive manner'. He quotes Green and Sherr in describing how helpers sometimes:

> come to feel that unless people experience certain feelings or deal with those feelings in certain ways they will suffer psychological of even physical harm. Trying to force what happens to real people into rigid prescriptive theoretical models is at best unhelpful, at worst it prevents counsellors seeing what is really happening and makes them see only what they *expect* to see. (1989, p. 207)

Of course, there is not only the matter of the way that one works with people facing death or adjusting to the loss of a loved one. There is also the matter of belief, and this in turn will be governed to some degree, and sometimes largely, by cultural factors. Most people believe in some form of continuity of consciousness after death. Whether it is defined in terms of a Heaven, a Paradise or back on Earth in another body, this notion of continuity is the belief that most people carry with them on a daily basis. Some also believe in a Hell, a state of eternal damnation. Yet others take the view that this is it, one life, one death and nothing more. Death at the end of life is existential death.

Some people claim to have memories of past lives; others dispute this and question the validity of such ideas. In truth, death is a conundrum, and people make sense of it, and find ways of handling the thoughts and feelings that become present when they consider death and dying, in many different ways. I myself, as a counsellor, would hope to feel able to respect each person's belief system. Any person's inner world, within which their beliefs about life and death are a significant feature, has been constructed by them as an expression of how they make sense of the world, themselves and the concept of death.

Having said that, I do not want to suggest that it is always a free choice. Some people do experience an indoctrination as to what they should or should not believe in. When confronted by death and dying, the person may cling more desperately to these beliefs, yet they may also find themselves facing the unravelling of their beliefs as they are found not to satisfy the questions and experiencing they pass through. I believe that people should feel able to reflect freely on the different views of death and what may or may not follow, and draw their own conclusions based on their own life experience and what, for them, feels instinctively right or satisfies the questionings they may have in their own minds, or what simply enables them to make sense of what it is to be a human being.

Recent years have seen a growth in thinking and understanding of the psychological processes associated with death, dying and bereavement. Many individuals have contributed to the development of approaches to working with people who have suffered bereavement, or who are facing death, in particular Elizabeth Kübler-Ross. More services are now provided for people experiencing bereavement, for instance the national bereavement counselling service Cruse. The hospice movement has had a profound impact on the provision of care for those who are dying or who are in acute pain, and with this has also come advances in, and expanded provision of, palliative care services.

So it seems timely to present a person-centred approach to counselling for death and dying. Parts 1 and 2 of *Counselling for Death and Dying* deal with the process and application of the person-centred approach to working with clients for whom death and dying have become a significant factor in their lives. In Part 1, a client faces up to the effects of, and the adjustments he needs to make following, the death of his father. In Part 2, a client faces her own death – after a late diagnosis of cancer – and must come to terms not only with this, but also the loss of her future role within her troubled family.

The rest of this introduction provides an introduction to the theory of person- or client-centred counselling and psychotherapy. It is presented in general terms deliberately, with occasional references to the theme of this book, so that the reader gains a more general overview of person-centred theoretical principles and their application before engaging more fully with its practice in the context of this book's theme.

The person-centred approach

The person-centred approach (PCA) was formulated by Carl Rogers, and references are made to his ideas within the text of this book in relation to the theme of death and dying. However, it will be helpful for readers who are unfamiliar with this way of working to have an appreciation of its theoretical base. This section provides a general overview of person-centred theory.

Rogers proposed that certain conditions, when present within a therapeutic relationship, would enable the client to develop towards what he termed 'fuller functionality'. Over a number of years he refined these ideas, which he defined as 'the necessary and sufficient conditions for constructive personality change'. These he described as:

1   two persons are in psychological contact
2   the first, whom we shall term the client, is in a state of incongruence, being vulnerable or anxious
3   the second person, whom we shall term the therapist, is congruent or integrated in the relationship
4   the therapist experiences unconditional positive regard for the client
5   the therapist experiences an empathic understanding of the client's internal frame of reference and endeavours to communicate this experience to the client
6   the communication to the client of the therapist's empathic understanding and unconditional positive regard is to a minimal degree achieved (Rogers, 1957, p. 96).

The first necessary and sufficient condition given for constructive personality change is that of 'two persons being in psychological contact'. However, although he later published this as simply 'contact' (Rogers, 1959), it is suggested (Wyatt and Sanders, 2002, p. 6) that this was actually written in 1953–54. They quote Rogers as defining contact in the following terms: 'Two persons are in psychological contact, or have the minimum essential relationship when each makes a perceived or subceived difference in the experiential field of the other' (Rogers, 1959, p. 207). A recent exploration of the nature of psychological contact from a person-centred perspective is given by Warner (2002).

Contact

There is much to reflect on when considering a definition of 'contact' or 'psychological contact'. We might think of this in terms of whether the therapist's presence is, to some minimal degree, impacting on the awareness of the client; that, if you like, the field of awareness of the client is affected by the therapist. And, of course, the opposite holds, that the client's presence is also impacting on the field of awareness of the counsellor. It is the first condition given, and arguably the foundation for therapy. It does not necessarily mean, however, that client and therapist are sitting together in the same room, hence telephone and internet counselling also involve contact. Whatever the situation, contact or psychological contact is indicated by each having awareness of the other.

In terms of therapeutic significance, are there degrees of contact? Is it true that contact is a matter of being either present or not, or is there a kind of continuum of contact, with greater or lesser degrees or depths of contact? It seems to me that it is both, that rather like the way in which light may be regarded as either a particle or a wave, contact may be seen as either a specific state of being or a process, depending on what the perceiver is seeking to measure or observe. If I am trying to observe or measure whether there is contact, then my answer will be in terms of 'yes' or 'no'. If I am seeking to determine the degree to which contact exists, then the answer will be along a continuum. In other words, from the moment of minimal contact there is contact, but that contact can then extend as more aspects of the client become present within the therapeutic relationship, which itself may at times reach moments of increasing depth.

Empathy

Rogers defined empathy as meaning 'entering the private perceptual world of the other ... being sensitive, moment by moment, to the changing felt meanings which flow in this other person.... It means sensing meanings of which he or she is scarcely aware, but not trying to uncover totally unconscious feelings' (Rogers, 1980, p. 142). It is a very delicate process, and it provides a foundation block for effective person-centred therapy. The counsellor's role is primarily to establish empathic rapport and communicate empathic understanding to the client. This latter point is vital. Empathic understanding has therapeutic value only where it is communicated to the client.

I would like to add another comment regarding empathy. There is so much more to empathy than simply letting the client know what you understand from what they have communicated. It is also, and perhaps more significantly, the actual *process* of listening to a client, of attending – facial expression, body language and presence – that is being offered and communicated and received *at the time that the client is speaking, at the time that the client is experiencing what is present for them*. It is for the client, the knowing that in the moment of an experience the counsellor is present and striving to be an understanding companion.

Unconditional positive regard

Within the therapeutic relationship the counsellor seeks to maintain an attitude of unconditional positive regard towards the client and all that they disclose. This is not 'agreeing with', it is simply warm acceptance of the fact that the client is being how they need or choose to be. Rogers wrote, 'when the therapist is experiencing a positive, acceptant attitude towards whatever the client *is* at that moment, therapeutic movement or change is more likely to occur' (Rogers, 1980, p. 116). Mearns and Thorne suggest that:

unconditional positive regard is the label given to the fundamental attitude of the person-centred counsellor towards her client. The counsellor who holds this attitude deeply values the humanity of her client and is not deflected in that valuing by any particular client behaviours. The attitude manifests itself in the counsellor's consistent acceptance of and enduring warmth towards her client. (Mearns and Thorne, 1988, p. 59)

Both Bozarth (1998) and Wilkins assert that 'unconditional positive regard is the curative factor in person-centred therapy' (Bozarth and Wilkins, 2001, p. vii). It is perhaps worth drawing these two statements together speculatively. We might then suggest that the unconditional positive regard experienced and conveyed by the counsellor, and received by the client as an expression of the counsellor's valuing of their client's humanity, has a curative role in the therapeutic process. We might then add that this may be the case more specifically for those individuals who have been affected by a lack of unconditional warmth and prizing in their lives.

Congruence

Congruence is a state of being that Rogers has also described in terms of 'realness', 'transparency', 'genuineness' and 'authenticity'. Indeed Rogers wrote that '. . . genuineness, realness or congruence . . . this means that the therapist is openly being the feelings and attitudes that are flowing within at the moment. The term transparent catches the flavour of this condition' (Rogers, 1980, p. 115). Putting this into the therapeutic setting, we can say that 'congruence is the state of being of the counsellor when her outward responses to her client consistently match the inner feelings and sensations which she has in relation to her client' (Mearns and Thorne, 1999, p. 84). Interestingly, Rogers makes the following comment in his interview with Richard Evans that with regard to the three conditions, 'first, and most important, is therapist congruence or genuineness . . . one description of what it means to be congruent in a given moment is to be aware of what's going on in your experiencing at that moment, to be acceptant towards that experience, to be able to voice it if it's appropriate, and to express it in some behavioural way' (Evans, 1975).

I would suggest that any congruent expression by the counsellor of their feelings or reactions has to emerge through the process of being in therapeutic relationship with the client. Indeed, the condition indicates that the therapist is congruent or integrated into the relationship. This indicates the significance of the relationship. Being congruent is a disciplined way of being and not an open door to endless self-disclosure. Congruent expression is perhaps most appropriate and therapeutically valuable where it is informed by the existence of an empathic understanding of the client's inner world, and is offered in a climate of a genuine warm acceptance towards the client. Having said that, taking account of Rogers' comment quoted above that congruence is 'most important', it is reasonable to suggest that unless the therapist is congruent in themselves and in the relationship, then their empathy and unconditional positive regard would be at risk of not being authentic or genuine.

Another view, however, would be that it is in some way false to distinguish or rather seek to separate the three 'core conditions', that they exist together as a whole, mutually dependent on each other's presence in order to ensure that therapeutic relationship is established.

Perception

There is also the sixth condition, of which Rogers wrote:

> the final condition ... is that the client perceives, to a minimal degree, the acceptance and empathy which the therapist experiences for him. Unless some communication of these attitudes has been achieved, then such attitudes do not exist in the relationship as far as the client is concerned, and the therapeutic process could not, by our hypothesis, be initiated. (Rogers, 1957)

It is interesting that he uses the words 'minimal degree', suggesting that the client does not need to fully perceive the fullness of the empathy and unconditional positive regard present within, and communicated by, the counsellor. A glimpse warmly accepted, accurately heard and empathically understood is enough to have positive therapeutic effect, although logically one might think that the more that is perceived, the greater the therapeutic impact. But if it is a matter of intensity and accuracy, then a client experience of a vitally important fragment of their inner world being empathically understood and warmly accepted may be more significant to them, and more therapeutically significant, than a great deal being heard less accurately and with a weaker sense of therapist understanding and acceptance. The communication of the counsellor's empathy, congruence and unconditional positive regard, received by the client, creates the conditions for a process of constructive personality change.

The vital importance of contact and of the client perceiving the presence of the counsellor's unconditional positive regard and empathic understanding towards them cannot be understated. Conditions one and six of the necessary and sufficient conditions for constructive personality change as formulated by Rogers have become a focus for theoretical discussion and debate, and rightly so. While they may not represent 'core conditions' insofar as the attitudinal qualities of empathy, congruence and unconditional positive regard are concerned, they provide the relational framework through which these attitudinal qualities can have therapeutic value and effect. Indeed, without the presence of contact and perception as described by Rogers (1957, 1959), there would be no relational framework for the therapeutic process to occur. It leaves us in the position that perhaps conditions one (contact) and six (perception) are in reality the 'primary core conditions' as they define the presence of a relationship. Then, unconditional positive regard and empathic understanding might be seen to define the quality of the relationship, while client incongruence and counsellor congruence define the state of being brought into the relationship. Taken together there emerges the existence of what we might then term a 'person-centred therapeutic relationship'.

Earlier, I drew attention to the notion that 'unconditional positive regard is the curative factor in person-centred therapy' (Bozarth and Wilkins, 2001, p. vii). Is one element the curative factor? Or is it the combination of factors? Or is it perhaps more complex than this, and the curative factor is actually more closely linked to the person or the client coming into therapy? Does the need of the client define the nature of the curative factor?

The suggestion that I want to make is that, yes, for clients whose difficulties lie in experiencing an absence of love, then unconditional positive regard may well be the most important relational experience for them and the one that carries or conveys the greatest healing potential. But what of the person whose psychological distress is linked to early (or later) life experiences in which they have been affected by people not listening to them, not trying to understand them, who have been left feeling that they are not understood, cannot be understood? Could it be that for them the presence of empathy within the therapeutic relationship might be the most significant healing factor, enabling them to redefine themselves in the context of feeling heard and understood? And if this is so, then could this same line of thought be extended to the person who was always lied to, who was never given straight answers, or whose early life experience was one in which significant others, through their own states of incongruence, constantly gave confusing and contradictory messages, leaving the person unable to know who to trust, what to trust and, in extreme cases, how to trust? Could it not be that for such a person, the presence of congruence, of authenticity and genuineness, might be the factor that carries the greatest curative or healing influence? And what of the child who was ignored, left to watch videos or play on their own, with little quality human relational experience? Could psychological contact be particularly important for them, the sense of another person offering them quality attention and relational interaction?

This is not to suggest that any of these alone would be enough, they need to be present alongside the other therapeutic conditions, but perhaps some are more significant or important than others in the context of what has been the core damaging factor in the experience of the client. To state it simply, those who have not been loved most need to feel loved, those who have not been heard or understood most need to be listened to, those who have been impacted on by the incongruence of others most need to experience a relationship full of authenticity, and those who were isolated and ignored need to feel contact and attention.

When it comes to counselling for bereavement or those facing death, their experience is likely to be affected by the conditioning effects of their past experiences. A history of loss, or significant loss at impressionable ages, may make the loss aspect of bereavement more unbearable. For someone else there may be unrealistic, yet acutely felt, experiences of regret for actions not taken, words not spoken, potentialities not realised. Someone who has lived a life in which they have felt little autonomy may acutely fear the process of dying from the angle of having no control over the physical process. Another person will find the prospect of dying alone unbearable. The nature of the structure of self that has developed and of the client's self-concept will shape their reactions and the areas of particular concern that arise for them. From the person-centred perspective, the presence in a therapeutic relationship of a companion offering the attitudinal qualities of the person-centred approach will help that person make the adjustments they need, inwardly and outwardly, to the grieving or dying process that they are faced with.

Relationship is key

PCA regards the relationship that counsellors have with their clients, and the attitude that they hold within that relationship, to be key factors. Cooper (2004) has reviewed findings from a range of studies from researchers and theorists to argue that 'there is growing support for a relationship-orientated approach to therapeutic practice' (p. 452). Among the evidence he cites is a vast review of research on the therapeutic relationship commissioned in 1999 by the American Psychological Association Division of Psychotherapy Task Force, which, citing Norcross (2002), was the largest-ever review of research on the therapeutic relationship, with its distillation of evidence coming to over 400 pages. To quote from Cooper: 'Its main conclusion was that "The therapy relationship ... makes substantial and consistent contributions to psychotherapy outcome independent of the specific type of treatment" (Steering Committee, 2002, p. 441).' (The 'therapy relationship' is defined here as 'the feelings and attitudes that therapist and client have towards one another, and the manner in which these are expressed' (Norcross, 2002, p. 7).)

Further conclusions Cooper (2004) cites from this study include, 'Practice and treatment guidelines should explicitly address therapist behaviours and qualities that promote a facilitative therapy relationship' and 'Efforts to promulgate practice guidelines or evidence-based lists of effective psychotherapy without including the therapy relationship are seriously incomplete and potentially misleading on both clinical and empirical grounds' (Steering Committee, 2002, p. 441). Also the recommendation is made that practitioners should 'make the creation and cultivation of a therapy relationship ... a primary aim in the treatment of patients' (Steering Committee, 2002, p. 442).

In my experience, many adult psychological difficulties develop out of life experiences that involve problematic, conditional or abusive relational experiences. This can be centred in childhood or later in life. What is significant is that the individual is left, through relationships that have a negative conditioning effect, with a distorted perception of themselves and their potential as a person. Patterns are established in early life, bringing their own particular problems. However, they can be exacerbated by conditional and psychologically damaging experiences later in life, that in some cases will have a resonance to what has occurred in the past, exacerbating the effects still further.

An oppressive experience can impact on a child's confidence in themselves, leaving them anxious, uncertain and moving towards establishing patterns of thought, feeling and behaviour associated with the developing concept of themselves typified by 'I am weak and cannot expect to be treated any differently' or 'I just have to accept this attitude towards me, what can I do to change anything?'. These psychological conclusions may rest on patterns of thinking and feeling already established, perhaps the person was bullied at school, or experienced rejection in the home. They may have had a lifetime of stress, or it may be a relatively new experience. Either way, they may develop a way of thinking typified by 'it's normal to feel stressed, you just keep going, whatever it takes'.

The result is a conditioned sense of self, with the individual then thinking, feeling and acting in ways that enable them to maintain their self-beliefs and meanings within their learned or adapted concept of self. This is then lived out, with the person seeking to satisfy what they have come to believe about themselves: needing to care either because it has been normalised, or to prove to themselves and the world that they are a 'good' person. They will need to maintain this conditioned sense of self and the sense of satisfaction that this gives them when it is lived out, because they have developed such a strong identity with it.

The term 'conditions of worth' applies to the conditioning mentioned previously that is frequently present in childhood, and at other times in life, when a person experiences that their worth is conditional on their doing something, or behaving, in a certain way. This is usually to satisfy someone else's needs, and can be contrary to the client's own sense of what would be a satisfying experience. The values of others become a feature of the individual's structure of self. The person moves away from being true to themselves, learning instead to remain 'true' to their conditioned sense of worth. This state of being in the client is challenged by the person-centred therapist by offering them unconditional positive regard and warm acceptance. Such a therapist, by genuinely offering these therapeutic attitudes, provides the client with an opportunity to be exposed to what may be a new experience or one that in the past they have dismissed, preferring to stay with that which matches and therefore reinforces their conditioned sense of worth and sense of self.

By offering someone a non-judgemental, warm and accepting, and authentic relationship (perhaps a kind of 'therapeutic love'), that person can grow into a fresh sense of self in which their potential as a person can become more fulfilled. It enables them to liberate themselves from the constraints of patterns of conditioning. Such an experience fosters an opportunity for the client to redefine themselves as they experience the presence of the therapist's congruence, empathy and unconditional positive regard. This process can take time. Often the personality change that is required to sustain a shift away from what have been termed 'conditions of worth' may require a lengthy period of therapeutic work, bearing in mind that the person may be struggling to unravel a sense of self that has been developed, sustained and reinforced for many decades of life. Of course, where it has been established more recently, then less time may be needed.

Actualising tendency

A crucial feature or factor in this process of 'constructive personality change' is the presence of what Rogers (1986) termed 'the actualising tendency', a tendency towards fuller and more complete personhood with an associated greater fulfilment of their potentialities. The role of the person-centred counsellor is to provide the facilitative climate within which this tendency can work constructively. The 'therapist trusts the actualizing tendency of the client and truly believes that the client who experiences the freedom of a fostering psychological climate will resolve his or her own problems' (Bozarth, 1998, p. 4). This is fundamental to the application of the person-centred approach. Rogers (1986, p. 198) wrote:

> the person-centred approach is built on a basic trust in the person [It] depends on the actualizing tendency present in every living organism the tendency to grow, to develop, to realize its full potential. This way of being trusts the constructive directional flow of the human being towards a more complex and complete development. It is this directional flow that we aim to release.

Having said this, we must also acknowledge that for some people, or at certain stages, rather than producing a liberating experience, there will instead be a tendency to maintain the status quo, perhaps the fear of change, the uncertainty or the implications of change are such that the person prefers to maintain the known, the certain. In a sense, there is a liberation from the imperative to change and grow, which may bring temporary – and perhaps permanent – relief for the person. The actualising tendency may work through the part of the person that needs relief from change, enhancing its presence for the period of time that the person experiences a need to maintain this. The person-centred therapist will not try to move the person from this place or state. It is to be accepted, warmly and unconditionally. And, of course, sometimes in the moment of acceptance the person is enabled to question whether that really is how they want to be. But that is another part of the process.

Configuration within self

It is of value to draw attention, at this point, to the notion of 'configurations within self'. Configurations within self (Mearns and Thorne, 2000) are discrete sets of thoughts, feelings and behaviours that develop through the experience of life. They emerge in response to a range of experiences, including the process of introjection and the symbolisation of experiences, as well as in response to dissonant self-experience within the person's structure of self. They can also exist in what Mearns terms as ' "growthful" and "not for growth" configurations' (Mearns and Thorne, 2000, pp. 114–16), each offering a focus for the actualising tendency. The former seeking an expansion into new areas of experience with all that that brings, the latter seeking to energise the status quo and to block change because of its potential for disrupting the current order within the structure of self. The actualising tendency may not always manifest through growth or developmental change. It can also manifest through periods of stabilisation and stability, or a wanting to get away from something The self, then, is seen as a constellation of configurations, with the individual moving between them and living through them in response to experience.

Mearns suggests that these 'parts' or 'configurations' interrelate 'like a family, with an individual variety of dynamics'. As within any 'system', change in one area will impact on the functioning of the system. He therefore comments that 'when the interrelationship of configurations changes, it is not that we are left with something entirely new: we have the same "parts" as before, but some which may have been subservient before are stronger, others which were judged adversely are accepted, some which were in self-negating conflict have come to respect each other, and overall the parts have achieved constructive integration with the energy release which arises from such fusion' (Mearns and Thorne, 1999, pp. 147–8). The growing acceptance of the configurations, their own fluidity and movement within the self-structure, the increased, open and more accurate communication between these parts is, perhaps, another way of considering the weaving together of the threads of experience to which Rogers refers (1967, p. 158)

From this theoretical perspective we can argue that the person-centred counsellor's role is essentially facilitative. Creating the therapeutic climate of empathic understanding, unconditional positive regard and authenticity creates a relational climate that encourages the client to move into a more fluid state, with more openness to their own experience and the discovery of a capacity towards a fuller actualising of their potential.

Relationship re-emphasised

The therapeutic relationship is central in addressing these factors. A therapeutic approach such as a person-centred one affirms that it is not what you do so much as *how you are* with your client that is therapeutically significant, and this 'how you are' has to be received by the client. Gaylin (2001, p. 103) highlights the importance of client perception. 'If clients believe that their therapist is working on their behalf – if they perceive caring and understanding – then therapy is likely to be successful. It is the condition of attachment and the perception of connection that have the power to release the faltered actualization of the self'. He goes on to stress how 'we all need to feel connected, prized – loved', describing human beings as 'a species born into mutual interdependence', and that there 'can be no self outside the context of others. Loneliness is dehumanizing and isolation anathema to the human condition. The relationship,' he suggests, 'is what psychotherapy is all about.'

Love is an important word, although not necessarily one often used to describe a therapeutic relationship. Patterson, however, gives a valuable definition of love as it applies to the person-centred therapeutic process. He writes, 'we define love as an attitude that is expressed through empathic understanding, respect and compassion, acceptance, and therapeutic genuineness, or honesty and openness towards others' (Patterson, 2000, p. 315). We all need love, but most of all we need it during our developmental period of life. The same author affirms that 'whilst love is important throughout life for the well-being of the individual, it is particularly important, indeed absolutely necessary, for the survival of the infant and for providing the basis for the normal psychological development of the individual' (Patterson, 2000, pp. 314–15).

In a previous volume in this series I used the analogy of treating a wilting plant (Bryant-Jefferies, 2003a, p. 12). We can spray it with some specific herbicide or pesticide to eradicate a perceived disease that may be present in that plant, and that may be enough. But perhaps the true cause of the disease is that the plant is located in harsh surroundings, perhaps too much sun and not enough water, poor soil, near other plants that it has difficulty in surviving so close to. Maybe by offering the plant a healthier environment that will facilitate greater nourishment according to the needs of the plant, it may become the strong, healthy plant it has the potential to become. Yes, the chemical intervention may also be helpful, but if the true causes of the diseases are environmental – essentially the plant's relationship with that which surrounds it – then it won't actually achieve sustainable growth. We may not be able to transplant it, but we can provide water, nutrients and maybe shade from a fierce sun. Therapy, it seems to me, exists to provide this healthy environment within which the wilting client can begin the process of receiving the nourishment (in the form of healthy relational experience) that can enable them, in time, to become a more fully functioning person.

Of course, it raises the question of what does 'fully functioning' mean for the person facing their own death? Perhaps it concerns reaching a state or way of being that is in some way satisfying to the person themselves. Perhaps it is concerned with gaining a fuller understanding of themselves, of what death means and of finding ways to resolve those aspects of themselves, or relationships with others, that are in some sense problematic. Perhaps it is about making peace. Perhaps it is about experiencing greater authenticity and facing up to the reality of a life that has left the person with profound regret.

The process of change from a person-centred perspective

Rogers was interested in understanding the process of change, what it was like, how it occurred and what experiences it brought to those involved – client and therapist. At different points he explored this. Embleton Tudor *et al.* (2004) point to a model consisting of 12 steps identified in 1942 (Rogers, 1942) and to his two later chapters on this topic (Rogers, 1951), and finally the seven-stage model (Rogers, 1967). He wrote of 'initially looking for elements which would mark or characterize change itself'; however, he summarised what he experienced from his enquiry and research into the process of change: 'individuals move, I began to see, not from fixity or homeostasis through change to a new fixity, though such a process is indeed possible. But much the more significant continuum is from fixity to changingness, from rigid structure to flow, from stasis to process. I formed the tentative hypothesis that perhaps the qualities of the client's expression at any one point might indicate his position on this continuum, where he stood in the process of change' (Rogers, 1967, p. 131).

Change, then, involves a movement from fixity to greater fluidity, from a rigid set of attitudes and behaviours to a greater openness to experience variety and diversity. Change might be seen as having a certain liberating quality, a freeing up of the human being – heart, mind, emotions – so that the person experiences themself less as a fixed object and more of a conscious process. The list below is taken from Rogers' summary of the process, indicating the changes that people will show.

1   This process involves a loosening of feelings.
2   This process involves a change in the manner of experiencing.
3   The process involves a shift from incongruence to congruence.
4   The process involves a change in the manner in which, and the extent to which, the individual is able and willing to communicate himself in a receptive climate.
5   The process involves a loosening of the cognitive maps of experience.
6   There is a change in the individual's relationship to his problem.
7   There is a change in the individual's manner of relating (Rogers, 1967, pp. 156–8).

This is a very partial overview; the chapter in which he describes the process of change has much more detail and should be read in order to gain a clear grasp of the process as a whole, as well as the distinctive features of each stage as he saw it. Tudor and Worrall (2004) summarise this process in the following terms: 'a movement from fixity to fluidity, from closed to open, from tight to loose, and from afraid to accepting' (p. 47).

In Rogers' description, he makes the point that there were several types of process by which personality changes and that the process he described is one that is 'set in motion when the individual experiences himself as being fully received' (Rogers, 1967, p. 151).

Does this process apply to all psychotherapies? Rogers indicated that more data were needed, adding that 'perhaps therapeutic approaches which place great stress on the cognitive and little on the emotional aspects of experience may set in motion an entirely different process of change'. In terms of whether this process of change would generally be viewed as desirable and would move the person in a valued direction, Rogers expressed the view that the valuing of a particular process of change was linked to social value judgements made by individuals and cultures. He pointed out that the process of change that he described could be avoided, simply by people 'reducing or avoiding those relationships in which the individual is fully received as he is' (Rogers, 1967, p. 151).

Rogers also took the view that change was unlikely to be rapid, making the point that many clients enter the therapeutic process at stage two, and leave at stage four, having gained enough during that period to feel satisfied. He suggested it would be very rare, if ever, 'that a client who fully exemplified stage one would move to a point where he fully exemplified stage seven', and that if this did occur 'it would involve a matter of years' (Rogers, 1967, pp. 156). He wrote of how, at the outset, the threads of experience are discerned and understood separately by the client but as the process of change takes place, they move into 'the flowing peak moments of therapy in which all these threads become inseparably woven together'. He continues:

> in the new experiencing with immediacy which occurs at such moments, feeling and cognition interpenetrate, self is subjectively present in the experience, volition is simply the subjective following of a harmonious balance of organismic direction. Thus, as the process reaches this point the person becomes a unity of flow, of motion. He has changed, but what seems most significant, he has become an integrated process of changingness. (Rogers, 1967, p. 158)

It conjures up images of flowing movement, perhaps we should say purposeful flowing movement, as being the essence of the human condition, a state that we each have the potential to become, or to realise. Is it something we generate or develop out of fixity, or does it exist within us all as a potential that we lose during our conditional experiencing in childhood? Are we discovering something new, or rediscovering something that was lost? And does facing death, of ourselves or of a loved one, sharpen our focus and experiencing such that such processes can become heightened to some degree?

Supervision

The supervision sessions are included in this volume to offer the reader insight into the nature of therapeutic supervision in the context of the counselling profession, a method of supervising that I term 'collaborative review'. For many trainee counsellors, the use of supervision can be something of a mystery, and it is hoped that this book will go a long way to unravelling this. In the supervision sessions, I seek to demonstrate the application of the supervisory relationship. My intention is to show how supervision of the counsellor is very much a part of the process of enabling a client to work through issues that in this case relate to coming to terms with the death of a loved one, or facing the prospect of one's own imminent death.

Many professions do not recognise the need for some form of personal and process supervision, and often what is offered is line management. However, counsellors are required to receive regular supervision in order to explore the dynamics of the relationship with the client, the impact of the work on the counsellor and on the client, to receive support, to encourage professional development of the counsellor and to provide an opportunity for an experienced co-professional to monitor the supervisee's work in relation to ethical standards and codes of practice. The supervision sessions are included because they are an integral part of the therapeutic process. It is also hoped that they will help readers from other professions to recognise the value of some form of supportive and collaborative supervision in helping them become more authentically present with their own clients.

Merry describes what he termed 'collaborative inquiry' as a 'form of research or inquiry in which two people (the supervisor and the counsellor) collaborate or co-operate in an effort to understand what is going on within the counselling relationship and within the counsellor'. He emphasises how this 'moves the emphasis away from "doing things right or wrong" (which seems to be the case in some approaches to supervision) to "how is the counsellor being, and how is that way of being contributing to the development of the counselling relationship based on the core conditions"' (Merry, 2002, p. 173). Elsewhere, Merry describes the relationship between person-centred supervision and congruence, indicating that 'a state of congruence ... is the necessary condition for the therapist to experience empathic understanding and unconditional positive regard' (Merry, 2001, p. 183). Effective person-centred supervision provides a means through which congruence can be promoted within the therapist. Merry gives a succinct overview of all of this: 'person-centred supervision is concerned with how you, the counsellor, form relationships with your clients, and how you can deepen your empathic understanding of them whilst remaining as congruent as you can and experiencing unconditional positive regard towards them', and adds that this places the onus on the therapist to be as open and non-defensive as they can be when discussing the way they think and feel about themselves in relationship with their clients (Merry, 2002, p. 170).

Tudor and Worrall (2004) have drawn together a number of theoretical and experiential strands from within and outside the person-centred tradition to develop a theoretical position on the person-centred approach to supervision. In my view, this is a timely publication, defining the necessary factors for effective supervision within this way of working, and the respective responsibilities of both supervisor and supervisee in keeping with person-centred values and principles. They contrast person-centred working with other approaches to supervision, and emphasise the importance of the therapeutic space as a place within which practitioners 'can dialogue freely between their personal philosophy and the philosophical assumptions which underlie their chosen theoretical orientation' (Tudor and Worrall, 2004, pp. 94–5). They affirm the values and attitudes of person-centred working, and explore their application to the supervisory relationship.

There are, of course, as many models of supervision as there are models of counselling. In this book, the supervisor is seeking to apply the attitudinal qualities of a PCA.

It is the norm for all professionals working in the healthcare and social care environment in this age of regulation to be formally accredited or registered, and to work to their own professional organisation's code of ethics or practice. For instance, counselling practitioners registered with the British Association for Counselling and Psychotherapy are required to have regular supervision and continuing professional development to maintain registration. While professions other than counsellors will gain much from this book in their work, it is essential that they follow the standards, safeguards and ethical codes of their own professional organisation, and are appropriately trained and supervised to work with them on the issues that arise. Also, in the context of the workplace, they should follow guidelines and policies specific to that particular organisation, and be mindful of health and safety issues.

Dialogue format

The reader who has not read other titles in the *Living Therapy* series may find it takes a while to adjust to the dialogue format. Many of the responses offered by the counsellors, Chris and Nicola, are reflections of what their respective clients, Billy and Barbara, have said. This is not to be read as conveying a simple repetition of the clients' words. Rather, the counsellors seek to voice empathic responses, often with a sense of 'checking out' that they are hearing accurately what the clients are saying. The client says something; the counsellor then conveys what they have heard, what they sense the client has sought to communicate to them, sometimes with the same words, sometimes with words that include a sense of what they feel is being communicated through the client's tone of voice, facial expression or simply the relational atmosphere of the moment. The client is then enabled to confirm that they have been heard accurately, or to correct the counsellor in their perception. The client may then explore more deeply what they have been saying or move on, in either case with a sense that they have been heard and warmly accepted. To draw this to the reader's attention, I have included some of the inner thoughts and feelings that are present within the individuals who form the narrative.

The sessions are a little compressed. It is also fair to say that clients will take different periods of time before choosing to disclose particular issues, and will also take varying lengths of time in working with their own process. This book is not intended to indicate in any way the length of time that may be needed to work with the kinds of issue that are being addressed. The counsellor needs to be open and flexible to the needs of the client. For some clients, the process would take a lot longer. But there are also clients who are ready to talk about their situation and their feelings almost immediately, sometimes not feeling that they have much choice in the matter as their own organismic processes are already driving memories, feelings, thoughts and experiences to the surface and into daily awareness.

All characters in this book are fictitious and are not intended to bear resemblance to any particular person or persons. These fictional accounts are not intended to encompass all possible processes that people may go through as they experience being faced with death and bereavement; they simply highlight some of the behavioural, emotional, cognitive, psychological, spiritual and social factors that can be associated with this.

Person-centred approach today

I am extremely encouraged by the increasing interest in PCA, the growing amount of material being published and the realisation that relationship is a key factor in positive therapeutic outcome. There is currently much debate about theoretical developments within the person-centred world and its application. Discussions on the theme of Rogers' therapeutic conditions presented by various key members of the person-centred community have recently been published (Bozarth and Wilkins, 2001; Haugh and Merry 2001; Wyatt, 2001; Wyatt and Sanders, 2002). Mearns and Thorne (2000) have produced a timely publication revising and developing key aspects of person-centred theory. Wilkins (2003) has produced a book that addresses most effectively many of the criticisms levelled against person-centred working (2003), and Embleton Tudor *et al.* (2004) have produced an introduction to the person-centred approach that places the theory and practice within a contemporary context. Mearns and Cooper (2005) have recently presented 'working at relational depth', while Vincent (2005) draws together a rich mix of Rogers' references on the theme of being empathic, along with his own thinking in this area, and Levitt (2005) has edited a timely book exploring the theme of non-directivity. It seems there is an increasing stream of publications presenting and exploring the approach and its application in counselling and psychotherapy

Recently, Howard Kirschenbaum (Carl Rogers' biographer) published an article entitled 'The current status of Carl Rogers and the person-centered approach'. In his research for this article he noted that from 1946 to 1986 there were 84 books, 64 chapters and 456 journal articles published on Carl Rogers and the person-centred approach. In contrast from 1987 to 2004 there were 141 books, 174 book chapters and 462 journal articles published. This is a clear trend towards more publications and, presumably more readership and interest in the approach. Also, he noted that there were now some 50 person-centred publications available around the world, mostly journals, and there are now person-centred organisations in 18 countries, and 20 organisations overall. He also draws attention to the large body of research demonstrating the effectiveness of person-centred therapy, concluding that the person-centred approach is 'alive and well' and 'appears to be experiencing something of a revival, both in professional activity and academic respectability' (Kirschenbaum, 2005).

It is worth highlighting at this point that within the person-centred community there are various divisions or 'tribes', as they have been referred to (Warner, 2000). Practitioners have sought to develop different approaches to practice, placing greater or lesser emphasis on particular areas of theory. There are those who present what has been termed 'classical' person-centred practice, which for many is regarded as conveying the purity of the approach. This, along with other forms of practice, is explored by Sanders (2000) who, in this important paper also identifies three 'primary principles' of the approach, focusing on 'the primacy of the actualising tendency', the necessity of therapeutic conditions [defined by Rogers in] 1957 and 1959 and therapeutic behaviour based on '*active inclusion* of these', and 'the primacy of the non directive attitude *at least* at the level of content but not necessarily at the level of process'. As well as 'classical client-centred therapy/counselling', Sanders (2000) also makes reference to 'experiential psychotherapy', 'process-experiential psychotherapy', and 'person-centred integrative therapies'. It is beyond the scope of this volume to explore these further, however, suffice to say that this volume seeks to demonstrate an application of a more classical approach, though I am not sure that I would position it completely at the classical end of the person/client-centred spectrum of practice.

This is obviously a very brief introduction to the approach. Person-centred theory continues to develop as practitioners and theoreticians consider its application in various fields of therapeutic work and extend our theoretical understanding of developmental and therapeutic processes. At times it feels as if it has become more than just individuals, rather it feels like a group of colleagues, based around the world, working together to penetrate deeper towards a more complete theory of the human condition, and this includes people from many traditions and schools of thought. Person-centred or client-centred theory and practice has a key role in this process. Theories are being revisited and developed, new ideas speculated upon and new media explored for presenting the core values and philosophy of the person-centred approach. It is an exciting time.

Part 1

CHAPTER 1

Counselling session 1: Silences and emerging emotions

Billy sat staring ahead of him. He was feeling numb. Sometimes that was how it was. At other times he felt surging sensations of sadness and grief that tore through him like a highly charged emotional wave, leaving him burning and aching inside. But today, in this moment, he was feeling numb. He was grateful for that.

He sat in his car; the rain was falling, he could see the droplets running down the windscreen. It was dark beyond. He was tight-lipped, his head shaking slightly from side to side. He wasn't aware of the movement. He did feel himself take a deep breath, and then his breathing returned to its shallow rhythm. He still couldn't believe it. He took another deep breath, but this time consciously, and moved his shoulders back a little. They had become stiff. He stretched his back and reached for the car keys in the ignition, taking them out and noting the clunk as he did so. Somehow it seemed loud. Perhaps it was the silence. It was quiet. He felt quiet as well. Yes, sometimes that was how he felt. He welcomed those times.

He hesitated. Counselling. Not something he'd ever anticipated needing. But he needed to talk. He needed to talk to someone. Friends had been good, but he didn't want to burden them. His partner had been supportive as well, but she'd made it clear that she felt he needed someone else to talk to. He hadn't agreed at first, preferring to simply say nothing and just carry on. But somehow that wasn't working. He felt low; dispirited was the word that often came to mind. It all seemed to him to be an over-reaction, somehow. Yes, he had been close to his father, and yes, it had been sudden – a heart attack. Well, yes, he'd been a smoker and hadn't maybe had the best of diets, but it had still taken him by surprise. In fact he had taken it worse than his mother, who now seemed to be getting on with her life after a few months of struggling to make sense of what had happened. She'd been to counselling. It was her who had finally convinced him to try it where his partner had failed.

He'd phoned to make the appointment the previous week. The counsellor's name was Chris. He'd found his name in the yellow pages.

Billy took a deep breath and opened the car door. The rain had eased a little. He got out, closed and locked the car door and made his way through the gate and up to the front door, ringing the bell and taking shelter under the canopy. The door opened after only a few seconds.

'Hello, I'm Billy, we spoke on the phone.'

'Yes, yes, we did, please, come in. It's horrible out there.'

'Thanks.' Billy came in. The hallway was warm.

'The counselling room is here, on the left, please come in.'

Billy went in.

'So, have a seat, whichever you prefer.' Billy chose the seat facing him as he came through the door into the counselling room. Chris sat down in the chair opposite him.

'So, we talked about counselling on the phone and, well, have you any questions?'

Billy shook his head. He suddenly felt unsure of himself, unclear as to what he was doing there. He felt anxious.

'Well, I want to give you a place here to talk about whatever you feel you want to talk about. And I hope that listening to you, responding to you, will help you.'

Billy nodded. 'Hard to know where to start, really. It's not something I'm used to, you know, talking like this.'

'No, it often isn't. Take your time.'

Billy sat staring down, wondering quite what to say next. Here he was, 42 years old, no reason to feel like he did, not really, and yet somehow ... somehow things just didn't feel right.

'Well, like I said on the phone, things were OK until recently and, I don't know, it's like everything feels like an effort. Just feels like, well, what's the point?'

'Mhmm, what's the point?' Chris responded simply and directly to what Billy had said, and waited for Billy to continue.

'I mean, I don't know. I suppose it does sort of relate to Dad dying.' Billy took a deep breath and pushed the emotions aside. They were often close but he wasn't going to show them, not now.

'Mhmm, your dad dying seems linked to how you're feeling.' Again Chris sought to be clear and straight in his response. He wanted Billy to feel heard. He wanted him to find his own way, realise that he could decide what he wanted to say and how he wanted to say it. Chris recognised that counselling was often an unusual experience for people. Talking and being listened to, really listened to, wasn't what happened in everyday life. Usually one person talked, and while the other listened often they were simply waiting to say what they wanted to say. But counselling was different. And counselling was not about being friends. Yet it was about forming a person-to-person relationship. Not everyone understood the difference.

In a friendship, while one person may be talking and in need of being listened to, the other person may not want simply to listen. They may have thoughts, feelings, experiences that they also want to share with their

friend. Friendship is a mutual relationship. However, the therapeutic relationship requires the therapist to be a disciplined listener, responsive to
the client, offering the therapeutic conditions and putting aside personal
thoughts and feelings that have nothing to do with what emerges within
the therapeutic process. Friends can be good listeners, and often that is
enough. But there are also times when someone needs somebody outside of
their circle of friends to talk to, to take their inner world to, someone who
can give them the time and space to be themselves, to explore, to express
themselves freely in the knowledge that what emerges and is expressed in
the room, stays in the room.

'We were sort of close, I mean not really close, but, well, we got on well.' Billy
lapsed into silence; a number of memories seemed to come flooding into his
mind. His dad had been a great woodworker, built most of his own furniture,
and he'd learned a lot from him. They'd built a few things together over the
years. He had a lot of his dad's tools now. His mother wasn't going to have a
use for them. Some of them he'd brought back to his own shed, the rest were
still in his dad's shed. Somehow, though, he didn't really feel like going over
there and using them. Wasn't the same, somehow.
'Got on well together.' Chris nodded and smiled. He felt a sense of warm compassion arise within him. Something about the way that Billy had spoken. His
voice had gone soft. He added, 'Sounds like he was important.' The words
simply formed and he felt he wanted to express the impression that he had
been left with. In a way he knew that might have sounded a bit obvious, but it
felt right somehow given the way Billy had spoken.
'Guess he was, well, yes, I know he was. I mean, he was sort of easy-going,
you know? Can't remember him shouting at us as kids. My sister and I, in a way
she was probably closer to him, fathers and daughters. I suppose I was closer to
my mum in some ways, and yet, I don't know, seems to have hit me harder
somehow.'
'Mhmm, his death has hit you harder than your sister?'
Billy nodded. 'Strange that, but, yes.' He took a deep breath. 'But umm, well, now
I've got to get on, you know?'
'Mhmm, get on with your life, yes?'
'Mum's doing well. She seems to have come to terms with it, I don't know how.
I mean, she's got good friends, and that's helped, and she had counselling, saw
a bereavement counsellor for a while. That seemed to help her. She was the one
that persuaded me to come along.'
'So she found counselling helpful and suggested you come?'
'Yes.' He thought back. Yes, it had been tough for his mum to start with. She had
been totally shocked by what had happened. But now, a year on, just over, she
was getting herself organised. She spent a lot of time with his sister, they
seemed closer now, somehow. He felt sort of, he wasn't sure, like he didn't
know who he was. That was a bit heavy, bit extreme, he thought to himself,
but it was something like that. 'So, well, here I am.'

'Well, it's a difficult time and I'm glad you're here, and I really hope that counselling is helpful for you, I really do.' Chris felt wholly genuine in what he was
saying. He felt connected to Billy, listening to what he was saying and the
way he as speaking, and he still felt that warmth for him, a man in his middle
years suddenly losing his father – he recalled the phone call with Billy when he
had said that it had been the sudden death of his father that seemed to have
affected him.

Billy looked up and looked into Chris's eyes. He only held the eye contact for a
short period, feeling he needed to look away. It didn't feel right to be looking
into the eyes of another man, and yet. . . . Somehow he did feel that Chris was
genuine, he couldn't quite put his finger on why, he just seemed, well, seemed
to care somehow.

'Not sure what to say now.'

'Sometimes it can seem like you don't have anything to say, or know where to
begin.' Chris wondered whether that had been a very helpful response.
He hadn't really empathised with Billy, hadn't really just let him know what he
had heard. Rather he'd made an assumption about what Billy might be struggling with. No, he wasn't sure that it had been helpful.

Chris may be avoiding sitting in a silence with Billy. He's offering him
options to encourage him to speak. This is not a person-centred response.
It might be facilitative, but it could be emerging from the counsellor's discomfort and, if he is unaware of this, or unaware of the cause of it, then he
is being incongruent and is therefore being therapeutically unhelpful.

Not knowing what to say seemed true enough, although, well, he had lots of
things he could say, but he didn't actually know what to say. What were you
supposed to say? 'I feel sort of, I don't know, sort of "what's the point?".'

'What's the point?' Chris let his tone of voice allow his empathic response to have
a questioning tone.

'It's like, I mean, he hadn't been retired that long. Sort of makes you think, you
know?'

'Makes *you* think.'

'It does. I mean, you work all your life and finally get some time for yourself and,
well, that happens.' He shook his head. His thoughts went back to his mother.
'She's doing great, my mother, that is. She seems to be getting on now. Yes, she
misses him, we all do. The first Christmas was difficult, and his birthday, and
hers as well. We haven't had a second of anything yet. I don't know, maybe
it's because she's sort of more religious than I am, says it's her faith that has
helped. I can't really accept that. I mean, I do accept that it's helping her, but I
don't know. I don't think I ever really believed in anything much, you know?
Never really felt I needed to think about it. But I don't really think . . . , well,
when you die, that's it. That's how I see it, anyway.'

Chris nodded. It wasn't his belief, but he wasn't there to express his beliefs. 'So it feels as though her faith is helping her, but you can't, don't see things the way that she does. For you when you die, that's it.'

Billy nodded. 'Mhmm. Just seems a waste. I don't know, I mean it helps her, but ...'. He shook his head. 'Not how I see things. I just see someone who worked all his life and finally gets time to relax, and that's it. Certainly doesn't make me believe in a God or anything.'

'Not how you see it, and it doesn't encourage you to believe in a God.'

'No. Just ..., I don't know, maybe if ..., no, no, can't see it. This is it, this is me.' Billy opened his hands out and looked down at his body. 'And when I've gone, that's it, you know?'

'When you've gone ..., that's it.' Chris kept with what Billy was saying, seeking to empathise with his words while also matching his tone of voice, which seemed to Chris to be conveying a kind of resignation, as if he was resigned to his fate in some way. That was how it was, and you had to get on with it, and it didn't make sense, it didn't seem fair, but ...

'Makes you kind of wonder, though ...'.

'Wonder?'

'Whether it's all worth it, I mean, you know, you sort of plan ahead, work for the future, but, well, what's the point. I kind of wonder. Is it all worth it?'

'Is it really all worth it.' Chris spoke slowly, holding the focus on what Billy had said.

'And it is, of course it is.' Billy was thinking of his children, Sarah and Tara. And yet he knew as well that sometimes he wondered, even when he thought about them. Billy lapsed back into silence. He felt strangely detached once again. Yes, it did give him things to think about and he was tired of thinking about them as well. He felt that familiar numbness creeping up on him. That question still went through his head, 'what was the point?'. He had no answer, in fact he wasn't really trying to find an answer. Sometimes he did, but at other times it was all too much. There was no answer. It didn't make sense. The only sense to be made of it was that life could be bloody unfair. He felt angry. He took a deep breath, the anger passed, the numbness became more present. He'd never felt like this before his dad had died, well, you didn't think about death and dying. At least he hadn't, not like it was going to happen to someone close to you. Not yet. Now, well, now he didn't know what to think. Truth was he didn't really want to think. Stay numb, that was the best way. A few whiskies of an evening, that helped. Clare didn't like it, but she didn't understand. It wasn't her dad. Her parents were alive. She didn't understand. It felt like no one understood, not really, what it was like, what he felt.

He thought about Chris, the thought just appeared in his mind. Would he understand? Could he? He was a counsellor. That's what counsellors were good at, weren't they? But how could he know? It all felt too much, too overwhelming. He was looking down and thought about looking up, to check what Chris was doing, but he didn't want to, he'd rather stay in himself, in his own world. Not that he was thinking of it quite like that. He just kept his head down, his eyes on the carpet, not that he was seeing the patterns, they were there, but in a way he wasn't. It sort of felt safe to stay in his own head, his own world. It was out there that troubled him. Yes, he was safe in his own head somehow. The numbness had returned. He was thinking, but somehow not thinking. Thoughts, but he didn't feel like he was thinking them, like they were being projected into his head somehow. They weren't his, and yet . . .

Chris sat in the silence, feeling a degree of intensity. The atmosphere felt, well, it wasn't so much tense in an uncomfortable kind of way. It didn't feel awkward or strained. It didn't feel like Billy was trying to find something to say; maybe it had been like that, maybe earlier, but now it felt different. Often, in his experience, you could sense a change during a silence. The sense of awkwardness could pass and often such shifts were indicative that the client was thinking or feeling in a way that was absorbing them. That they were engaging with their own inner world, as it were, being what was present, focusing on what was emerging. The awkwardness was often associated with not knowing what to say, feeling embarrassed, being uncomfortable with silence or being with a stranger, all quite reasonable reactions.

Chris believed that during silences, as a person-centred therapist it was important for him to maintain his therapeutic attitude. Just because the client wasn't outwardly communicating didn't mean that he could let his attention wander. It was part of the discipline of being a therapist. And it was a discipline, a self-discipline. Not everyone appreciated this. He was contracting with a client to offer his availability for the therapeutic hour, to provide for that relational therapeutic climate that he knew was facilitative of constructive personality change.

He also believed that somehow his interior attitude made an impact, even during silence. He believed that somehow it made an impact on the client – was impact too harsh a word, maybe impression was better, softer – even though there was no visible or verbal form of communication occurring. He felt genuinely accepting of Billy's need to be outwardly silent, and he was grateful for feeling that way. He believed that his warm acceptance of his clients had to be felt, that it wasn't something you thought about feeling towards your client, it had to present at a visceral level in experience.

Chris was also aware of what was present within his own experiencing and felt accepting of the sense of receptivity that had developed. It was as though he felt open to whatever emerged, both inwardly and outwardly, and that there was a sort of alert expectation. He felt no urge to speak, to break the silence.

Billy, meanwhile, continued with his own thoughts. He wasn't aware of it but he had begun to shake his head slightly from side to side. The thoughts that were coinciding with this movement were linked to a deep sense of resignation. There didn't seem any point. It felt like a heaviness. He felt tired. He felt himself yawning. His eyes were gritty. He hadn't been sleeping well. Couldn't settle. He'd wake up feeling distinctly uneasy, hot, sometimes sweating. It could be a dream. He seemed to keep dreaming of trying to get somewhere, but never arriving. Always some other obstacle would arise in the dream. He'd wake up, often looking at the clock and it seemed like it was always 2.30am. He didn't know why. But often it seemed to be that time.

He'd have to get up, cool down, try and settle. He'd watch TV, read a magazine. Sometimes it helped, sometimes it didn't.

Chris noted Billy shaking his head. He still didn't want to disturb the silence, yet he also felt that he wanted – or was it needed – to make contact with him, remind him that he was there for him. He spoke gently, wanting Billy to perhaps hear his words but without them pulling his attention too forcibly away from what was preoccupying him. 'Leaves you shaking your head.'

Billy heard Chris's words. They seemed distant. They didn't disrupt his thoughts. Yes, yes, it did leave him shaking his head. He had no answers. There weren't any. He took a deep breath and nodded, 'Yes', closed his mouth and tightened his lips. He felt an uneasy churning in his stomach and his head felt odd, sort of fuzzy.

Chris didn't say any more. He had clearly said something that had meaning for Billy, that had conveyed an empathy for what he had observed. He waited, maintaining an attitude of openness and alertness to whatever Billy might want to say.

Billy moved in his seat. It had begun to feel uncomfortable. He began to wonder what Chris made of him. He was suddenly conscious of the silence. It felt awkward. He felt uncertain. Seemed like he should be talking, that maybe he shouldn't have come. He wasn't sure what to say but he wanted to say something. The discomfort was increasing. He moved again in the chair.

'Uncomfortable?'

'Sitting too long in the same position, I guess.' He paused.

The thought ran through Chris's mind that it can get uncomfortable psychologically, too, when you're stuck in the same way of thinking for too long.

'Is it always like this?' Billy was wondering whether what he was experiencing was typical of counselling.

'Can you say a little more?' Chris didn't simply empathise with what Billy had asked. In truth he wasn't sure quite what Billy meant specifically, and felt it might help him to respond if Billy was able to be a little more specific.

'Well, just sitting, I mean, I feel like I should be saying something but I don't know what. That's why I'm here, but now I'm here I don't know what to say, or even if it's worth saying anything.' Billy looked up and made eye contact with Chris.

'Can be difficult. From what you are saying you came here to talk, but now you're here it seems really difficult.'

Billy nodded, aware that hearing Chris speak left him even more aware of how difficult and uncomfortable it seemed. It didn't make sense. Why was he here? How could this possibly help? He felt cheated, pissed off. It was a waste of time. 'Doesn't make much sense *just* sitting here.'

'That how it feels, like you're *just* sitting here?' Chris empathised with the emphasis that Billy had placed on the word 'just'. He also responded with a questioning tone to his voice. Yes, he had heard what Billy was saying, but was that all he was experiencing? He wanted to hear what more Billy might want to say.

'I feel frustrated.'

'Being here, like this, leaves you feeling frustrated?'

'I want to feel different. I don't want to keep feeling like this. I want this to end. I want to get on with my life. I want to feel like I did ...'. He hesitated. 'Like I did, you know ..., before ...'.

Chris nodded, feeling a warm compassion in his heart for Billy in response to the impassioned statement that he had just made. Billy's words had been spoken with such emotion, a real yearning, it was palpable. From being so flat, the words had sort of burst out, full of energy. They touched Chris deeply. He felt the emotion within himself rise in response.

'You want to feel like you did before.' Chris didn't say any more. He guessed it was 'before his dad had died', but these were words that Billy was choosing not to utter. Maybe they were the words that he needed to find and voice for himself, when the time was right. Or did he need to hear them from Chris, a sign that he, Chris, understood what Billy was trying but was unable to say. He took the view that Billy might need to say those words for himself, it was a split-second decision, as they often are. He accepted that at this moment Billy had said what he needed to say in the way that he needed to say it.

'I was OK then, just getting on with my life, you know? Just thought, well, I mean, just sort of expected things to continue as they were.'

Chris nodded, aware of feeling that perhaps 'things' was an easier word to say than 'people'.

'Things just carrying on as they were.'

'Well, you don't think about it all being different, do you? I mean, you don't. Everything was sort of settled; me, Clare, the girls, Mum and Dad being grandparents. It was like, you know, sort of what you expect.' Billy looked away.

Chris nodded again, feeling in himself a sadness, a sense of how this stable family unit that must have seemed as though it would just go on like that, if not forever then certainly as long as Billy wanted to imagine it. That the family could be suddenly broken up by the death of Billy's dad was something that was not expected.

'Yeah, everything feels settled, you knew what to expect, how it was going to be, and then ...'. Chris noted that he had picked up on Billy's style of ending the sentence before actually stating what had happened directly.

'And then .... You don't think, do you?'

'Not something you thought about at all.'

Billy looked back and again made eye contact. It felt to Chris as though he was looking for something. His eyes seemed intense, searching in some way. 'It's just so hard to believe.' Billy shook his head again, swallowing and then taking a deep breath. 'Just ..., oh, I don't know. I just can't seem to accept it somehow.'

'Just can't seem to accept what has happened.' Chris was very aware of maintaining his empathy, of keeping to the way Billy was expressing himself. He was still not mentioning his dad directly and Chris continued to speak in the same way. He trusted Billy's process, that he was still saying what he needed to say, what he could say, in the way that he needed. He wasn't going to start introducing the missing words. He found himself taking a deep breath as the thought struck him that Billy's missing words sort of paralleled the fact that they were references to the person that was missing. He noted this but let the thought go. He could appreciate that Billy was not yet able to speak directly of his father or that he had died, or at least not able in the context of the counselling. He had to make no assumptions beyond that. Billy was expressing himself, his thoughts, his feelings in his own language. He was describing the contents of his inner world, or at least those contents that he felt able to express, or wanted Chris, or himself, to hear.

Sometimes words have too much painful emotion attached to them to be voiced. Come counsellors might choose to supply the words that Billy is not using. This might have a place. Some might say to also not use those words was a collusion, and some schools of thought take a negative view of this. From a person-centred perspective, however, this is not collusion, but empathy and respect. Empathy for what the client is saying, and respect for their choice as to what they are choosing not to say. The person-centred counsellor does not seek to get ahead of their client. They are a companion, walking beside them, sometimes a step behind them, allowing the client to point out what they see, feel, think. It is not for the counsellor to point out to the client what the counsellor sees within the client's inner world. At least, not early on in a therapeutic relationship. Maybe later, when the relationship is well established and there is a much deeper connection, there may be times when the therapist is able to draw attention to what they sense to be present in the client's inner world that the client is barely aware of. But not early on. Too much empathy, however well meaning and however sure the counsellor may feel they are right, can lay bare experiencing to the client's awareness before its time, with potentially damaging results. The person-centred counsellor trusts the client's process. The degree of incongruence within the client can leave them vulnerable to the effects of empathic responding that have advanced beyond what they are experiencing or want to have made visible.

'And yet it did, it has, and I have to accept it. And in a way I do, I mean, I know it, but I can't sort of, I don't know, it's like I can't sort of believe it.'

Chris felt the urge to respond in a particular way. He knew he hadn't much time to decide what response to make, and he didn't want to get himself caught up in thinking about it and lose touch with the flow and with what Billy had said. Was it appropriate to say it, or not? The words in his head were, 'Can't believe it, or don't want to believe it?'. He made his decision. He stayed with Billy's inner world, with what Billy had chosen to reveal, and how he had described it. 'It's hard to believe, you can't quite believe that it happened.'

Billy was taking another deep breath and once again his lips tightened. He had also tightened his jaw but was unaware that he had done this. He couldn't believe it had happened and yet he knew that it had. And it had been over 12 months ago now, of course he knew that, and yet .... He still half expected his dad to call round, or be on the phone. Those had been the hardest times, coming back from something, a day out with the girls perhaps, or a football match – in the past they'd gone together, but his dad had lost interest. 'Too much money. It's not a sport, it's a business. I'm not paying to watch a business' was what he would say. Billy agreed to a degree, but he still liked to go now and then, and his dad always liked to hear about what Billy had thought of the match. Anyway, he'd come back and catch himself thinking about telling his dad about how 'the City' had got on, or what the girls had been up to at the beach, or wherever they'd gone. He'd really loved them, he had been such a good granddad to them both. And he'd realise that he wasn't there to talk to. And it could really eat him up. Such a small thing and yet . . . . It still got to him. It was getting to him now as he heard his dad's voice. He always called the girls his little angels. He suddenly felt very emotional. He closed his eyes, feeling them filling with water, and looked away.

'Sorry.'

'A lot of feelings.'

Billy nodded, and swallowed hard. He didn't want to describe what he had been thinking, or what he was feeling. He knew he'd find it hard to say, that he'd end up feeling more emotional. He didn't want that; felt he had to be in control. 'Gets to me sometimes.'

Chris nodded, 'Yeah, some memories . . .'.

'Too painful . . .'. Billy took a handkerchief from his pocket, his eyes still closed tight. He wiped his eyes and blew his nose. 'Sorry.'

'It's OK, there's a lot to feel.'

Billy was taking a deep breath. 'Yeah, that's for sure.' He sort of expected Chris to say something more. Somehow he had this idea that counsellors were sort of in the business of making people cry, but it didn't feel like Chris was like that. Yes, he was feeling emotional, but Chris was allowing him to be how he was, no pressure. That felt good. He felt a bit relieved too.

Chris smiled warmly.

'I guess I need to feel like this.'

Chris nodded.

'Just have to come to terms with it, I guess. Not easy, though. I think I'm realising he was more important to me than I thought.'

'More important than you thought.' Chris nodded as he responded.

Billy took another deep breath and pursed his lips. 'This is tiring, you know.' He spoke as he felt a yawn coming on. 'Oh dear. I feel really drained.'

'Emotions can take it out of us.'

'They take it out of me. But it's strange, I sort of feel a little clearer somehow, but still tired.'

Chris glanced at the clock. 'Just a few minutes left. Do you think this is helpful? Do you want to continue with counselling?'

'Twenty minutes or so ago and I might have said no. I wasn't sure. But I feel different now. Feel like I have to come back, I need to say more, don't I? Haven't really said much this week. It's not easy. Do I have to . . . , I guess I do, come to terms with it, with what I feel, how it's affecting me.'

Not all clients will express emotions so early in counselling, but some will. Clients may attend counselling for bereavement at very different stages in their process of coming to terms with their experience. Here, Billy is still feeling very emotional, there are memories of his dad that still bring feelings to the surface, painful feelings that cause tears to flow. Not everyone will express themselves like this in a first session. Equally, not everyone will experience such lengthy silences. This first session captures some of what can occur, but should not be taken as a typical first session. In truth, there probably isn't such a thing, except in textbooks! Clients come with whatever feelings and thoughts are present, each able to express them to varying degrees. For the person-centred counsellor, the early sessions are very much concerned with forming the therapeutic relationship and allowing the client to feel increasingly free to be as they need to be.

The session drew to a close and they agreed to meet again the following week. Billy left, spending a few minutes sitting in his car in the silence before driving away. He felt as though he had a lot to think about. His dad seemed to be more present to him, somehow. He felt a kind of relief from having had that first session of counselling. He still wasn't sure what to make of it. But he felt pleased to have talked a bit, though sorry that he hadn't maybe said more. 'Well Dad, I don't know quite what to make of it, but I've got to do this. I don't want to forget you I couldn't do that but I've got to find my way forward.' He shook his head, wondering at himself. He'd never spoken like that, and certainly not out loud. And yet it had somehow felt natural and right. He turned the ignition and headed into the night, feeling a mixture of lightness and bemusement. He'd started something. He wasn't sure what it was, or what it was going to lead to. But somehow, in some strange way, it felt like he was doing the right thing.

Points for discussion

- How would you describe Billy if you were describing this first session to your supervisor? What impression has he made on you, and why?
- What responses from the counsellor seemed particularly facilitative to you, and why?
- How do you respond to silences? Would you have responded differently from the counsellor in this session?
- Do you feel that the counsellor demonstrated person-centred practice? What were particularly clear examples, and were there times when you felt the counsellor was less than empathic in his responses?
- What specific issues might you take from this session to supervision?
- Write notes for this session.

CHAPTER 2

Counselling session 2: Loss of past, loss of future

Billy walked up to the door. He'd had a strange week. His emotions were
still very present and he was still finding it difficult to sleep. He wanted to talk
about it. Every night, it was wearing him out. He wasn't concentrating too
well at work either.

Chris answered the door and Billy went into the counselling room.

'So, how do you want to use our time this evening, Billy?'

'Just not sleeping. I wake up, can't settle. I don't know. Crazy dreams. Every
night.'

Chris listened. 'Mhmm, dreams, disturbing, unsettling?'

Billy nodded. 'I keep waking up, same time, just about every night. I know the
time now before I open my eyes.'

'So you get off to sleep and then wake up after having these crazy dreams?'

'Mhmm. I seem to get to sleep OK, a few stiff whiskies, you know, settles me down.'

Chris nodded and was aware of feeling some concern, wondering how much Billy
might be turning to alcohol to relax, or to cope. But he wasn't there to address
this, but to accept what Billy had to say. 'So the whisky helps you sleep, but you
wake up and then you can't settle.'

'And then I dream, and I'm always trying to get somewhere, usually driving, but I
never make it. Always something stops me. I get lost, get distracted, something
happens and I'm always, I don't know, it's like sometimes, hmm, sometimes I
do get there but when I do I'm too late, but I don't know why. I don't know
what I'm late for.'

'So, you either don't arrive, or you do arrive but you're too late for something.'

The person-centred response to clients who share dream experiences
is not to start interpreting the dream, but to listen, empathise, warmly
accept what the client is saying. The person-centred counsellor thereby
helps the client explore the dream in whatever way the client wishes.
It's an exploration, but the client leads and makes their own interpreta-
tions and meanings.

Billy nodded. 'And I often think of Dad. Something about the silence at night. And not just about me. I see him with our daughters, Sarah and Tara. He was so good with them. Not surprised really. He was always good with children. He thought the world of them, and they thought the world of him. They still get sad, but they believe he's gone to Heaven. They've drawn pictures of him with God.' He shook his head. 'It's not been easy for them, for any of us, but it feels like everyone else has come to terms with it except me. Why am I so stuck?'

'Feels like you're stuck, and everyone else has sort of moved on?'

'Something like that. I mean, yeah, he was my dad, we had good times, and, yeah, difficult times as well. I probably wasn't the most understanding teenager, did my rebelling, settled down. But it's ..., I don't know, I just keep coming back to the senselessness of him dying. Worked all his life. Looked forward to retirement. He used say he'd earned it. Within two years and he's ...'. Billy shook his head.

Chris noted that again Billy was unable or unwilling to finish his sentences when they related to his father's death.

'Seems so senseless. Just doesn't seem fair. Lives his life and then, just when he gets to some time for himself, it's taken away.'

'Doesn't quite get there.'

'No. He was digging in the garden, Mum was busy in the kitchen, didn't hear him. Maybe he called out, maybe not. We don't know.' Billy shook his head again. 'He wasn't very fit, I know that, and I know, well, people have heart attacks, but you just don't think it's going to happen, not to someone close to you.'

'No, you know it happens, but not to someone that close to you.'

'I need to talk, I know I do. I don't know if I can make sense of it, I don't think I ever will, but I need to talk. I spend too much time thinking, I can't be like that. It's not good for me, or for anyone around me. But ..., I don't know, why is it affecting me like this? Why? I mean ...'. Billy stopped speaking. He had been about to say something and it sort of didn't come out. He felt suddenly strange again, sad, anxious, emotional.

'Take your time, no rush.' Chris sensed that there was something Billy had meant to say but hadn't been able to get out. He wanted him to feel supported and unpressured. He knew it could take time and that everyone had to work through their experiences at their own pace.

Clients must express themselves at their own pace. Often it takes time for all the experiential elements to be present in the client's awareness to enable them to communicate the fullness of their experience. There may also be times when what is communicated will be in small parts, gradually building up a fuller picture. As each part is heard and understood, the client is enabled to move on to the next one. The person-centred counsellor will wish to be sensitive to the client's process.

'I was going to say ...'. Billy swallowed, the emotions were coming to the surface again, he could feel them, it was as though they were rising up inside him, into his chest, his throat, he breathed out, trying to keep some control. 'This isn't easy.'

'No. No, just take it slowly.'

'I want to say this but ..., my heart is thumping. But I've got to say it.' He felt a cold sweat breaking out. 'You know, I do wonder sometimes what he thought about me. He was proud of the girls, but I don't know about me. We never really sort of talked about how we felt about each other. Well you don't do you? And now, now, well, now ...'. He paused again, composing himself. His throat burned and it felt as though there was a huge, hard lump in it.

'Things that you never said to each other, and now it's ...'

'... too late.' Billy remembered after the last session. 'Strange, haven't done it before, but after the last session here I sat in the car and I talked to him.' Billy stopped for a moment, thinking back to what he had said. 'I don't do that, but I did. Told him I didn't want to forget him, but I had to find a way forward. I'm sure he'd understand. I know he would. He just took things in his stride, somehow. I've never really been much like that. Sometimes his relaxed kind of attitude towards things irritated me. But that was how he was. And he still ...'. Another pause. 'I don't know.'

'Something you don't know?'

> The counsellor responds to the not knowing, rather than the content. The client does not need an empathic response that reflects what he has disclosed, but to hear his moment of not knowing. That – having been heard – allows the client to then say more, sharing further his perception of his father. In a sense, the client's father is gradually becoming more and more present within the therapeutic relationship.

'Mhmm. He worked, well, he had different jobs over the years, but mainly in retail, and mainly do-it-yourself, you know? Managed people at one of the big stores, and was around to give people advice. He loved it. Work wasn't stressful. He had a pretty normal lifestyle really. Liked a few beers. Never got drunk. Can't remember him being drunk. Bit merry sometimes, you know, Christmas, birthdays, celebrations, but never that bad. But he was overweight. He probably ate too many of the wrong things. But he knew what he liked and wasn't going to change. He used to get a bit breathless at times. He'd smoked as a younger man, but had given it up about twenty years ago. That was when his weight had increased. Though it wasn't just the smoking. He didn't take much exercise apart from his garden. He loved his garden.' Billy paused again, he could see his father pulling up carrots he'd grown. 'Always proud of his vegetables.'

'You have lots of good memories.'

'I'm grateful for that. But however good it was, there could have been so many more good times ahead. And I think about the girls, but it isn't just them.

It's me, I know it's me. I miss him. And I can't really make sense of how much it seems to have affected me.'

'Yes, he was special, you miss him, and it's really affected you.'

'He was special. I suppose everyone says that. But he was. He was ready for a joke, have a laugh. He'd completely lose it sometimes, tears would stream down his face about something. And it was infectious. It would get us all going. End up not knowing what on earth we were laughing at. Just great to have around, you know?'

Chris nodded, aware of not feeling there was anything to say in response. Billy had his memories, they were his and he was revisiting them now. Chris felt that his role at this point was to, in a sense, be there as a kind of witness to what Billy needed to relive.

'It's different to last week, you know. I didn't know what to say. Now, I don't seem to know when to stop.'

'And that's OK too.'

'I guess so. I feel kind of different. Hmm. Hard to describe. This'll maybe sound strange but, yeah, I'm glad he was my dad.' Billy paused as words came into his mind. He felt an upwelling of emotion again. 'You know what's hard, really hard?'

'No.'

Billy wanted to speak but his lips were closed tight. His heart was thumping in his chest again, and he could feel the tears building up in his eyes. 'I never really told him how I felt.'

'How you felt?'

'About him. You just don't do you? I should have done. I could have done, but I didn't. Now it's too late. I can say it but ...,' Billy shook his head, '... but he can't hear me.'

'Things you wished you'd said and still want to say, but he can't hear.' Chris kept his response focused. He was aware of feeling incredibly concentrated. Something about the way Billy was talking demanded his total attention. He was glad he felt like that and was responding in the way that he was. It was quite natural and unforced. He felt the depth to what Billy was saying. Every word seemed to carry emotion. Everything related back to some memory, something that remained alive to Billy, in his heart, in his mind. He felt privileged to be listening.

'It's too late, isn't it?'

'That's how it feels?'

'Yeah.' He smiled, slightly wryly. 'You know, sometimes I wish I did believe that you lived on or went to Heaven or something. But I can't, I don't.'

You mean you think that would make a difference?'

'I think so. It wouldn't feel so permanent, so ..., I don't know, I'm sure it would feel different. But, well, I don't know ...'.

'It's something that you just don't know.'

'No. Suppose not.' Billy could feel the emotions building once again. 'He was a good dad and a good granddad, he really was.'

'Mhmm, good to you, to your daughters.'

'He was just so good to have around, you know?' The tears had formed in Billy's eyes again, driven there by the rising emotions.
'Yeah, so good to have around.'

> This kind of simple, focused, empathic response can be so powerful. It goes direct to what is being said. And in these kinds of response tone of voice, facial expression and body language are such powerful contributing factors. Where a client is engaging with painful feelings, it is so important that they not only hear that they are being heard, but that they also feel it, and arguably the latter is more important.

'Just something about knowing he was there, somehow; he was always there for us, always.' Billy closed his eyes as the surge of emotion tore through him. 'Always there. Always had time.'
'That was important, him being there, having time for you all.'
Billy had screwed his eyes up, they burned with emotion. 'I miss him.' Billy swallowed, his breathing coming in short, sharp intakes. 'He was always just so full of life. I think that's partly what makes it so hard to accept. He wasn't someone you could imagine not being there. And then, now, he isn't and I just don't seem able to accept it. I don't want to. I want him to still be here. Is that crazy? Is it? Sometimes I think, what's wrong with me? That I can't, I don't know . . . , I just.' Billy was shaking his head again.
'It seems sometimes as though there's something wrong with you because of the way you feel?'
'I can't . . . . I just . . .'. Billy looked at Chris. 'I can't accept he's gone.'
'No, it seems he was such a part of your life, and it just feels like you can't accept he's not there any more.'

> There are too many words in the response; it could have been much briefer and more focused. A nodding of the head and 'can't accept he's gone' would have sufficed. And there would have been, perhaps, a more prolonged moment of eye contact, an opportunity for something deep to have been conveyed or shared between them, a holding of the client in his sensed inability to accept that his father has gone. This would arguably have been more therapeutic.

Billy looked away. 'I really respect him, you know, for who he was, how he was. He was a good man, it doesn't seem fair, doesn't seem right. And I know life isn't always fair, people die and you wonder why, why them? He just had so much life, such a presence. It's like there's a big gap, big hole, nothing to fill it.'
'Nothing to fill that gap he's left behind.'

'I'd talk to him about, you know, different things. He'd always give you good advice. He just ..., I don't know, he was just there, always there. I just miss talking to him, you know. But it's more than that. It's him just not being there. He's a memory and yet ..., he's so much more than a memory. Hmm. I look at his tools and I can remember him using them. The different things he's made, we made together. We used to joke that maybe we should have gone into business together. We never did. I mean, we did a few jobs for other people, him more than me, but it was always more of a hobby for him. He loved working with wood. I don't know why. I guess he picked that up from *his* father.'

'Something that ran in the family?'

'Mhmm, something like that. I just, I don't know, we built our kitchen together, and at the time, well, yes, it was something we did. We did a good job, though I say it myself. Now I sit in the kitchen and I can remember us doing it. It's like I'm surrounded by him and yet he isn't, but he is, you know?'

'Mhmm, the things that he did, that so remind you of him, just make him feel so present.'

'And that's maybe why it's hard to accept he's not there because there are so many things that remind me. Hmm. So many things.'

'And things that you did together.'

'Yeah, yeah, we did a lot of things together. Mhmm. Glad we did, glad that's how it was, and yet somehow, is it possible that it can make it more difficult?'

'It seems from what you are saying you were really close, really shared some good times.'

A number of the preceding empathic responses might have been briefer and may not have come across with enough feeling tone. Is the counsellor a little detached? Could the responses have been influenced, perhaps, by the counsellor's own feelings, maybe in relation to his own father?

'Mhmm, we did. And it's, yeah .... Hmm. We did. Hmm, yeah. Yeah.' Thoughts, feelings were rising up once again. A particular line of thought had become more present in Billy's mind. It wasn't an easy thing to say. He could feel the emotion again, his throat, his eyes, burning. He took a deep breath and slowly blew the air out through his mouth. 'Ohh.'

'There's a lot that you miss.'

'Mhmm, and it's not just about the past. I mean it is, the memories, the reminder, you know? It's something else as well, and it feels important, really important.' He swallowed, he could feel it wasn't going to be easy to say. His voice felt as though it was wavering with the emotion.

Chris nodded gently, slowly. 'Mhmm?'

Billy was taking a deep breath. 'It's the thought of not doing those things again, together. Just knowing that we'll never, you know, work on something. It's not just about the past, not really. I mean, yeah, it is, but it's also about the future. Hmm. Feels like that's quite important, you know?'

'It's not just about the past, what you did together, the memories, the reminders, it's as much about the future, the things you won't do, can't do together.'
'I think that's what I'm missing, in a way missing more. Things that haven't happened, that can't now happen. I suppose I sort of had . . . , well, you know, just thought that things would carry on. You do. I suppose I saw him being around and we'd carry on as we always have. I guess we did spend a lot of time together in many ways. Hmm, a lot of time.'

> Bereavement is, if you like, a two-directional process. Yes, there is what has been lost in terms of the person who is not now there, and there is the loss of the future involvement with that person. Clients may find that they need to engage with each at different times. For some people one will be more important than the other. The person-centred counsellor will allow the client to focus on what is most pressing for them.

'And that's why there's that big gap, all the time you spent together.'
'And now, now it's like, hmm, I sort of feel a bit lost somehow.'
'Mhmm, lost, not having him around.'
'Mhmm.' Billy's voice had softened. The intensity of the emotion had quelled. Chris's tone of voice reflected this, there was a stillness in the room, it felt to Chris as though Billy had become calmer, more reflective somehow. He did not wish to disturb that.
Billy lapsed into silence. It was a different kind of silence. There was something calming about it, almost as though there wasn't anything more to say. As though a kind of natural pause had arisen. 'Hmm.' He sat, still thinking of his father. The moments passed.
Chris sat, respecting the quiet. Yes, that was the word for it, it was quiet rather than a silence. He wasn't sure quite what that meant, but it seemed somehow significant to associate quiet rather than silence with what was being experienced, what he was experiencing. He gently voiced his experience. 'It feels quiet.'

> An interesting contrast. What might this difference be? Silence is what happens when there is no sound; however, quiet may be thought of as something more deep and profound. At least in this case. Other people may use these words to mean something different. Empathising with a word does not mean the counsellor has empathised with the experience that the word has been chosen to represent. In this case, as we shall see, the client attaches his own meaning to the word that the counsellor has used, and whether or not they are meaning the same thing somehow does not matter.

Billy nodded, he felt it too. It was like the quiet that arises when there is no need to say anything further. It sort of felt as though he had said what he needed to say. And it was quiet, and his life was quiet without his father being around. That was something else. Yes, he was quieter, life was quieter. 'It's as much about the future. It's not just the past, it's the future, I think that's what's hard. Yes, being reminded of the past, of him, what he did, of things we did together, yes, that's not easy, but that feels like that's sort of OK, somehow. That sort of, I don't know, I can make sense of that. It's, yeah, tangible, you know? I see something, reminds me of him, or brings a particular memory to mind. And yeah, I can feel good about the memory, it's not that so much that gets to me, makes me feel sad. It's when I think that it's gone in the sense that it won't happen again. It's, it's that. It's that knowing, yes, yes, that's what's so hard to accept, knowing that I can't have those experiences again.'

'Mhmm, can't have those experiences, with him.'

'No, no I just have the memories, and they're important, and I'm glad I have them, but the future, no more memories, in a way. I only have what I have, but I sort of want more.' Billy smiled, a little weakly. 'Hmm, no more memories, no new ones. Not of him, of being together.'

'No new memories, that thought of no new memories to be created in the future, of him, of being together.'

'It's like losing the future is harder than losing the past? Does that make sense?'

Chris nodded. 'Yeah, it makes sense to me, that the loss of what might have been feels more present than the loss of what was.'

It was Billy nodding now. 'That's exactly it. Mhmm, hearing that, yeah, that really makes, really does sum it up somehow. It is the future, isn't it, that I'm missing? The things that can't happen, the things I still want to do with him, or with him around. Hmm, that's, hmm, that's not easy.'

'No, the things you won't now be able to do together.'

'I mean I know he's not there, I know it, and I know I can't dwell on how things might have been. I know that, but it's like I know it up here?' Billy touched the side of his head. 'But that's not enough. It's like, yeah, I know it, but I don't, um, I was going say I don't feel it, but I do, yes, of course I do. I do feel it, but what I don't, um, what I can't seem to do, no, it's what I don't want to do. I don't want to accept it. That's, yeah, that's what it is. I really don't want to accept it.'

As we have seen, bereavement can be as much if not more about the future that can't now happen as about the past that is ended. Of course, it varies from person to person, and can be greatly dependent on how much of a future the bereaved person feels they would have had with the person who has died. Here, Billy clearly has a long history of spending a lot of time with his father and, clearly, he had naturally expected that to continue, possibly expecting more time once his father had retired. Coming to terms with that future now having to be different is in many ways likely to be the main focus for him. He sees something that reminds him of the past, but it is also going to remind him of the future that now cannot be. Loss runs behind and before us. The things we never did and now cannot do with the person who is no longer there.

'You don't want to accept that your dad's not there and that the future you'd assumed would happen, can't now happen.' Chris sought to be clear in his response. Billy was working his own way towards an understanding of where the emphasis lay in his sense of loss and bereavement. He didn't want to influence it. It was Billy's inner world after all, and Billy needed to find his own words, his own meaning, for what he was experiencing.

Billy listened in part to what Chris was saying, but also he was still very much with what he had said himself. 'Yeah, I don't want to accept it.' He was talking more to himself than to Chris. It was like he was verbalising his own internal dialogue.

Chris picked up on the reflective tone of Billy's voice. He didn't want to draw him away from his internal process. He made sure the tone of his response was unlikely to feel invasive or disturb what was occurring for Billy. 'Yeah, not something you want to accept.'

They both lapsed into silence. But the silence was very different to what had occurred in the first session. Then it was more of a silence about not knowing what to say, or not being, or feeling, able to say things. Now it was more a matter of things that needed to have been said, had been said. There was a kind of natural silence that followed. It was more a time to assimilate what had been said, and thought and felt, a kind of moment in which to draw together the threads of what had occurred, of allowing the experiences and insights to come together creating, perhaps, a new sense of how things were.

The session continued, though it maintained a reflective tone, and Billy left early, saying that he felt somehow that he had a lot to think about, that he felt as though he had done as much as he wanted, or needed, to do that day. The stillness, the silence, the quiet was still with him as he left. It sort of felt protective, somehow. He wasn't quite sure what it meant, or why it was there, but he felt calmer as he drove away.

Chris, meanwhile, had returned to the counselling room and was sitting with his own thoughts. The quietness had felt profound. It was with him too. He honoured it. It somehow didn't feel right to suddenly start doing something else. He had time to sit, there was nothing pressing. He didn't have another client to see that evening. He felt as though he just simply wanted himself to be in that place, that space that somehow both he and Billy had entered and shared during that session. He thought about himself, his own expectations of the future. He thought about his partner and the assumptions he had about their future together, aware that, yes, they were assumptions. But then, who wanted to think about a future that you didn't want? He knew they wanted to be together, and you didn't dwell on a future not being together. It was too painful. Yet you also knew that, yes, things could happen. Always that tension, or potential tension, between wanting continuity and knowing that life is wracked with uncertainty. He smiled. How we try to make the uncertain certain. And we can't. And we get so attached to what we want, hope, expect, assume, and then it doesn't work out, then it hurts, then it can hurt so much. He took a deep breath and began to write his notes for the session.

Points for discussion

- What elements of counselling session 2 made the most impression on you, and why?
- Evaluate Chris's responses in terms of 'the necessary and sufficient conditions'. How would you describe the strengths and weaknesses of his application of the person-centred approach?
- What were the key elements to session 2, and why?
- Does the reference to 'quiet' have meaning to you? Reflect on the differences in a therapeutic context between silence, quiet, stillness and calmness.
- What might you take to supervision had you been Chris?
- Write notes for this session.

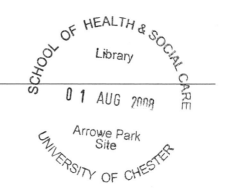

Counselling session 3: The pain of knowing that he has gone

Billy was sitting in the counselling room. The session had already begun with him saying a little about his week. Chris had listened and responded to what, at times, had begun to feel a bit like a list of events. And yet as Billy spoke Chris just felt that the way he was speaking, it seemed as though each event hadn't been fully lived. It was like there was no enthusiasm, everything sounded flat. He found himself thinking that it was like something was missing, something important.

'Things just don't seem to have the same . . . , I don't know how to describe it, but it's like things sort of don't have any shine, if that makes any sense. And yet, after last week, I left here feeling different. I can't describe it. It faded as the week went on, but I felt sort of easier somehow, a little more alive, I suppose. But I couldn't maintain it.' Billy paused, wondering if that was maybe how it was with counselling, but that perhaps eventually it sort of stuck, stayed with you, became more permanent. Something like that.

'Like you couldn't maintain that feeling that you had as the week went on, it sort of faded.'

'It wasn't that I tried to maintain it; more I was aware it was there and then, well, then it had gone. Funnily enough I slept better that night. And I sort of felt OK the next day, but the next night was back to usual, waking up, unable to settle.' Billy actually felt quite desperate about his lack of sleep. It was leaving him feeling irritable at home, but he didn't feel like saying any of this to Chris. He just had to learn to handle it a bit better.

'So, a night of sleeping OK, and the next day OK, but then back to the usual pattern.'

'Seems so, though I'm not dreaming as much, not waking up quite so unsettled, but still waking up. It's different. I think about things more, I mean, yes, well I did before, but it's different. I feel different somehow. It's like when I wake up now I suppose rather than my thoughts being sort of anxious, I'm thinking more without that reaction.' Billy wasn't too sure how to describe it, he just knew that it felt different. 'Does that make sense?'

'Let me check that I'm understanding you, Billy. It's like when you wake up your thinking feels different, not so anxious.'

Billy nodded. 'I think about the past mainly, but then about the future too. I sort of feel like I need some kind of a direction and you know I got to thinking about the dreams, it's sort of easier to do when you're not so anxious and unsettled. That journey, always trying to get somewhere but never arriving. It's like I'm not sure what my direction is and maybe I'm looking for a direction somehow. But then, I get to think about my family, they're my direction, and my job, you know, but there's that gap, a sort of . . . , I don't know, something missing. And I know that's my dad, or at least, it must be partly that, but I need something else, something else in my life, but I don't know what.'

Chris listened attentively to what Billy was saying. He seemed quite on edge as he was speaking. It seemed like it was really important for him to find that direction. He could appreciate this. He wanted to show his empathic understanding for what Billy had been saying, and the tone of it as well. 'It feels, I don't know, like there's a sort of urgency – is that the right word? – in the way that you speak of wanting to find a direction, fill the gap. Is that how it is?'

Billy thought. 'Sort of, something like that. It's like I've got to, yes, I suppose it is a kind of urgency, sort of. Not sure.'

Chris recognised that probably he'd used the wrong word. It hadn't been a word that Billy was relating to easily, so it was probably from his, Chris's, frame of reference. 'May not be the right word, the right idea.'

So long as what is being suggested by the counsellor is genuinely felt, then it is less likely to be problematic in terms of its impact on the therapeutic relationship. Constantly using words that don't make sense to the client would leave the client distrusting the counsellor's ability to empathise or understand. But getting it not quite right, if the attempt has been sincere, can enable the client to feel encouraged to explore more deeply and seek to convey what is present for them in some other way, which may then be caught and understood by the counsellor. Through this process, the client becomes more accurately aware of what they are experiencing, and more able to accurately communicate it to the counsellor. As this is achieved more and more consistently, the client enters into a more congruent state. It is helped by the fact that the counsellor's attempt to understand is authentic, they genuinely want to understand what the client is experiencing and seeking to communicate. This genuineness is a vital component of the therapist's attitude and of the therapeutic process.

'It's like, you know, I can't replace my dad, I know that, I sort of wouldn't want to and, well, that wouldn't make sense. But I have to fill that gap, it sort of, well, it's there, I can feel it, particularly at night, though not only then. And I don't know if I can, maybe I can't, but it's like there's a sort of hole inside me, and I want to fill it, but I don't know how to or what with. And then I wonder if it's

just normal and something I have to get used to, sort of accept it. But I can't, I don't want to, not yet, not really.'
'So something about filling the gap left by your dad, like a hole inside you, and it's whether you can accept that he's no longer there to fill it. And not wanting to fill it.' Chris wasn't sure about what he was saying. It felt difficult to get hold of. He had a sense of what Billy was saying, but somehow it felt sort of hazy. Yes, he could understand it logically, and yet somehow it wasn't clear. And he appreciated that as it wasn't clear for Billy then maybe what he was experiencing was the sort of hazy experience that Billy was having and trying to find the right words for.
'Can I?' Billy paused, lost in own thoughts and uncertainty. 'Can I? How? How do I fill it?'
'Mmm. Comes down to "how can I fill the gap in me?".'

> Responses such as this in the first person can be very therapeutic. However, it is a form of empathy that is not offered all of the time. Often it is most appropriate when there is a strong sense of 'I' in what the client is struggling with.

Billy knew how he should be responding. 'And you know I know that it should be my family, of course it should, and being there for my mother as well. But, I don't know, whenever we do things as a family, he's there, with me, sort of, yeah, and I'm, you know, saying things like, "Dad would have enjoyed that", or "wish he was here to see this", things like that.'
'Things that feel like they're about what he has missed.' Chris felt himself frowning, he still didn't feel connected somehow with Billy.
'Yeah, what he's missing. And, yeah, what we're missing too, you know?'
Chris nodded. 'And, yeah, you really miss his involvement and you sort of bring him into the picture, so to speak, aware that he hasn't experienced things that are happening now.'
'And it affects me, how things are for me. It's not that I'm always thinking of him, but in a way I do, particularly when we're together as a family, and particularly when Mum's with us. My thoughts turn to him really easily. Mmm.'
'Like he's a kind of reference point in some way, sort of when the family are together he sort of has to be there too?'
'Mhmm. Yes, it doesn't feel right otherwise. It just doesn't.' Billy took a deep breath. He felt stiff. He hadn't moved in the chair for a while and his back was stiff. He moved his shoulders a little to try and free it. 'Oh, I don't know. I can't stop thinking about him, I don't want to stop thinking about him, but I want to sort of, I don't know . . . , I just don't know.'
'You think about him, you don't want to stop that, but . . .'.
'But, yes, very much "but . . ."'. Billy sniffed. 'Mum's been good. She can see that I'm hurting and I don't want it to be difficult for her because of how I am. She

tells me it really is OK, he's gone, he's at peace, and that we all have to make the best of our lives. She's moved on. She spends time with us, but she has her own life as well, with her friends. But I just can't seem to be like her. I know she has tough times, she's told me that there are times when she can feel very lonely and lost. But that it isn't as bad now as it was to start with. But for me, somehow, I don't know, it feels like it's getting worse, not easier.' Billy was shaking his head. Can't seem to get my head round how she's coped and I just, well, I just feel like I'm going nowhere.'

'Can't understand how she's able to be the way that she is.'

'Yes, and, well, it's an awful thing to say maybe, but sometimes I think that she didn't care. How could she have cared and then get on like she is. I know how difficult it is, maybe she didn't care like I do. And that's not fair. They loved each other, I know that, but sometimes I do think that way. I know she has to move on. But ...'.

'But?'

'Makes me wonder.'

'Makes you wonder how much she cared?'

> The client does not confirm that the counsellor's response is correct, but builds on it. Sometimes this can be an indication that the counsellor has summed something up in a powerful and accurate way. And it immediately releases the client to move on in their process.

'And that's crazy thinking, it really is, but I get like that. I know she loved him, and still does. It's me. I suppose everyone should feel like I do, but they don't, at least they don't seem to. Maybe that's a good thing. If everyone was like me, well, don't suppose it would be too good. I don't want everyone feeling like I do. But, and this'll sound crazy I'm sure, but it can feel like I'm the only one keeping his memory alive.' Billy felt confused. He felt as though he was rambling. He didn't understand, he couldn't make sense of it all, he didn't like how he felt, but he didn't want to let go of thinking about his father.

'Feels like it's all down to you.' Chris paused, aware of his own sense that it all felt like quite a burden for Billy. He decided to share his experience as it felt strongly related to what Billy had said and how he had said it. 'And that feels like quite a burden, a heavy burden to carry, that's how I'm experiencing what you are saying.'

Billy smiled weakly, and sniffed. 'S'ppose it is. But, it's like something that I have to do.'

'Mhmm, it's important, you want to keep his memory alive.'

'But it gets in the way and that's what's so difficult. I want to not forget, I want him to be part of my life ...'. He paused. 'Maybe that's what I'm doing.'

Chris nodded slowly, it felt as though Billy had realised something important and he left him the space to be with his thoughts, his feelings.

There is empathy towards what the client is experiencing and communicating, and it seems there is also a need for a kind of situational empathy, and in this case the counsellor is sensitive to the client's need to be with his thoughts and feelings. The client has spoken reflectively. That can be a powerful indication that the client needs a moment or two, perhaps longer, to be with that reflective process. The counsellor warmly accepts how the client needs to be and does not intrude into the process that is sensed to be occurring within the client.

'Hmm, I'm trying to keep him in my life, trying to make him a part of things. And I do remind everyone about how Dad would enjoy something that we're doing. And the children, particularly them. And they sort of agree. They seem to like that and they'll talk about him, maybe share a memory, particularly Sarah. Somehow she was closer to him, I don't know why. Tara sort of seems to be able to relive the memory or whatever and then switch back to what she's doing. Sarah will go quiet for a bit, maybe she's a bit like me. And sometimes Mum'll say something afterwards, and Clare. They've both pointed out that it may be upsetting the children, that I do it too often. Maybe they're right, I don't know, but it feels like I need to make him be part of things, you know?'

'I'm just aware of my sense of how important it is for you to bring your dad into the experience.' Chris knew he wasn't responding empathically to what Billy had just said, but felt that he was acknowledging something that felt strongly present through what Billy had been saying.

Billy was nodding. 'They don't understand, Chris, they really don't.'

Chris was aware that this was probably the first time Billy had used his name when speaking to him. He sensed the importance of what was being said and that the way Billy had spoken was expressive of this. He wanted Chris to hear, that what he was saying was somehow more directed at him by using his name.

'They just don't understand, that it's different for you.'

Billy stared ahead of him, his own thoughts beginning to crowd in on him. 'No, they don't. They don't know what it's like. Feels that they just forget him. Maybe it's their way. I can't be like that. It's not right. It's not how I want to be.'

'No, you need to keep his memory alive, in your thoughts, in your heart, in the family, is that what you mean?'

Billy nodded and looked at Chris. 'Yes. Yes, that's exactly it. That's how it is.' It sort of felt a relief somehow. 'I need to keep him alive.' Chris noted that it was now not just the memory, now it felt like it was more than that. 'Yes, I mean, I know, well, you know ..., but that's how it is. It doesn't feel right to not keep him a part of everything.'

'Mhmm, that in some way it just wouldn't be right to not keep him part of everything.'

'Yes.' Billy took a deep breath.

'Mhmm. I'm really struck by the strength of your feeling in this, Billy, it really feels very present to me.' Chris spoke as he felt. There was a real intensity in what Billy was saying and Chris felt strongly that he really wanted Billy to know that he was hearing and experiencing this.

Sometimes this kind of response can be the effect of a build-up within the counsellor. It can almost be a kind of release for the therapist, a making visible of what has become present within them. Yet it is very much a congruent response. It is more than simply acknowledging what a client tells you they are feeling, it is making visible to the client that the counsellor, too, is really experiencing something of what is present for the client. The focus is more visceral.

'Well it's certainly present for me.'

'Keeping him alive, keeping him present.'

'Can't let him go. I can't.' Billy looked away again.

'No, can't let him go, keep him alive.' Chris nodded. The atmosphere was changing, he felt a familiar quietness emerging. He felt as though he was suddenly more alert. Something was happening. He recognised the experience. Often it could occur when something deep was emerging for a client. The silence had a certain electric feel to it. He kept his concentration and his openness, sensing that something important was happening. He needed to be open, ready and responsive.

'Keep him alive.' Billy's words seemed to float from a distance.

Chris sat quietly, maintaining his attention and focus on Billy. Not wishing to in any way disturb the internal process that was occurring for him. He responded, his tone of voice gentle. 'Trying to keep him alive.'

Silence. A very, very quiet silence. Chris waited.

Billy felt himself go cold. He had stopped thinking. A kind of blankness had sort of descended on him. A kind of nothingness. Nothingness. Emptiness. So quiet. So quiet. Billy closed his eyes, he felt a churning in the pit of his stomach and it seemed to rise up his body. It wasn't a sick feeling, but more of a sickly unease. His arms felt strangely heavy, numb, and yet he could feel them as well. His shoulders were tight and quite raised, but he was oblivious to this. He was also holding his breath. It was as though everything had stopped, for a moment. He had no sense of time. He wasn't thinking, he just was. The thought came clearly into his mind. He didn't know where it came from, it was just suddenly there, like a quiet voice but seemingly with no one speaking. *You can't keep him alive.* He remained still, hearing the words in his head, feeling the surge of emotion that now tightened his throat, his eyes filling with tears. He took a deep breath and dropped his head into his hands, the emotion continuing to pour through him. His breath started to come in short bursts. His eyes, his face, felt so wet. He sniffed and swallowed. 'Oh.' He continued to hold his head in his hands.

Chris reached over and placed his hand on Billy's shoulder. He pressed gently, wanting to reassure him, convey his presence, but not take his focus away from what was happening, from what was clearly being released.

> Physical contact, sensitively offered, can be extremely powerful. It should be firm. Often it is to provide a kind of reassurance. It connects at a physical level and can be particularly helpful where a client's thoughts and feelings are inducing a strong physical reaction. In a sense, physical contact becomes an empathic response to the physicality of what the client is experiencing. Through touch, the counsellor can convey a genuine warm acceptance of the physical expression of the client, empathic sensitivity to the physicality of the client's experiencing and a grounded quality of authenticity.

Billy didn't move, except for a gentle rocking to and fro. Chris heard him taking a deep breath, and another 'oh' that was more of a deep, deep sigh, coming from somewhere in the depths of his being. The sound of emotion. The sound of a man experiencing something of himself, a hurt, a pain, a horror, a realisation that was unwanted, and yet which had burst upon him. A knowing, a genuine knowing, that his dad was gone and however hard he tried, he couldn't bring him back, couldn't keep him alive. Only memories. Only memories. And the pain of the absoluteness of his having gone, and his never coming back.

Chris continued to sit closer to Billy, maintaining the slight pressure on his shoulder. He didn't want to interrupt the release of emotion. It had to come out. To say something or do something that might hinder the flow in some way would not be helpful. It is one of the hardest moments for a client, and for a therapist, sitting and knowing that the person you are with is facing up to a pain that they have tried to avoid, to keep away from, the pain of loss, absolute loss. The pain that comes from knowing, finally knowing and accepting, that someone special is no longer there. A hurt that can emerge soon after the loss, or weeks, or months later. Chris felt his heart open to Billy and maintained his attitude of caring, compassion, call it what you will – love, perhaps? Love, the kind of love that bearing witness to the suffering of another human being pulls out of you. Billy, still hunched over, groaning with the pain of his loss, and there was nothing to be done to relieve that pain. It had to be sat through. For Chris it felt like his own emotions were going through a wringer, being squeezed out, yet how much more was Billy experiencing?

Billy just sat there, he wasn't thinking about how he felt, he just was what he felt – a groan of pain, of loss, of heartache, of emptiness. He'd never felt anything like this before, and had no idea that he had the capacity to feel what he was feeling. It was like a tidal wave of hurt that filled his whole being, bigger than his body, enveloping him. 'Oh God.' Billy felt his eyes and throat still burning, he swallowed, the lump in his throat seemed huge. He took a deep breath. He could feel Chris's pressure on his shoulder more clearly now. The pain was subsiding a little. He felt strange, not quite in himself. It wasn't a feeling he could have described. He just knew he felt weird.

Chris pressed Billy's shoulder a little more, sensing that Billy was emerging from his experience. 'Take your time, no rush. You've had a shock, it'll be OK.'

Billy was taking a deep breath and as he breathed out drew his hands down his face a little, blinking over his fingertips as he did. He closed his eyes again as another surge of emotion flowed through him, less intense, but setting off another flow of tears which spilt over his eyelids as he closed his eyes once more.

He kept his left hand over his face as he fumbled in his pocket for his handkerchief, finally releasing it from his pocket and taking it in both hands burying his face in it. He rubbed at his eyes through the handkerchief. They felt puffy and gritty and still burning. He rubbed his handkerchief across his face and looked up, breathing deeply once more as he did so, and blew the breath out of his mouth as he dropped his hands, resting his chin on his fingertips. He blinked, looking across at Chris, still feeling somewhat disorientated from his experience. Chris, meanwhile, had squeezed Billy's shoulder once more and had drawn his hand back as Billy's face had emerged from behind his handkerchief.

'You OK?'

Few words have been spoken during Billy's emotional release, yet Chris's warm and supportive presence has been communicated. Billy may have felt lonely within himself, but he would also, to some degree, have experienced not being alone. Chris has maintained his focus and his openness. He has remained responsive not only to Billy but also to his own experiencing. He has, one might say, stood by his client, a companion, a fellow human being, allowing himself to be affected by the pain that has emerged within the client. It is highly likely that while that openness within the counsellor is purely subjective to them, such a state of being does make an impression on the client. More is probably communicated by this openness than by words, body language or even physical touch. Perhaps in moments of sensitive contact like this, there is a more subtle touch involved at an emotional level that may have some kind of energetic basis.

'I think so.' He swallowed, and blew his nose. 'Ooohh, I feel knackered.' The emotions were still very close, he could feel them and he knew it wouldn't take much for them to spill out again. 'He's gone, hasn't he? I mean, I can't keep him alive, can I? That's what I've been doing, but I can't. I can't.' He breathed out heavily as he finished speaking, a sigh of resignation, of perhaps a final acceptance of some kind.

'No, you can't keep your dad alive, not any more.' Chris was very aware that he used the word 'dad' in his response. It felt right to do so. It was instinctive.

'Hmm. No. No, he's not here any more. I mean, I've known it, but I guess I haven't been able to accept it.'

'Maybe haven't wanted to accept it?'

'Mhmm. That's closer. Yeah. Hmm.' Billy was taking another deep breath. 'Mmm.' He paused. 'I feel wretched. Is that what I mean? Wrecked maybe. Where do all the feelings come from?'

Chris nodded. 'We can carry so much'.

Billy shook his head. 'I've had that locked up inside me?'

Chris nodded. 'Probably trying to keep away from it, or keeping it away from you.'

Billy was shaking his head. 'I still feel very, very fragile.'

'You will. It's a shock. It can feel quite shattering.'

'It's certainly a shock, and very tiring. My eyes, they just feel like sandpaper, so does my throat.'

'Have some water, please.' Chris poured some from the jug beside him and handed the glass to Billy.

'Thanks.' He sipped it, it felt refreshingly cool. It was what he needed. He took the glass from his lips, which he tightened. Another deep breath. 'It's like, I just, hmm. I need to have time with this. Got so many feelings inside me. Just need to try and settle back down.'

'Yeah, do what you need to do, Billy, take your time, no rush, just be how you need to be.'

'I feel like I . . .'. He shook his head, unsure what to say, unsure quite what he was feeling.

'Mhmm?'

'I feel wiped out. He's gone' Billy shook his head. 'I know it, I suppose I've always known it, but now I know it differently. Hmm.' Billy paused, he wasn't thinking. It was like he just had to sit. He wasn't trying to make sense of anything, in truth he really didn't have the energy. For now he just needed to sit. He took another sip of water. 'Hmm.'

'Like you really know.'

Billy nodded. He looked up at Chris, and then looked down again, still nodding slightly and breathing quite deeply.

Chris made no response other than to maintain his focus and attention on Billy. There were about ten minutes of the session left. Chris trusted that Billy would use the time as he needed, maybe to say something about what he had experienced, maybe to sit quietly, maybe to prepare himself for heading home. It was Billy's time and Chris would be there with him as he sat being as he needed to be. He'd check out that Billy felt OK to head off, happy to offer a little more time if he needed it. He knew that while he still felt alert himself, he would also feel drained after the session. His own emotions had become powerfully present in his experience and he knew he would need time to settle back down himself.

One thing Billy did do before the session ended was to thank Chris. 'I knew you were there, it wasn't that I was thinking about you being there, but you were and, well . . . ,' Billy nodded, 'it helped. I'm grateful.'

Chris smiled, slightly tight-lipped, 'Thanks, thanks for that. I'm glad I was able to respond in a way that you experienced as helpful. That was how I wanted to be.'

Points for discussion

- How has the session left you? How do you deal with the feelings and thoughts than can arise during an intense session like this?

- What do you feel facilitated Billy in the emotional release that occurred?
- Evaluate the accuracy of Chris's empathy during this session. Were there occasions when you would have responded differently? What would have been your responses, and why? Justify your responses in terms of person-centred theory and practice.
- Does empathy always have to be accurate to be effective? How accurate is necessary and sufficient for therapeutic effect?
- What would you be taking to supervision from this session?
- Write notes for this session.

CHAPTER 4

Supervision session 1: Beliefs about death and dying

Chris was quite relieved to be in supervision. His last session with Billy, the previous evening, was still very much with him. He had found himself reflecting on it during the night. It had been a very deep experience for Billy and it had certainly made a strong impression as he had sat there listening to him, trying to offer him support but without distracting or invading the psychological and emotional space that Billy needed. He was also aware that he wanted to reflect on the whole counselling process so far, not just that particular interaction.

He had supervision once a month for his client work, and the same for his supervision practice. He preferred to keep this separate from his therapy work. He knew that not everyone took that approach, it was really just how it had developed, and he preferred it that way. Yes, there was a similarity and there were overlaps. He remembered in one supervision session exploring how different he was as a supervisor to how he was as a counsellor. That had been particularly helpful. He realised that there wasn't so much a difference in how he was – he was still seeking to offer the therapeutic conditions for his client or supervisee to experience – but as a supervisor he was also carrying the agenda of checking that his supervisee was effectively able to offer the therapeutic conditions, and recognising that there may be times when he would need to offer support to help restore the supervisee.

Often he found it was a matter of helping his supervisee restore congruence as often it was an emergence of incongruence that seemed to block accurate empathy and genuinely felt unconditional positive regard. And this was what he found as well, when he came to supervision. It was an opportunity for him to reflect on what was happening, on the process, on the effect it was having on him. An opportunity to reflect on whether he was offering the therapeutic conditions, or whether there was material from the client that was impacting on him in such a way that it was making this difficult.

He thought of Billy. It wasn't difficult to feel for him, although he was also aware of the intensity that he had been expressing before the emotional release, that had felt almost unnerving in some way. He was also aware on reflection, how easy it might have been to have started to feel some sympathy for Billy's family. He hadn't felt that, but he recognised that that might have emerged for him.

Lucy came in, she had just been making a hot drink.

'So, what do you want to bring today?' She spoke as she set his cup of tea down on the table beside him.

'Well, I really want to review a couple of my supervisees, but before that I really want to spend a bit of time processing a new client and the impact he is having on me.'

Lucy settled herself into the chair and prepared herself to listen and to be fully present and available.

'You remember last time that I was planning to see a new client, Billy. He'd phoned to make an appointment. A bereavement issue.'

Lucy remembered and nodded. 'Yes, you said you had a new client who you were about to start working with.'

'Well, I suppose, no, I know we've come a long way and in quite a short space of time. But that's how it is sometimes. And other times, as we know, the process can feel much slower.' He frowned and shook his head. 'Not sure that's really how I want to think about it. It's not a matter of fast or slow, it's about the pace that the client needs to go at. And people come for counselling at different stages in their process as well. What I would say, though, is that the first sessions were full of silences and, well, I stayed with them, allowing Billy to be how he needed to be, minimally letting him know that I was there, but really letting him have his own space. He seemed to be quite focused on his own thoughts. Some of the silences seemed awkward, uncomfortable, him not knowing what to say. But we seemed to work through that, really by my maintaining my focus and attention and I'm sure experiencing in myself a trust in the process. I am sure that helps to create a supportive atmosphere, although others may think that too subjective.'

'Your own inner attitude affecting how the client experiences the situation, do you mean?'

Chris nodded. 'I think that's important. Or maybe it just affects me, keeps me focused and alert. There is something about that attitude of trust. It's not that I am trusting something specific to happen, but it feels linked to acceptance and openness. I don't know, but I think it's a deeply facilitative attitude to have. There's no anxiety, and that can be unnerving sitting with someone who's anxious – I'm thinking about this from the client's perspective. I know as a client myself I always want my therapist to feel, well, present in a kind of solid sort of way, dependable, reliable, you know?'

Lucy nodded, briefly wondering if that was how Chris experienced her, but decided that was her curiosity and let it go, wanting to let Chris continue with what he wanted to say about Billy.

'Anyway, we've had three sessions. In the first I recall Billy saying that he didn't know what to say, but by the end of the session I did feel more of a sense of connection. Things had moved on. Yeah, more of a connection, more communication, verbal communication, but he felt more present, and maybe I was in response to this as well. I don't know. I felt present. Anyway, there was more of a connection.'

'OK, so, by the end of the session, after initial awkwardness and silences, you felt more connected.'

'Yes, but I think we both did. He said something, I think, yes, I'm sure he did, something about being unsure at one point during the session as to whether counselling was right for him. Yes, at the end, I was checking out whether he wanted to continue. Yes, that's right, that was when he told me about his mother having had counselling after his father had died. And she encouraged him to come along. But he was still so very focused on his father. It has been over a year since his death, but it seems they were close, doing things together.' It was difficult to remember back to the first two sessions, the last one was so present. He wasn't sure whether he was remembering what had happened accurately. It wasn't clear.

Lucy continued to sit and listen, seeking to maintain her openness to both what Chris was saying and how she was experiencing him. She was struck by a sense of the seriousness of how Chris was speaking. In a sense she wasn't surprised, she knew he took his counselling work seriously, and in an appropriate and professional manner. No, more than professional, it was personally important. She smiled inwardly, knowing that that was perhaps not the way others might see it. But for her, being a therapist was a personal commitment, and seriously personal because she was using herself as a therapist. 'Sorry, headed off into a train of thought there. I was thinking that you sounded serious, I mean, I know you take your work, your clients, being a therapist seriously, but there was something about the way you were speaking that struck me as conveying a particular seriousness. I don't know if that has meaning to you.'

In these situations it is important, from a person-centred viewpoint, to voice these 'inner journeys'. They may have relevance to the supervision process. And disclosure does demonstrate openness, which is important within the supervisory relationship. In this instance the train of thought was linked to a perception that the supervisor has had towards her supervisee's way of expressing himself. For some reason, it made a particular impression, strong enough for her to find herself dwelling on it. Where these inner journeys stem from a sense of connection with the client, then there is a high likelihood that they have relevance and meaning, and should be offered, but with an openness to the possibility that they may not have meaning for the supervisee.

Chris frowned, he wasn't sure what Lucy might be picking up. 'Can you say more?'

'Just that the way you were talking, something about ..., I don't know, it felt more serious than I've heard you speak about other clients. No, I'm not sure it's about contrast, it just struck me that there's something serious, a seriousness to what is happening for Billy, between you and Billy. Does that make sense?'

Chris felt himself taking a deep breath as he thought about what Lucy had said. Serious. It did feel serious. Did it feel unusually serious? He wasn't sure. It had certainly been intense that last session and, yes, in a way it had felt serious, it was an important and highly significant session and experience for Billy. 'I suppose that I do feel serious. The session yesterday evening was a very intense and emotional experience for Billy, well and for me, and I know that today.'

'Something about that session made a particularly strong impression on you?'

Chris nodded. 'I want to talk about that but I also want to put it in context, say a little more about those earlier sessions and the lead-up to the last session. Although those two early sessions now feel a little hazy, like they're obscured by yesterday's experience.' He smiled, wondering if that was how Billy might be feeling. Could last night have left him less sensitive to things that happened before? He began to describe the first two sessions in more detail, mentioning the silence and Billy's difficulty in referring directly to his father's death. 'He talked as well, and particularly in the last session, about how he needed to keep his dad's memory alive. That is important, was important.'

'Was? Is?' Lucy was struck by what Chris had just said and wondered where the emphasis needed to be placed.

'I think it is important to him, but maybe something will have changed from the last session. But I'll come back to that.' Chris paused, collecting his thoughts. 'Seems like he mentions his dad a lot at home, particularly when the family are together, bringing him into the conversation. That had started to become an issue for his mum. Seems like his mother is moving on but Billy, well, in the last session he was struggling with this, with whether people would move on like that if they really cared for his dad, cared like he did.' Chris frowned as he reconnected with the experience of listening to Billy as he had talked, so intensely, about how he couldn't understand them, and they couldn't understand him.

'Something come to mind?' Lucy had picked up on his change of expression.

'There was such an intensity. I mean, he really did seem intense. I could sense it, well, I don't like to label, but I could see it could have been seen as being almost to a point of obsession. You know how an obsession can almost take on an otherworldliness?' Chris was thinking how he had felt, and about how when someone is so locked into a way of seeing things that are clearly an expression of their reality, but which can seem so at odds with what someone looking on may be experiencing.

'And that was what you sensed?'

'It was heading in that direction. There's an uneasiness about it.'

'Makes you feel uneasy, you mean?'

Chris nodded. 'Yes, the person themselves is clearly, well, I suppose in a sense they are simply being what they are experiencing in awareness. I suppose, hmm, that's an interesting one, I guess there's a kind of congruence as far as they are concerned.'

'Maybe, maybe not. They may be aware of what they are experiencing, but is it a full and accurate awareness of what it is that is urging them to that obsessive degree?'

Congruence is more than being aware of what is being experienced. There is the matter of accuracy and a sense of knowing and understanding the nature of what has become present. So, for instance, something might cause a person to feel intense anger, but the reality may be that the intensity of the anger is not totally linked to the trigger in the present. There may actually be some other conditioning experience that, at an experiential level, is associated with what has occurred, but this other conditioning experience is not present in awareness or known to be associated by the person. Yes, they are aware of what they are experiencing, but we might say they do not know the full picture.

'I don't know, but it's just the intensity of what Billy was saying and how he was saying it, of his need to keep his father's memory alive and then, well, then he went quiet. Maybe the intensity was linked to what happened, a kind of precursor, or a final struggle to hang on to his need. The atmosphere changed, went quiet, I could feel myself becoming more alert. And, well, there was a huge emotional release.' Chris shook his head as he thought back to Billy sitting there, his face in his hands, and that painful, almost an otherworldly, again that word, groan coming from the depth of his being.

'Something released.'

'Something very deep, very deep, very intense and very overwhelming.'

Lucy felt her own alertness intensify as she heard Chris speak. It felt as though the atmosphere in the room now had changed. She could feel a kind of electric silence. She knew how experiences within therapy sessions could seemingly be carried into supervision, almost relived in some way. It felt that way.

'I can feel the intensity.' She spoke softly, not wanting to disrupt the silence, the quiet, the kind of hush that had descended in the room.

Chris nodded. He felt it too. It was having a humbling effect on him. He tightened his lips, and immediately saw Billy doing the same thing in the session. 'It's very present.'

Lucy nodded, feeling OK about simply being with it, allowing what had emerged in supervision to be, to exist. She could not explain the experience, she didn't really feel she needed to. She accepted that such things could happen, particularly where deeply human experiences had occurred. It seemed to her that there was a depth of human experiencing that took people into a place that seemed ..., she wasn't sure, but sort of outside of time and space, outside of the day-to-day awareness. And those kinds of experience made a deep impression on those who witnessed them, or who were in some way connected to the person having the experience, such as Chris would have been. And when Chris relived it in supervision, something of it's tone re-emerged, like an echo, yet more than an echo. Coming to terms with death, engaging with the deep pain associated with human tragedy and hurt, and abuse, was an experience that could have this kind of effect.

In talking about a client's deep, visceral experiences, sometimes reactions from the counsellor (or supervisor) that have a connection or resonance to them can emerge in supervision. It is like a retuning in to what passed in the session. It is somehow brought into the supervision relationship. This can be particularly so in relation to death and dying, where deeply held feelings are likely to have been present within the therapeutic relationship and which, at times, may affect the counsellor more than they are aware of. Supervision is, in part, an opportunity for such an effect to be made visible. Such processes will help to restore congruence. Where a counsellor is affected by what a client is saying or experiencing, but is not fully aware of the depth or nature of the effect it is having on them, then the counsellor can be considered to have entered into an incongruent state.

Chris was still with his image of Billy and with the feelings that had become present within him as he saw him groaning in the chair. 'It came from so deep, so deep.'

Lucy nodded, and responded in a way that expressed her wanting to offer support to Chris for what he had gone through and what he was reliving. 'A lot of pain for you to have to be open to, Chris, a profoundly deep pain.'

Chris found himself instinctively taking a deep breath. His eyes were moist. Something so very human about the whole experience, of being with another person in pain, knowing that you could not take the pain away, just be there with them, for them, as best you could. Knowing that you could not reach into the pain, it was too intimately personal to the person experiencing it. 'Can we ever really understand another person's pain?'

Lucy was shaking her head. 'I don't think so. It's so personal, isn't it?'

'And somehow more so when it is emotional pain. And it can be more than emotional, I want to say *psychological*, because it can be more than emotion. My sense was that Billy's whole being was in pain, he was not just in pain but being pain.' He stopped and shook his head gently as he thought about the awesome nature of what he had just said. It wasn't something that he felt he had experienced, but maybe through Billy he had in some sense glimpsed its shadow, he couldn't think of any better way of putting it. He could not feel what Billy had felt, but he could feel his own reaction to what he experienced Billy as experiencing. 'And then there was a shift. Well, it was embedded in his experience. From talking about how he needed to keep his dad's memory alive the realisation just hit him that he had actually been trying to keep his dad alive, but that he couldn't, his dad was gone. All he had was the memory, but he said something about realising that he had been actually trying to keep his dad alive, keep the hope alive that his dad hadn't gone. The pain was realising, knowing, really knowing, that he had gone.'

'Like a deeper knowing.'

'I want to say a *knowing knowing*, if that makes sense.'

Lucy nodded, she did understand that. It reminded her of the death of her twin sister. Her death had been a terrible experience, like part of her had been wrenched away. It had taken her a long time to come to terms with it. And she had come to a place of knowing, but it had been soon after her death. She had not been able to really deny that her sister was no longer there, though she did have some psychic experiences afterwards that left her feeling that her sister's presence was close. And that was comforting. It fitted her belief about death, that the soul lived on and, well, it had felt like she was still around. And then there was that one day, she could remember it quite clearly. It was like her sister had gone. Her presence was no longer there. And she knew, and it was a total knowing, that her sister had moved on in some way. But it still wasn't the sort of 'gone' that she sensed Chris was describing Billy as having connected with. Or maybe it was, she didn't know.

'It put me in touch with my own thoughts about my twin sister's death. That does make sense.'

Chris sensed from the way that Lucy spoke that she had her own understanding. He didn't need to say anything further.

'He said about how his mum tells him that his dad is at peace now. She clearly has beliefs that Billy finds difficult. I don't know if he said this, maybe it's my assumption, but I think he said something at some point about believing that death is the end, that's it, nothing more. And maybe that's why the revelation that his dad has gone had such a potent impact. He knows, in line with his belief, that he will never see his dad again. While his mother, well, maybe she does believe she will see him again, and that's helping her through. There is loss, but not a total and utter end.'

'You can understand why people want to believe in something more. It helped me, but it wasn't for that reason, it's just how I've always seen it somehow. I just can't see life as being just a one-off. It just doesn't feel right. I cannot imagine myself not existing. Now maybe I'm fooling myself, but I just don't think so. But that's me. It's not something religious or anything like that. I don't think of it like that, Heaven, Paradise, whatever. No, religion doesn't attract me. What impact do our beliefs have on the way we work, or simply the way we are, when working with clients who have suffered a bereavement or are facing their own death? Can they get in the way?'

Chris thought about what Lucy was saying. He, like her, had a sense of continuity. He didn't know exactly what her beliefs were, but he did feel as though he had been in touch with Billy in his pain. But he knew as well that, yes, he couldn't actually imagine what it would be like to feel that someone had gone forever, because he simply didn't feel that was how it was. He respected those who did feel that way, but he just couldn't imagine thinking that way about life, and death.

'That's a tough one to call. It sort of makes you wonder, does an atheist need an atheist bereavement counsellor? Do people need to be matched to counsellors with a similar faith? Or is it something that doesn't matter? Empathy, unconditional positive regard, authenticity, when present in the counsellor and experienced by the client, do they make the question of faith or belief less important?'

'I guess there is no definite answer, it will vary from person to person. And I'm aware that we're kind of getting a little bit into a discussion on belief, which is fine, but what about Billy and how you are relating to him as he faces what, for him, is the absolute certainty that his dad has gone, forever?'

'Yes, well, I do feel we connected. I mean, I wasn't thinking about my beliefs when I was with him. I was totally focused on his and what he was experiencing and how it was affecting me. I was not having his experience but relationally I was in there with him.'

'Mhmm, and that's important.'

'And he did say at the end that he was grateful that I was there, that it helped. So, yes, he was aware of my presence. It actually felt good to know that. I'd touched him on the shoulder, just maintaining a gentle pressure, wanting to offer something reassuring but not disrupt or break into his experiencing. I was glad to have done that.'

Lucy smiled back, touched by the emotion in Chris's voice. 'I can hear how important that was for you.'

'It's, yeah . . .'. Chris's eyes had watered up. 'It's tough being a witness to someone else's pain. Gets to you. I'm glad it does. What was it I read somewhere, "how can they feel our love if we cannot feel their pain", I think that was how it went. And perhaps as well our clients need to glimpse something of the effect of their pain, and somewhere in that there's a place for compassion. And I think of that book by Peggy Natiello, that wonderful title: *The Person-centred Approach: a passionate presence*. And you know, somehow I want to also say something about the healing power of compassionate presence. And I don't exactly know what I mean by that, but somehow it feels important.'

They both lapsed into silence for a few moments, the words having individual meaning for them both.

Points for discussion

- What does 'the healing power of a compassionate presence' mean to you?
- What is your reaction to the supervision session? Was it helpful, unhelpful, appropriate in its style and content?
- How would you have felt had you been the counsellor. Would you have got what you would have wanted? If not, what else would you have wanted from supervision?
- What is your belief in relation to the beyond-death experience? Do you think it impacts on how you would work with someone facing death and coming to terms with bereavement?

- If you were the supervisor, what might you feel a need to take to your own supervision from this session?
- If you were the supervisee, what would you be taking away from this supervision session, and how might it change you or inform your next counselling session with Billy?

CHAPTER 5

Counselling session 4: Exploring change and tackling the alcohol

Chris sat in the counselling room waiting for Billy to arrive. A few more minutes to go, and it gave him time to reflect. The last supervision session had been helpful, although he had realised afterwards that he hadn't really processed his feelings towards the silences that had occurred with Billy early on. It wasn't that there was anything pressing, but he remembered that he had planned to discuss them, and the role of silence. But then, well, the last session had taken his focus away from that. Hmm. He wondered whether that had some kind of significance for the therapeutic relationship that they were building. Maybe that was it, the focus was much more on what was pressing and present, the 'here and now', as it were. Billy's present was so very much linked to his past and the memory of his father. He wanted to move on. That meant letting go of aspects of the past. Letting go but not forgetting.

He thought of the bereavements in his own life. There had not been many. He wasn't a member of a large family. There were his grandparents. Only his grandfather on his mother's side was still alive. Yes, he had memories, fond memories, particularly of his mother's mother. He guessed that was because they had spent a lot of time together when he was a child. It all seemed so distant now and his memories nowadays seemed more linked to images on photographs than actual memories of events and 'live' interactions, as it were.

Chris brought his thoughts back into the present. He liked to spend a couple of minutes silently preparing himself with his eyes closed, to really let go of any of the thoughts that were in his mind and might distract him from his therapeutic work. Time to affirm to himself his intention to be sensitive and open for the next hour, putting his own cares and concerns aside to be fully present for his client.

The doorbell rang and he went out into the hallway. It was Billy.

'Hello Billy, come in.'

'Thanks. Thanks a lot.' Billy came in and waited for Chris to close the door.

'Go on through.'

'Thanks.' Billy went in, took off his jacket, which he put over the back of the chair, and sat down.

'So, what is with you today?' Chris liked to keep his first comment very open. He knew that it would have been tempting to have said something about the previous session, but that would have immediately directed Billy to a particular focus, and that may not be what Billy wanted to talk about, or at least not straightaway. He believed, in line with person-centred theory, that his client needed to have the opportunity in therapy to experience their own autonomy, to experience the reality that the therapeutic hour was their hour, for them to use as they wished, with the focus that they wanted to bring.

'I'm not sure. I was thinking on the way here about, well, how I was feeling actually. I was contrasting what it was like coming over today with how it had been previously. I don't know why I was thinking like that, but I was.'

'Mhmm, something about the contrast.'

'I guess it was because I was aware of feeling different. I suppose, yes, it's like when I had come over before, yes, I wanted . . . , no, wasn't so much wanted, more a sense of needing to come. I knew I sort of had to. Yes, knew I had to but maybe wasn't really wanting to, and that bit felt different.'

'So, aware that in the past that while you knew you had to come, there wasn't a sense of wanting to come.' Chris nodded as he spoke and as he felt himself appreciating what Billy was saying.

'And while it was hard last week, and painful, and I sort of don't want to go through that again – and I don't think I will. I'm seeing things differently, and feeling differently as well – I sort of felt good about coming today. Like I wanted to.'

'Feeling good about coming to therapy, feeling like you want to be here.' Chris maintained his close empathy for what Billy was saying.

'And that's sort of different. Got me thinking. I mean, I still think of Dad a lot, and I do feel sad, I miss him, you know? And I seem sort of more emotional somehow, like after last week I sort of feel more tearful. And yet at the same time – and this doesn't feel like it makes sense but I feel somehow sort of better in myself.'

What Billy was saying seemed particularly important somehow. It was the way Billy was speaking, exploring and making sense of himself as he spoke. 'Let me check I am hearing your correctly. You miss your dad and you feel more tearful, but at the same time you're feeling better as well, almost in spite of the upset.'

> The counsellor has sought to clarify his understanding, motivated to do so perhaps because it felt important and he wanted to be sure that he had heard Billy correctly and, by confirming this, that the client was aware that he had been heard and understood.

'Yes, in spite of, yes.' Billy paused. 'Like I'm somehow, hmm, in a sort of strange way I feel more alive. Hmm, something like that. I don't know.' He paused again. 'One thing I've done this week, I decided after last week that I had to face my reality, that somehow seems important. It was right what I said, about trying to keep my dad alive. And I can't do that, I hadn't accepted he had gone. It hurt too much to be able to accept it and I didn't want to hurt. I was thinking about that when I was driving back last time. It got me thinking about the whole idea of hurting too much, and yet I had been avoiding the real pain, the pain I felt here last week.' Billy lapsed into silence as his thoughts went back to that last session, and the pain he had felt. Not just a pain, it was hard to describe still. He didn't really have the words for it that seemed to capture the nature of what he had gone through.

'Mhmm, how you had avoided the real pain.'

'A sort of underneath pain, I don't know how else to describe it. Anyway, I realised that I needed to cut back on my drinking. I know why. As I was driving along I was aware of thinking that I needed a drink. That it would settle me down. And somehow that seemed to feel wrong. I don't mean wrong in some sort of judgemental way, but it didn't feel right, that it was, well, I don't know. It's hard to describe. I just knew that I felt different about what I needed to do.'

Chris was nodding. He had a sense of what Billy was struggling to describe. Clearly, his experience in the last session had been profound. He knew that people didn't always change 'just like that', in an instant, as it were. But deep experiences could make a huge impact, and it wasn't necessarily the experience that caused people to change, rather the experience was a sign, a symptom, an outward effect or expression of the change that was occurring. It isn't necessarily that a person feels different because they release the emotion; rather their emerging capacity to now release the emotion is itself the result of changes already taking place.

'As though you were seeing yourself, and in particular your drinking, in a fresh light?' Chris knew that what he had said wasn't using words that Billy had used, but it felt to him as though it summed up what Billy was saying, certainly how it was coming across to him. He felt in himself totally accepting of Billy, of what he was saying. It was good to hear his openness.

Billy was nodding, that felt so right. 'Yes, a fresh light. Yes, yes.' He nodded again as he thought about it. 'I knew I had to not do things to keep me away from feeling, yes, that's how it was, and how it is. Keeping my dad's memory alive had become an attempt to keep him alive, which was an attempt to avoid feeling the effect of his, well, his having died.'

Chris nodded, acknowledging that he was listening. He didn't say anything, letting Billy continue.

'And, yes, I realised when I thought about wanting a drink that actually that was for the same reason. I mean, to avoid feeling. I've cut back. I never used to drink like that in the evening. I want to cut back but it's, well, it's not easy, even though it's what I want to do.'

'You're finding it hard to cut back, you mean?'

Billy nodded. He felt a bit embarrassed. 'I'll be OK, but, well, I'm in control, it's not a problem, but, well, I haven't cut back as much as I had sort of planned.'

'Mhmm, like it's hard to break that habit of having a few drinks of an evening.' Again, Chris did not feel judgemental, just totally accepting of what Billy had experienced and was describing.

'Yeah, well, not just the evening. I was drinking during the day as well, and you hear so much these days about binge drinking – well I don't binge, but I do drink more than I should. I've sort of realised that, but it feels difficult to change somehow.'

'And it's something you would like to change?'

'I have to. I know I was drinking to sleep, to sort of stay a bit numb, I suppose. I've cut back a bit, but I'm not sleeping too well.'

Chris nodded. He was aware that people could drink to relax and sleep, but actually it was more alcohol-induced than a natural physiological switching off. That people who used alcohol could, when they tried to cut back, find themselves unable to 'switch off' naturally. He felt it was appropriate to share this, and to say something about how it could be dangerous to try and just stop drinking if you had become dependent on it.

In the above dialogue, the counsellor has shown how a non-judgemental and accepting approach can enable a client to explore what might otherwise be very difficult experiences to talk about. Any hint in his voice of being critical of Billy's drinking and it is likely that Billy would stop disclosing, or perhaps deny more strongly that he has any kind of problem. A lot is talked and written about denial. And yes, people do deny they have a problem with alcohol when in fact their drinking is causing them (or others) a problem. However, often the denial is a response to someone asking them in such a way, or a tone of voice, that makes it hard for the person to be open to the possibility that their drinking is a problem or a concern. Often there is a fear of criticism, of being labelled an alcoholic, of being made to feel worthless, weak-willed or a failure. Warm acceptance of the person and what they are tentatively describing is far more likely to encourage a person to explore their drinking than some kind of interrogation. I have sought to describe this elsewhere (Bryant-Jefferies, 2001, 2003b).

'Alcohol can get people to sleep, but it's not naturally induced, and, well, people can then wake up and find it difficult to get back to sleep again. That's when some people drink more for the same effect and, well, it can then get out of control. People have to keep drinking to maintain a certain level of alcohol in the system. And then you have to be careful cutting back. People can experience significant withdrawal symptoms. When it's like that you can't just stop, it's dangerous.'

Chris is aware that he is conveying information, that in one sense he has stepped out of his client's frame of reference. But he feels it is appropriate. He has information that is important, and he wants Billy to be aware of it. He cares about Billy, he sees sharing this information as an expression of his unconditional positive regard. And he is being authentic.

> This is information he knows, which he feels will help Billy to be more informed – though he realises he is making the assumption that Billy is not aware of the subtle, and sometimes not so subtle, effects of alcohol.

'Yes, I know you can't just stop if you're a really heavy drinker. I guess I'm aware of realising how it can creep up on you. I don't think I'm drinking enough to be not able to stop. But, well, I'm not finding out am I, because I'm not stopping? It just feels like it brings me, I don't know, a sort of relief.'

'Mhmm, that's how it feels, a relief.'

'And maybe that's OK for a while, but I don't want to continue like that. I don't want to rely on it. I have been, I can see that. Hmm. It blurs me. Cutting back, well, not drinking during the day. I didn't every day, but sometimes I would have a drink or two at lunchtime. Just got into the habit, I suppose. It's not a problem. But I've stopped that. I feel better for it. And I'm not drinking so much of an evening, but I do still like something last thing at night.'

'Mhmm, yeah, it's a kind of habit you slid into, but you realise now that it's not what you want to continue with, but like most habits it's not always easy to break, and more so when it's something that affects how you feel.'

'And that's the key, isn't it, that it affects how I feel? And I have to accept that I will feel upset, I do, I am more sensitive, I can feel it.' He shook his head, he was still in a way coming to terms with the immensity and the intensity of what had happened in that previous session.

'You're trying to be more open to what you feel, even when it is painful.'

Billy nodded. 'And I guess it's a human thing to want to avoid pain.'

'We don't generally choose it.' He thought of the fact that some people needed to feel pain, but often that was for other reasons. He let his thought pass.

'I think somehow the fact that I know . . . ,' he hesitated, feeling his emotions welling up, '. . . still not easy to talk about.' He swallowed.

'Take your time. The fact that you know . . .'.

'Yeah, thanks.' He swallowed again. 'The fact that I know he's gone, hmm . . .'. He blinked as his eyes filled with tears and he felt teardrops trickling down his cheeks. 'Somehow that's making me know that I have to get on with my life. I sort of knew he had gone, but couldn't, didn't want, to accept it. Now I'm, yeah, now I am beginning to accept it. And it's making me think differently. I've done a lot of thinking this week, different kind of thinking. Not just going back over the past. Some of that, remembering, you know?'

Chris nodded.

'But also thinking about the future as well.' He sniffed. 'I think I'm sort of understanding how Mum is moving on. Had a long chat with her over the weekend. We were both in tears, but we were smiling as well. That was different.' He felt the emotions rise as he recalled the conversation and how it had felt. 'It was like we cried together, and I don't think we'd done that, not like that. And it was OK. Mhmm. It was OK.' He smiled. 'Hmm, just, yeah, OK.'

Chris nodded again. 'Mhmm. An OKness about crying together, and smiling.' He smiled himself. There was something quite tender about what Billy was saying. It sounded like he and his mother had discovered, or rediscovered maybe, something quite precious that they could share.

It is not unusual in some families for the bereaved members to not necessarily show their feelings to each other, or to genuinely share their grief. Yes, things may be shown, but not always at a deeper level, and particularly across generations. But it can be so healthy, bringing people together and enabling people to gain strength from knowing that they are not alone in what they are experiencing. Of course, it is not something that can be planned or made to happen, it will spontaneously occur when those involved are ready and able to make visible to themselves, and others, what they are truly feeling. And yes, it may well feel quite tender when it is described. It is a precious moment, with often a strong sense of familial love emerging, sometimes for the first time for some while to the degree and depth that it does. The client will need to experience that what they have shared is warmly accepted, honoured, respected, and is responded to in a very human and heartfelt way. For that is what it is for the client, a genuinely heartfelt experience.

Billy took a deep breath and nodded himself. Yes, he thought, it had felt good. Somehow made them feel closer. 'Made me realise I'd distanced myself. Too wrapped up in what I was feeling all the time. Hmm. Yeah.' Billy paused, sniffed and swallowed as he thought about it. It had been a good experience. It had felt like they had connected again. He was glad that had happened.

'Wrapped up in your own inner world, leaving you distant from other people.'

'I feel bad about that now, and yet ...,' Billy was shaking his head, 'in spite of what's happened – and I know I can't keep Dad alive – there is still part of me that wants to.' The tears were back in Billy's eyes once more, and Chris found that his own were moistening too.

'Yeah, that part can't just disappear. You know you can't, but you still feel you want him alive.' Chris could feel the strength of the emotion between them. This felt so much at the heart of Billy's experience at this time. Knowing what was not possible but still wanting.

'That's what I have to come to terms with. Since last week it's really hard to think of him without feeling tearful. I've never felt quite like this. I mean, I don't feel tearful all the time thinking about him, but when I really think about him, memories, I feel different. I can't really describe the difference, but I feel, well yes, it's a sadness. A real sadness.'

Chris felt himself taking a deep breath, sensing the depth of sadness that Billy was communicating.

'And that sadness is with you now?'

Billy nodded. Chris's words seemed to cause the emotions to rise up again, his eyes filling with water. He couldn't speak, keeping his jaw firm and his lips tight. He breathed in, his breath coming in short, jagged bursts as the emotions tried to find a release.

Chris felt his heart going out to Billy. Clearly there was so much hurt and sadness within him. In one sense he was surprised and yet at the same time he wasn't. He knew how everyone's reaction to a bereavement was unique to them, with its own tone and intensity, and timing. For whatever reason, the death of his dad had really hit Billy hard, was still hitting him hard. He just had a sense that there was something more to it, but he had no idea what it might be.

Billy had taken out his handkerchief and was drying his eyes. His throat felt constricted. His eyes were burning a little from the saltiness of his tears. 'It's not just about the past, Chris, I can feel that it's not just that.'

'Something other than the past that's making you feel like this?'

'I sort of, well, since Dad retired we had begun to do work together. We had on and off, but, I don't know, it sort of takes me back to when I was a kid. He'd give me little jobs to do.' He smiled. 'I loved that. And he was always so encouraging. Just, yeah, he was a very patient man. He always had time, or made time. There was a kind of easiness about how he was.' Billy went silent. He was back thinking about his father's shed. 'You know, they've lived in their house, well, it was the house I was brought up in, from about the age of six anyway. That was when we moved there. So, yeah, it has a lot of memories. I suppose that's good in a way, but it also makes it sort of difficult. Mum's talked about moving to somewhere smaller, but she's not sure. It's so much her home, it would be hard for her to move anywhere else. I'm not sure that she will. And I'm not sure that I'd want her to, but that's not really fair. I know that. But it's sort of our house. I guess it's the place with so many of the memories and the thought of losing that . . .'. He sighed. 'There's a guy at work, his mother died. His father was already dead. He can't sell their house, it's just, well, empty except that it is full of his parents' belongings. And he goes there each week, mows the lawn, keeps it tidy. I don't want to get like that. I've heard him say about what he does, we got chatting about it after Dad died. In a way I could sort of understand him then, but now, now that feels like that's too much. Makes me wonder what I'd do if Mum died. I suppose it would be tempting, I don't know. I guess we're all different.'

'I guess we are, each having our own responses and ways of dealing with it.' Chris was aware that his response was more from his head than his feelings. He was aware of how the focus from which he responded changed at different times during sessions, depending on what the client was expressing, whether they were expressing thoughts or feelings.

'I think if I did that I'd have a real problem. But I can understand it. And I guess anyone like that would be doing it for their own reasons.'

'Mhmm.'

'It's like getting rid of someone's clothes. I mean, Mum sorted that out. But the tools, I couldn't give his tools away. I mean, they're useful anyway, but some of them are really old, they go back to when I was a child! I remember using them then. They're like a piece of him, somehow. I guess we all want to keep things to remind us . . .'.

Mhmm, for you his tools are what carries most meaning.'

'They do.' He smiled. More memories. 'He was a really meticulous carpenter, well, you have to be. He'd make a joint that was absolutely perfect, nothing else would be acceptable to him anyway.' Billy paused. 'That was how he was. And I'd make something that was, well, it would be all loose, but he was always so positive and encouraging. Yeah. I guess I was looking forward to sharing some more work with him in the future. I think that's a big part of what I've lost.'

Chris nodded, feeling that perhaps this was linked to the strength of feeling that Billy had expressed, that somehow his lost hopes for doing carpentry once again with his dad had a long history, rooted in childhood experiences that quite clearly had made a huge impression on Billy.

'Yeah.' Billy felt calmer as he spoke, as he thought about what he had just said, although his chest felt a bit tight and constricted. And his back was stiff again. He moved in the chair. 'How long have we got?'

'Few more minutes.'

'I don't think there's much more to say today. I think I need to head off, keep working at it.'

'At your own pace.'

With the earlier releases of emotion in the session and before, the client has moved to a place where he can now reflect on his father, his memories, but in a way that leaves him calmer. It is perhaps no longer quite so acutely painful to think about him because the pain has begun to be released. The release of feelings enables the thinking to change. The thoughts no longer attract quite the same intense reaction. This can take time. For some people there will be a long process of struggling with the pain, and there can be rage and anger as well as hurt and sadness that has to be released before the person can begin to think of the person they have lost in a new way. That isn't to say the pain has gone, or that they have ceased to feel or have become insensitive. Do we ever lose our hurt when we have lost a loved one? It depends. In a way, it may depend in some measure on how much of one's future was invested in the presence of that person. Hence it is perhaps harder to lose a child than a parent, or a parent than a grandparent. Perhaps, but not always. It also depends so much on the meaning and importance of the relationship to the person who has been bereaved.

The person-centred counsellor will not impose on the client an expectation of what they should feel, or what process they should go through in counselling for a bereavement. They will trust the client's inner process and accept the time that a particular client needs to try and reach what will be, for them, a satisfying place from which to continue to live their lives, or make the choices that, in full awareness, they wish to make.

Billy nodded, feeling himself instinctively taking a deep breath. 'I'm going to bring in a picture next time. I've talked about him so much, I sort of want you to see him. Is that OK?'

'Sure, that would be great.' Their eyes met and some deeper communication passed between them. In that moment it wasn't a counsellor-to-client contact, it became man-to-man.

Billy nodded. 'Thanks. I'm ready to head off.' As he got up he reached over to shake Chris's hand. It was a firm grip. Again a moment of connection passed between them. For Billy it was self-affirming, it felt good, solid. He was grateful to Chris for being how he was. He felt that he'd come to the right man. He knew he was going to come through it. He felt emotional. 'Thanks.'

'It's OK. Glad it's helping.'

Billy nodded. 'It is. It definitely is.'

After Billy had left Chris went back into the counselling room. That had felt important. There was something very human in what had passed between them, a kind of joint knowing in some way. No need for words, just that knowing. He felt quiet as he began to jot down his notes.

Points for discussion

- What were the significant moments or interactions in this session?
- How are you reacting to Billy's process? How does it differ from experiences you may have had, personally or in the context of therapy?
- Evaluate the session in terms of Chris's application of the person-centred approach. What do you feel are the strengths, and weaknesses, of his practice?
- Something man-to-man occurred at the end of session that was important for Billy. Consider what difference there might have been for Billy had he had a female counsellor.
- What would you take to supervision from this session?
- Write notes for this session.

CHAPTER 6

Counselling session 5: Coming to terms with his impact on his family

Billy's week had been a little better. He began the session by telling Chris how he was feeling.

'I seem to be a little easier now, easier in myself.'

'Easier?' Chris was unclear what Billy meant by this. He wanted to empathise with him, show Billy that he had an appreciation of what he was experiencing, yet he also knew that empathy was not simply concerned with reflecting back a client's words. That might be how counselling skills were taught, but that was not the empathy as defined within person-centred theory. He wanted to genuinely understand what was present in Billy's experience and awareness, if Billy wanted him to know, so that he could then communicate that back in such a way that Billy felt his inner experiencing had been heard.

Billy thought about it a little more. 'It's like, yes, it's like I am more able to talk about Dad. Hmm, no, I've been able to talk about him, it's something more than that. It feels different. I feel different. Clare tells me that I've changed as well. We had a long chat about it – actually, I've noticed we are talking more, that seems to be happening. Hmm.' He reflected for a while on this. It somehow felt important as he said it. 'Yes, that's something else that feels easier.' He thought back to a conversation he and Clare had had earlier in the week.

Chris continued to listen. He imagined that 'easier' might mean more openness, less tension, but that was his meaning. Billy hadn't clarified what he meant, maybe he wasn't able to, maybe he was still working his way towards communicating it. Anyway, he sensed that Billy had more to say and he didn't see any point, or feel any urge, to interrupt his flow. Billy was in process and it seemed to Chris that his process needed to be respected and given an uninterrupted space. Chris was aware of how, when a client was talking and then pausing to think, to collect his thoughts, or to take a moment to open to feelings that were emerging, some counsellors could take the silence as a cue to jump in with an empathic response. Chris knew that this was not always required. In fact, in a way, it showed a lack of empathy for the client, for the processing that was taking place.

There is something about being sensitive to the client's process. It can be quite delicate, having a certain fragility as the client struggles to get a clear sense of something present within them. The counsellor has to be able to discern between the client saying something that they need to have heard, and their saying something that is an expression of their own processing and which, the moment they have said it, they have then moved on to perhaps a deeper and different focus in themselves. Where a client is sensed as needing to feel heard, then some verbal response should be made. But where there is a processing process occurring, then the counsellor needs to allow it to flow, undisturbed, while sensitively waiting for the client to communicate what they next feel they need to put into words, and/or have the counsellor hear.

As a person-centred counsellor, Chris felt strongly that an important feature of relationship building in a therapeutic context lay in developing an understanding and a respect for his client's manner or style of processing and communicating. He waited for Billy to continue, maintaining his focus, feeling his warm acceptance for him as he sat, frowning slightly, clearly considering something about his conversation with Clare.

'What came out in our conversation was, well, hmm, she told me that actually it had felt like walking on egg-shells sometimes, that at times I had seemed impossible to cope with.' He paused. 'For her.' He paused again. He was aware of the mixture of reactions that he had felt when she had told him this. 'She told me I had become jumpy, edgy, unpredictable.'

Chris nodded, aware that the thought that was with him was how much of this had been purely down to Billy's relationship with his father, to the feelings he had, the loss he was experiencing and how much might simply be the effect of his alcohol use affecting his mood, and probably exacerbating the difficult feelings and emotions that were present within him. Billy was continuing to speak.

'She mentioned being very wary of mentioning Dad, or of any situation where he might be mentioned. I asked her why, and why hadn't she told me. She said she had tried to but I'd always reacted, clearly not wanting to hear what she was saying. Said she'd given up but she was torn, aware that it was all having an impact on our daughters.' Billy lapsed into silence. He was feeling emotional. That had been a hard thing to say. He loved his daughters and he felt sad and ashamed that he had affected them as well. He shook his head slightly.

'That was a tough thing to hear.'

Billy swallowed and nodded. 'In a way it was probably that which stopped me reacting against what she was saying. I mean, it wasn't a reaction like it had been before, but I knew I still didn't want to hear about the effects I had had on her, on them. But I also knew I had to, that she was right, that I probably had been a bastard, insensitive and oversensitive. And, well, coming here has helped me to listen somehow. That's what being listened to does to you, yeah?'

'Can do. So, whereas at one time you would have reacted and not wanted or been able to hear what Clare was saying. Now you were, are, able to do so.'

Billy nodded. 'Yes. And now I know that she's right. But I was being, well, I couldn't be any different. That's unnerving that you can be like that, that it seems perfectly reasonable to you, and yet it's affecting people around you.' His thoughts went back to something else Clare had said.

'People close to you.'

'And she told me, hmm, and this isn't easy to say. I'm so emotional at the moment, seem to get tearful so easily.'

'Take your time.' Chris wanted to reassure Billy. He could see the pain in his face. These were not easy things for him to say. He was having to, well, choosing to, talk about some very difficult feelings that were present for him towards those people most important for him. He wanted to reassure Billy that he didn't need to feel pressure to say anything.

Billy took a deep breath and sighed. His eyes felt watery. 'She told me that I might not have been able to see them, but she saw the expressions on our daughters' faces when I reacted, that sometimes it made them upset, that sometimes it had made them frightened, that she had had to reassure them, tell them it was OK, that what she did say was, "Daddy's finding it difficult at the moment, but he's still Daddy . . .".' He paused to swallow, the next bit was the really hard bit to say, his eyes were brimful of tears and his throat had what felt like the largest hard lump in the world in it. He swallowed again and his head movement triggered a release of tears. He sniffed, took out his handkerchief and dried his eyes, the emotions remaining very present.

Chris stayed calm, aware of feeling his heart going out to Billy, this man who had been so volatile and reactive, so unable to see the degree of reaction he was putting on his family as a result of his father's death, a man who had fought with himself to avoid knowing, and therefore feeling, that his father was dead, and gone. Now, here he was, unable to contain his emotions as he tried to describe and come to terms with what his partner had told him about his effect on them. He was aware that he had a lump in his own throat as well and his own eyes felt moist. He felt good that he was being affected, he'd be concerned if he wasn't, this was an acutely emotional time for Billy, he needed to be open to its effect on him not just as a therapist, but as a person and as a man.

Billy had dried his eyes, Clare's words were still within him, he was struggling to say them. It felt like they were a lid on another surge of emotion, that if he said them he'd be swamped by them. 'I'm sorry, I'm finding this really hard to say.'

Chris nodded. 'Yeah, these are really hard to say . . .'. He sought, through his tone of voice, to empathise with the difficulty Billy was having.

Billy had tightened his jaw and his lips. He nodded, his head movement slight and a little jerky. The emotions felt as though they were filling his whole being. He swallowed again. He knew what he needed to say, he knew that he needed to say them. He needed to hear himself say them. He couldn't swallow them back, there was no point to that, but he could feel the hurt that was trying to burst out. He took another deep breath and slowly breathed out, trying to compose himself a little. It made a slight difference, but not much. He swallowed again, and immediately felt another surge of emotion. He had to speak, he had to get it out. He was going to hate hearing himself say the words, and he was going to feel so awful and ashamed.

'She said that she had told them,' he swallowed again and closed his eyes, releasing more tears, 'that I was still their daddy.' Another sharp intake of breath and another swallow, 'And she told them, '' but we all still love him …'','' another sharp intake of breath, ' ''… don't we?''.' His shoulders heaved with emotion, his breathing again short and sharp. The lump in his throat had eased a little, but his eyes burned with tears. He felt the sadness and shame once again that he had felt when he had heard Clare's words. His face was buried in his handkerchief once more.

The tears continued to flow, his breathing remained erratic. Chris reached across and placed his hand on Billy's shoulder, as he had in that earlier session. He felt that he should say something, but what was there to say, what was there to say? He pressed Billy's shoulder slightly, he knew his words would probably sound hollow in contrast to the depth of emotion that Billy was experiencing.

'I don't know what to say, Billy, I'm just so deeply touched by the emotion of what you have been able to say.' He spoke softly, not wanting to take Billy away from his experience and into a focus of thinking about the effect it was having on his therapist.

Billy stayed with his head in his hands a little longer. He had heard Chris, and he appreciated what he had said. He appreciated that he had said something. Slowly his breathing became easier, and he took his hands away from his face. He felt Chris squeeze his shoulder again and take his hand away. He'd appreciated that contact. It had felt a lonely place in himself. He wanted to respond to Chris. 'There's nothing to say. It just …, that just …,' he shook his head, 'what she said just …,' he shook his head again, feeling so many emotions. He'd felt hurt but so deeply affected as well. 'Touched', the word Chris had used. The thought of their faces, listening to their mummy telling them how much they loved Daddy, what on earth had they been feeling. 'I've hurt them, Chris, I've hurt them all, and I have to make that up. And I've hurt myself, but I guess I deserve that.'

Chris found himself instinctively shaking his head. 'You feel like you deserve feeling hurt?'

Billy nodded. 'I lost it, Chris, I know I, you know, had every right to feel what I felt with Dad, you know, but I was out of order.'

'It was a difficult time for you.'

'I know, but …, that's no excuse.'

'From what you are saying, it's hard for you not to be hard on yourself.'

Billy sat tight-lipped, the emotions were easing. 'I knew it had got to me, but I hadn't appreciated how hard it was going to be to say what I just said.'

The counsellor has not been very empathic, he has sought to reassure Billy by encouraging him to think differently. He has moved away from a person-centred focus and an acceptance of what Billy is thinking and feeling. He now moves into expressing his own feelings, and then draws himself back to a focus on Billy. However, for Billy there is an appreciation for what Chris has said. In the moment, in the very person-to-person experience he has, perhaps, most needed a human response. He knows how hard it was to hear what he heard from Clare, and he knows how hard it was to tell Chris, but he managed it. Simple empathy, while it has its place, may not be enough, may not be what is therapeutically demanded. A very human experience may need a very human response from the counsellor. This Chris gives.

'What you heard from Clare, what you told me just now, was, I think, one of the most deeply human end emotional things I've ever heard. I really am touched. I can feel your hurt, I mean, I know I can't because it's yours, not mine, but in a way it feels like I can. I respect you for wanting to say it and to be able to. I genuinely feel quite humbled sitting here given what you have just gone through.' Chris felt absolutely authentic in his description of what he was feeling. And having acknowledged that he knew he must now step away from being at risk of getting more absorbed into his own feelings and reactions, and ensure that he was able to experience his empathy for Billy, for whatever Billy needed to say next.

Billy was taking a deep breath. He really appreciated hearing what Chris had just said. 'Thanks.' Another deep breath. 'Thanks I appreciate that. It's easier to not face these things on your own. And, well, I'm not on my own now. In a way, hmm, in a way I think I had become very alone. So preoccupied with my own feelings. But that's passed now, and I hope for good, certainly for the better, for us all.' His thoughts had returned to something else Clare had told him. 'Something else Clare said, about how she had felt utterly relieved when she knew I was coming for counselling. Apparently Mum was a great support, and when I'd said about going to counselling, she'd explored with her how good counselling had been for her, and how good it would be for me, but that she needed to be patient.' He looked down. 'I hated hearing it; something else that made me sad, the thought that Mum was having to support her because of me. I should have been there for her, not have to have her supporting Clare because of how I was.' He lapsed into silence, shaking is head, again tightening his lips and taking a deep breath as he did so. 'There were times when I wanted to defend myself, when I so didn't want to hear what Clare was telling me, but after she'd said about my daughters, I sort of just lost any desire to defend myself, I was too stunned, horrified, and yet deeply touched. I don't know, words don't seem enough sometimes. I guess I lost the will to defend, I just lost my energy, just had to listen, take it ..., like a man.' Another shake of the head. 'I wasn't too good at that, until now. She was right, everything she said. I know I couldn't have heard what she was saying a few months ago, I don't even know if hearing her say about what she'd had to say to Sarah and Tara, whether even that would have stopped me, made me think, I don't know. I just don't know. I'd sort of like to think that it might have, but I really don't know. I was in another place. I guess I was sort of blaming everyone else, in a way, nothing was my fault, it was the world, God, if I believed in one, whose fault it all was. I just wasn't handling it. And I'm pretty sure, well I know, anything she said to me during that time was, well, it was her problem, not mine. You know, I'd have just thought that she didn't understand, she didn't understand *me*. Just so centred on me, what I was feeling. I lost it. It wasn't like that throughout, Clare reckons it built up. I seemed OK to begin with, that was how she saw me, but as the weeks passed after Dad's death I gradually changed.'

There is a strong case for some form of family work where it is clear that a family member is really struggling to come to terms with a bereavement. The family system is placed under a lot of pressure, having to adapt and adjust to the changes in the person who has been so affected. They will begin by being supportive, doing what they can, realising it to be an effect of the loss. It is normal to feel loss, feel disorientated, depressed, angry, sad, so many feelings that naturally and normally arise. But over time the family may begin to lose their caring, the family may want to move on, but the person who is so strongly affected holds them back. Irritation and frustration can arise on both sides. And, of course, different people will be having different experiences and, if we think in terms of a bereavement process, may be at different stages. It may not be that there is a series of feelings people have to go through in a particular order, people move around, often in different places. Sometimes the family needs help and support to stay together.

Chris nodded, 'So, the change was gradual?'

'Yeah. And it has all just given me so much to think about, make sense of.'

Chris felt a strong sense of the soul-searching that Billy must have gone through, was still going through. So much hurt to hear the things that were said about the effect he was having on the family. 'Feels kind of soul-searching.'

Billy thought that, yes, that did sum it up. 'I can see now just how much I had become sort of "locked-up" in myself, that's how it feels, looking back. And yet to me, at the time, somehow it all seemed perfectly clear. They didn't understand – and maybe they didn't – but I couldn't listen, couldn't hear and couldn't understand them either. It really was like I was so caught up in what *I* felt, with what *I* thought, that there was no, I don't know, just no space left inside me to hear, let alone understand, what they were saying, to see things from their perspective.' Billy took a deep breath as he experienced the feeling that his words had brought back into his awareness. He breathed out slowly. 'I've learned a lot; I hope I have.'

The way Billy spoke, it seemed to be a summary of how his experiences had left him. He chose to empathise with what Billy had conveyed. 'A lot to learn from and you hope that you have learned.'

Billy felt a nod of agreement within himself, yes, yes he really did hope he had learned. Hearing Chris respond like that left him feeling that he had said what he needed to say and his thoughts moved on to one of the implications of what he had said. 'What's so shocking is the fact that it was so easy to slide into. I suppose it happens for lots of people. But it's when it happens to you.'

Chris nodded, 'Then it makes a bigger impression, the fact that it happened to you ...'.

'And that I wasn't aware of it, not like I am now. That's the part that really does leave you feeling, well, quite shocked really.'

'Shocking to know that you have the capacity to have that happen to you.'

'You think you're in control, you think you're doing the right thing, but then, well, I guess hindsight's a wonderful thing, but ...'

'... but?'

'But it's too late then. It's happened, you've caused other people misery and heartache, and needlessly ...'. A pause. 'If only I could have, I don't know ...'.

Chris noted the shift from second to first person in what Billy was saying. It had taken Billy back from general comment into engagement once more with his own experience. He spoke directly to Billy. 'If only I ...'.

Billy's thoughts and feelings were very much centred in a kind of disbelief and a certain sense of shame, and yet even as he allowed himself to think and feel these things, there was another part of himself saying, 'But your dad died. It's a tough experience to come to terms with.' And yet, in spite of this, he knew in himself that he was going to find it hard to accept how he had been. Guilt. That was something else.

'You know, and this is hard to describe, but I sort of feel guilty about how I was, but at the same time I want to say I don't as well. It's like I feel both at the same time in some weird sort of way that I can't explain.'

'Guilty and not guilty, you mean?'

'Guilty about how I was and yet not guilty as well because the cause was, well, I mean, reasonable, with Dad dying, but then I lost it. Then I got stuck. I don't know, it's hard to get my head around.'

'Sure, there are aspects to it all that you feel guilt about, and other things that you can say to yourself that I don't need to feel guilty about that.'

Billy nodded, he was taken by how Chris had worded that. 'Yes, I have things I don't need to feel guilty about. Hmm, don't need, yes, so maybe it's OK to feel guilty about some things and not feel guilty about others?'

'Feels like there's a kind of judgement in what you are saying.'

'I can feel guilty about trying not to feel guilty!'

'It's quite entangling, isn't it, guilt about not feeling guilty as well?'

'Somehow, what I need to do is to accept. I guess I can't help having feelings about it, and it will make me wary and I hope that I can find ways of sort of checking myself out in the future. I don't want to, I don't know, have to go through this again.' He thought of his mother. He knew that she was likely to die before he did and he didn't want to go through the same difficulty. At the same time he had a sense that he might not, their relationship was different. 'Hmm, just thinking about Mum, when she dies, which I hope won't be for a long while, but, well, will it be the same reaction, but then I don't think so. I don't know, and maybe it's because of what I have been through this past year, and what I've learned since, and the fact that I do have a different relationship with her.'

'You think you're different, your relationship with her is different?'

'Very much so. I haven't, I guess, the same, well, yes, I mean Dad and I did things together, you know, stuff that Mum and I didn't do, and, well, yes, I don't really have a sense of having sort of looked forward to doing things with Mum in the way that I did look forward to doing things with Dad.' He paused. 'And yet, well, you know, she's Mum.'

'And that would make it still a significant loss, you mean?'

Billy nodded. 'Significant, but different. I guess it comes back to realising that we're all different, relationships are different and, well, I guess we can't sort of second guess how we'll react. I like to think how it would be, but will it? If I'm really honest with myself, I really don't know.'

'And that's difficult, that not knowing. You know what you hope or expect, but . . .'.

'But, yes. You don't know, do you?'

'No.'

'I didn't expect to wind up here a year or so after Dad died, talking this way. I hope I learn from it, I really do. But I guess it does come back to the fact that we all react differently.'

'Mhmm.'

'And yet, why did I react the way I did? Why did it get so intense? I know I had hopes and plans for the future, and I know that these sort of were probably linked back to stuff as a child, and early adult life as well. But other people must be like that. It can't be unusual.'

'Your hopes, expectations, something that you would share with lots of others.'

'That's right. I don't think it was particularly unique. Yet, not everyone, surely, gets so caught up in themselves like I did. Just makes me feel there's something wrong with me.'

'Something wrong with you for reacting like you did?'

'I mean, how I felt was OK, I was sad, of course I was, but it slid away from me, got so intense. I can't be right to have allowed that to happen.'

'Like you feel there's something wrong with you because of how it got so intense?' Chris was aware of how this theme in different forms kept returning, clearly Billy was really struggling to fully come to terms with this.

Billy was silent, trying to think a way through his feelings, to make sense, to accept, but he couldn't. 'It's not that anyone else has said this, it's what I hear myself saying to myself.'

'Something wrong with me.'

'I've got to sort this or else it'll be the next thing that I get, I don't know, but it feels like something I need to resolve before I can move on.'

'Like it's sort of stopping you, holding you back in some sense?' Chris wanted to clarify what Billy was meaning and experiencing. It was clearly an issue that was important to Billy and if he was going to work through it then he really needed to connect with the detail of his experiencing. The right words were going to be important.

'It's like, I don't know, unfinished business. Why me? Why? And for so long? I can't seem to not think about that aspect of it.'

'Is it the what happened or the length of time, or the intensity, or some other feature that really sticks with you?'

Billy appreciated the question. It sort of opened up the landscape in a sense, gave him a number of angles to view it from. 'It would be easy to say "all of them", but I think it's the intensity, and then the length of time. I think I can accept that it was, yes, acceptable to go through the feelings that I had, but I got locked into them. And I couldn't see it. Hmm.' He paused. 'That's more what it's about, the not seeing it. How can you not see something about yourself?'

'How could you not see what was happening to you?' Chris spoke reflectively rather than trying to make his response sound like a specific question he was asking of Billy.

Billy nodded, knowing that this was the nub of it. Yes, the other factors were there, but this was what was standing out. 'That's why I think there's something wrong with me. I *should* have seen it.'

'I *should* have seen it. 'Chris kept the focus and the emphasis on Billy's words.

'I think so. Others did, but I couldn't hear them.'

'Mmm.'

'Yet, hmm . . .' Billy paused, feeling a wave of emotion as a thought came to mind. 'No one's actually blaming me. I mean, things have been said, but somehow they're not blaming me. Mum's been really understanding, and so has Clare now that we are talking about it all. It's more about concern. They still cared about me, Chris, even though I was out of order.' He shook his head, his eyes watering as he felt choked by what he was saying and feeling. 'Yes, in spite of me being how I was, they didn't abandon me or anything, they still cared, they just couldn't get through to me.'

'Mhmm, still caring for you, but unable to reach you.'

Billy had looked up. He needed to look into Chris's eyes. It was instinctive. He needed to see something. He didn't know what. He needed to, yes, somehow having just said, that he needed to *know* that Chris was listening, really listening, really hearing, really accepting.

Chris met Billy's eye contact. He felt himself smile slightly, but it was a tight-lipped smile. It felt like a very serious moment, something important was passing between them. He did not know what Billy wanted, but clearly he needed something. Chris felt warmth and acceptance for Billy, and he respected him. He respected his striving to be open within the counselling sessions, not just to his therapist, but to himself. This was important, and so hard. Facing ourselves, being open to what is present within us, really open, without making excuses, facing ourselves as we are, as we perceive ourselves to be, openly and honestly, is not an easy thing. And anyone who thinks therapy is an easy option has no appreciation of this process, or has not experienced it themselves first hand in order to be able to acknowledge what it can be like.

Billy saw a steadiness in Chris, and he experienced what he could only describe as a sense of OKness. He did not feel judged. It was as though Chris's expression seemed to convey an appreciation, maybe more than that, more an understanding of what Billy was going through. He needed that.

We see so much in the eyes of another person. Of course, we may not always interpret accurately what we see, but in a therapy session, where the counsellor is striving to be authentically present and transparent, and therapeutic relationship exists, so much is communicated and received through eye contact. When a person touches something deep in themselves and looks into the eyes of another person, and the eye contact is returned and held, what is present within each person gets across. We may not fully understand the process, but a mutual knowing can emerge into awareness. They are profoundly important moments.

'Mmm.' Billy nodded slightly. 'I have to come to terms with it. I can't judge myself, I have to accept that what happened, happened, make sense of it the best I can and move on, however much that feeling might be around, that uncertainty over whether it might happen again.'

'Move on, not judge yourself, in spite of that concern as to whether it might happen again.' Chris spoke in a reflective tone, and slowly, allowing his empathic response time to be present between them.

Billy's thoughts had shifted to another aspect of what had happened. He also had a sense that time was passing and looked over at the clock. Only a few minutes left. He took a deep breath. 'There's something else. Clare's told me that she thought my drinking hadn't helped. I felt myself react to that. OK, so maybe it did, well, I don't know, I guess it didn't help, though it felt like it has helped me, and I don't think it ever really got out of control.'

'Mhmm, didn't feel out of control to you but she experienced it differently, and you reacted to that.' Chris was glad in a way that Billy had introduced this. When the thought about his drinking had come to his mind earlier he had wondered whether it would be something that needed to be explored. But it wasn't for him to decide. As a person-centred counsellor he did not want to direct his client's focus, but at the same time a deeply felt concern that was present for him was something he would voice. It hadn't felt that way in this case. He believed that his clients should be allowed to explore what was most pressing to *them*. Yes, he appreciated that clients could sometimes avoid things that were pressing because they were uncomfortable, painful, but he also believed that by offering a genuinely non-judgemental relationship that the client experienced and could grow to trust, there was more likelihood that difficult material would be shared and could be explored in a timely and accepting manner. He didn't believe it was helpful, and certainly not congruent to the relational principles of his practice, to push issues out into the open because it had become in some sense his issue to address their issue.

'I suppose, well, it's back to normal now, but, yes, I guess it was, well, my drinking did increase. I'm just not so sure whether it was a problem.'
'Like it wasn't a problem to you but it had become a problem for Clare?'
Billy nodded. 'I guess so.'

While 'problem drinking' is not the theme of this book, I have dealt with this in other titles in the *Living Therapy* series (Bryant-Jefferies, 2003b, 2006), it is nevertheless worth reflecting on here in a bereavement context. Alcohol can suppress feelings and emotions for some people. For others it can release emotions. Elsewhere I have described alcohol as the lubricant that oils the hinge on a door into the emotions (Bryant Jefferies, 2001). For some people alcohol causes the door to swing open, for others it seems to cause it to swing shut. And, of course, if you drink enough then it takes you into uncon-sciousness, into oblivion, and as we know, with other drugs can prove a lethal combination taking one away from pain and discomfort permanently.

But when does alcohol use become 'problematic', and when is it an addic-tion? We can think of it in terms of whether the alcohol use causes problems. It is arguably problematic if it causes problems for anyone, unless, of course, the other person's threshold of tolerance is actually unreasonable. So, for instance, the person who is tee-total declaring that someone else's glass of wine is a problem to them is unreasonable. But if the person drinks a whole bottle and starts to become disruptive, then it is problematic. However, it is also about context. Two to three glasses of wine of an evening may not be viewed as problematic from a health perspective, and may not cause proble-matic behaviour, but if it means that for a low-income family money is then not available to be spent on adequate food or clothing for a child, then it is problematic. It is also a matter of context.

Addiction or dependency can be either psychological or chemical. Does the person need to drink to stave off physical withdrawal symptoms? If so then it is a chemical addiction. But if they need alcohol to cope emo-tionally or psychologically, for instance to face the day, cope with a difficult relationship or relax to deal with work stress, but they would not experience physical withdrawal if they stopped drinking, then that is psychological dependency. And, of course, the two can occur simultaneously, particularly if someone drinks increasing amounts over a significant period of time. This is where alcohol becomes a pertinent topic when considering bereave-ment. People can drink, or drink more, to cope. This can help over a short period, but it comes with the risk that if it continues and increases, then a genuine dependency can develop. Counsellors working with clients on bereavement issues need to have an appreciation of the risks associated with alcohol use (or other drugs). It is not appropriate to be judgemental, all people do what they need to do to feel better if they can. But when an addictive substance becomes a key feature of that coping mechanism, then dependency becomes a risk.

'Mhmm.'

'I don't know, but it's OK now, and, well, I need to head off, there's not much time left today. I just, well, I sort of mentioned it. I guess I'm not comfortable about it. I don't like to think it's a problem.' Billy wasn't sure that he was glad he'd mentioned it, but had felt that he needed to. It was something else that Clare had said and, well, yes, something else to make sense of.

'Not something that you like to think of as a problem.'

'I don't think it is. I guess it was a phase, caught up with everything else. It's not an answer, I know that. And, well, hmm, maybe it did affect . . .'. His thoughts went back to his daughters, what might they have thought? That was definitely uncomfortable to contemplate.

'Did affect?'

'Wondering how it might have affected my daughters.' He didn't like the thought. He needed to be sure. 'I've got to talk to Clare. I-I'm not sure I trust my memory of everything. And maybe Mum, but she wasn't around day to day, you know?'

'Sure, I'm sure you'll ask what you need to ask.'

'Hmm. As usual, I leave with something to think about. So many threads to all of this. I guess you can just keep going and going?'

'You can, people do, but others reach a point where they feel satisfied and want to sort of move on from therapy.'

'I guess I've thought about, well, coming here for as long as I need to, but not, well, not forever, you know?' He smiled.

'No, and I'm not sure that "forever" is good, but then I also know that for some people regular therapy is what keeps them going, some people are really affected by difficult experiences and they do need someone to talk to, someone to help them make sense of the problems they are experiencing.'

People can have extremely traumatic experiences, particularly in early life but not exclusively so, that can really 'disrupt' their development and impact on their emotional, mental and psychological state in profound ways. Mental health services categorise people in terms of 'borderline personality disorder' and 'personality disorder'. Certainly people can experience a greater deal of 'disorder' within their psychological functioning which then impacts on the external functioning as well. Often, people who experience such disorder have also experienced very problematic events in their lives, often during developmental phases when they are trying to make sense of who they are, of the world around them, when their sense of self is undergoing foundational development. Therapy characterised by the core relational principles of the person-centred approach can be a vivid contrast to the life experiences of people so affected, and it can take years of experiencing a genuinely healthy and healing relationship – or set of relationships – before inner change can occur to a significant and sustainable degree. We live in a 'quick-fix' society, but there is no quick fix for, say, 10–15 years of sustained abuse and rejection, or lack of heartfelt emotional nourishment.

In the context of this volume, a bereavement can bring back into awareness many of the memories of early life experiences associated with loss. The counsellor working with the bereaved must be competent to work with the range of presenting issues associated with the trigger event – the bereavement – that has brought them to counselling and therapy.

The session drew to a close and Billy left feeling in a sense glad that while his difficulties had been quite intense they were relatively surmountable. He was moving on. Yes, there were elements that he still needed to make sense of, but he felt sure that he would. He wanted to, he had to. His daughters were growing up. He needed to be there, play his part, experience being a father. Experiencing being a father. As he pulled into the driveway back at home and pulled up in front of the garage, the thought was very much with him, and the emotions that came with it. His eyes had watered again. Why was he so sensitive these days? But perhaps it was for the best. At least he felt things, and they were important things he needed to feel. Yes, it wasn't always easy, he understood why people avoided feelings, they could be so exquisitely sharp, and sweet, yet tinged with a stinging pain. The thought that had touched him was how much of the past year he'd missed out on. He didn't feel he had, but he guessed that in some way, at some level, he had missed out. He felt sure he hadn't taken the interest in his daughters' lives that he probably should have done, and if he was shutting out feelings related to his dad's death, what other feelings had he shut out? He thought of Clare. They had grown apart, but, well, that seemed to be being reversed now, and he was grateful for that. He felt the emotions rise again, and tears trickled over his eyelids and down his cheeks. 'Silly old fool,' he muttered to himself. And yet, somehow, even if he was a silly old fool, he was in some part glad that was what he was. He took a deep breath and dried his eyes, hoping that they weren't going to look too red. He had a home, he had his family, yes, his dad wasn't around to share in it, and his daughters didn't have their granddad, but they had their grandma, and he still did have so much to still look forward to, and be grateful for. 'Yeah.' He got out of the car, locked it up and headed for the front door. He could still feel the emotions, and his eyes watered again as he allowed himself to be grateful, once more, for what he had. He turned the key in the front door to let himself back in. Hmm, another surge of emotion, he blinked back the tears, something else to talk to Chris about maybe. No, something to talk to Clare about, that was the order it should be in.

Points for discussion

- How has the session left you feeling? Do you feel that you have a clear understanding of the nature of your feelings and their cause? In other words, is your experience congruently (authentically and accurately) in your awareness?

- What were the key therapeutic moments in the session?
- Which therapeutic qualities did you identify as being most present for Chris? Critically reflect on the quality and impact of his communication to Billy.
- In what ways might you have responded differently to things that Billy said? Support your ideas theoretically.
- What would you take to supervision from this session as the counsellor?
- Write notes for this session.

CHAPTER 7

Counselling session 6: Love, sensitivity and moving on

> When you came in my life, you changed my world, my Sarah
> Everything seemed so right, my baby girl, my Sarah
> You are all I want to know, you hold my heart, so don't let go
> You are all I need to live, my love to you I'll give
>
> When you begin to smile, you change my style, my Sarah
> When I look in your eyes I see my prize, my Sarah
> You are all I want to know, you hold my heart, so don't let go
> You are all I need to live, my love to you I'll give
>
> (Lynott and Moore, 1979)

Billy sat with tears in his eyes in the counselling room. 'I need to talk through something that just happened and, well, it links back to when I got home last week and most of my week really.'

'Sure, what's happened?' Chris could see the emotional state that Billy was in, not just his eyes, he could just feel it in the room. The moment Billy had come through the door, it was there.

'I got back, I was feeling emotional before I went in, thinking about what I might have done to my daughters with how I've been. And, well, as I opened the door, well, actually when I turned the key in the lock, something about *being let back in*, I don't know that really got to me. Like I was letting myself back in, but I was also being let back in to the family in some way. I don't know, it just sort of really hit me, and I sort of, yeah, I've just felt really emotional since, more so than before somehow. It's like, I don't know, I'm so sensitive at the moment and then just now, on the radio …'. He swallowed, 'I just heard a song, Thin Lizzy song *Sarah*, just got to me. Really got to me.' He took a deep breath as the tears returned to his eyes. 'And this is how I am at the moment, things set me off.'

'Left you feeling so sensitive and something about that particular song.' Chris knew the song, and he somehow wasn't surprised. He knew a little bit about

Phil Lynott, that he'd been brought up by his grandmother, called Sarah, but that the song was really about his daughter, Sara. Yes, he could imagine it getting to Billy, it was an incredibly touching song.

'You know it?'

Chris nodded.'

'The words, they just . . .', he closed his eyes as the emotions welled up inside him once more, pushing more tears into his already watering eyes.

Chris sat, feeling the emotions within himself in response to what Billy was saying and feeling.

'Yeah, . . . they just . . .'. He waited to see if Billy wanted to say more.

'I just, well, couldn't help thinking of my daughter. And, of course, the oldest is Sarah. My Sarah.' The words from the song were resonating in his head, but the feelings were in his heart. 'My Sarah'. 'Why am I so emotional?'

'Something you so want to understand, "why am I so emotional?".'

'It's like, I don't know, things affect me more. I just feel so sensitive. I don't think I've ever been like this before. Not as much, not as tearful. I mean, I sort of think of myself as sensitive, but this feels like . . ., it's just, well . . .'. He shrugged. 'I don't know.'

'Mhmm, hard to understand.'

'Hard to cope with. Don't get me wrong, I'm not complaining. I'm sort of glad I feel what I feel, you know, but it's like, I don't know, it takes so little to set me off.'

'Little?'

Billy had felt uncomfortable with the word the moment he had said it. And hearing it coming back to him made him more unsure if it was what he wanted to say. It wasn't little, not thinking and feeling about his daughters, his family. No, it wasn't little, far from it. But other things, he'd watched a cartoon, a *Tom and Jerry*, for goodness sake, and it was about the Jerry falling in love, and that had got to him. 'Anything involving love is getting to me.'

'Love is what's really touching you.'

Billy was taking a deep breath. 'Love, I just seem so sensitive to it at the moment. Is that normal?'

'It happens. People can find themselves sort of resensitised in some way, more open to feelings, to emotions that perhaps, for whatever reason, they haven't let themselves experience.'

Billy nodded. 'Love gets to me at the moment, I think of my daughters, and Clare. I don't know, everything seems so much more precious, all of a sudden. I think I felt that way after Dad died, but I think I lost it somehow, and it's back with me. It's like life is precious, it's, well, we can't take it for granted, can we? We have to make the most of it, and I have so much to make the most of.'

'Mhmm, life's precious and that preciousness is something you are really aware of at the moment.'

'Mhmm. We booked a holiday together, get away. I think we all need it, off to Madeira for some sunshine. Got a good deal at a hotel, all-inclusive and, yes, we're heading off over the Easter break.' Billy was pleased they'd arranged it. He was looking forward to it. Although they had had time away since his dad died, looking back now he hadn't really got away from anything, just took it with him. Now he felt different, felt that he could enjoy himself, and, well, enjoy being with Clare and the girls.

'Great, I hope it's a wonderful experience for you all.'

'Thanks. So do I! I'm sure it will be.' He paused. 'And I've just got to get used to being so sensitive, so easily affected by things.' His mind went back to the cartoon. He knew it sounded silly but he felt like he needed to say it. 'I even got emotional over a *Tom and Jerry* cartoon the other day – the girls had a video on.'

Chris smiled, 'Sounds like you really are sensitive at the moment.'

Billy lapsed into silence. What a thing to admit to. Still, he felt comfortable with Chris. He'd shown Chris a lot of emotion, a lot of himself. But that did feel OK. Over a short period of time he had come to respect Chris a great deal. He was good at what he did, but what a thing to do for a living.

He wasn't too sure what to talk about. He'd said what he wanted to say about his sensitivity. He felt sure he'd get over it, and now he wasn't sure. Nothing felt too pressing. Life seemed back on track. 'I don't know what to say, now. Feels like I've said what I want to say in a way. Nothing feels sort of, I don't know, urgent.'

'As you said that, my mind recalled something you said earlier, not today, something about feeling easier. It just came back to me.' Chris wasn't sure why it had come to mind, but it had done so and in quite a clear way. It felt natural, 'easy', to say it.

'I guess it is, well, I know it is, except for accepting how I have been and how I am with the emotions. But, yeah, I feel, hmm.' Billy thought for a moment about the sentence that had come into his mind. It did seem to sum it up somehow. 'I sort of feel on top of things, rather than feeling things are on top of me.'

Chris nodded, 'That sounds very clear, you feel on top now.'

'I do, and I know that so much of this is down to you, to this. I had no idea what to expect when I started, but now, well, now I can really understand why Mum found counselling so helpful. She probably went at the right time for her. Maybe I should have come earlier, I don't know, I really wasn't in a place to really make best use of it, I don't think.'

Chris wondered briefly whether to continue in the almost conversational style that seemed to be developing, or maintain a more disciplined, empathic focus. He chose the latter. 'Mhmm. Wondering if it would have been the right time for you to have come sooner.'

'But I didn't see a reason. I don't know. I can't sort of imagine myself sitting here as I was, you know?'

'Mhmm, it would have been different but hard to imagine.'

'Well, I guess I'll never know. But I am grateful and I suppose, well, we kind of touched on it last time, but I am wondering how long to keep coming.'

'Well, that's really up to you. From my perspective it's about coming for as long as you feel it is helpful.'

They continued to discuss this and agreed that rather than stop, to have another session in two weeks before the holiday and another when he got back and at that point review whether to stop. Both men felt comfortable with that arrangement. The rest of the session was spent with Billy talking more about his past. It was strange, he felt more able to talk about it without feeling the way he did in the past. Yes, some memories did bring his emotions to the fore, but he was also able to somehow appreciate, yes that was the word that made sense to him, he could appreciate his past. At one point he made the comment, 'You know, I guess in a way I always did appreciate the past, but never really dwelt on it because I had the present and the future to look forward to. Then, with Dad dying, I couldn't appreciate the past and I sort of lost the future, and I suppose I was simply all over the place in the present. They're all bound together, aren't they?'

Chris had nodded in response. It was very perceptive. They then explored this a little more. Chris had noted again the tendency towards a more conversational tone. He was comfortable with this. In his experience counselling processes could become more conversational as they reached their natural conclusions. Billy headed home and Chris was left to reflect on the session and write his notes. His mind went back to the song that Billy had mentioned and found he couldn't get the tune out of his head. He hunted down the CD, and found one that had the song on it, although it was a different CD to the original. His eye caught another song, one he hadn't listened to for a long time. He played it. One line struck him forcibly, it had in the past, but it somehow seemed to have more presence as he listened to it now, 'Death is just a heartbeat away' (Moore, 1985).

Chris found himself pondering on that all-too-pertinent statement. Just a heartbeat away. We all assume that we will have another heartbeat as we all assume that the next breath will follow the current one. To live accepting that either might be our last – would that make us feel more alive, or more depressed? To live each moment as if it was all we had. Could we sustain it? He changed the focus of his speculation.

Death. What was it, is it? What does it mean to die? What happens? He thought of the people who he had known who had died. Well, he thought to himself, they all know. If something lives on then they know. And if nothing, well, it doesn't matter. There's nothing to make sense of. He didn't believe in a God, or a Heaven or Hell. The dice was too loaded against some people for that to feel right or just. And if there is no God, then evolution and what we call 'life' is chance, no purposeful design, just a rather unlikely emergence within the vastness of the cosmos. Is that all we are? Or, if there is a God, are there laws and some designed purpose to it all that is somehow hidden, known only to that God. Could we know? Science? Religion? Are there prophets, sages, people who have glimpsed? Do they have to be religious? Could they be scientists? Or people from any walk of life? Were there people who saw more, knew more about life, and death? He didn't know. It was a nice thought but was it all simply a way of avoiding facing the prospect of existential death. His intuition said life goes on. But was that because he couldn't imagine non-existence?

He sighed. So many questions, so much to consider. What he *did* know was that death was something we all faced, that we all had to find our own ways of dealing with it. And he believed, wholeheartedly, that within a therapeutic relationship founded on the principles of the person-centred approach, people could allow the full extent of their hurt to emerge and to experience it being heard and accepted; they could experience the warmth of another human being, a companion, on their journey into their often painful and confusing inner world; and that they could emerge different, maybe still hurt, but more able to function more fully, and maybe with more meaning, and certainly with greater authenticity. He thought of how the death of those closest to us often heralded the death of a part of ourselves. Sometimes it was the part in which we had invested out hopes for the future, sometimes it was a part more associated with the past. And sometimes the loss was very much of the present. He picked up his pen and wrote his notes.

Points for discussion

- Consider Billy's process in response to his dad's death. What are the significant features?
- What aspect of the counselling do you think proved most helpful for Billy, and why?
- What does death mean to you? How does your belief affect the way you live your life?
- How are you feeling towards Billy? Do you feel that has changed as you have travelled with him on the therapeutic journey?
- Write two paragraph's describing Chris's qualities as a counsellor.
- What do you think was most important for Billy to experience from Chris: empathy, unconditional positive regard, genuineness or contact? And why?
- What would you take to supervision from this session?
- Write notes for this session.

Reflections

From the counsellor

I have found working with Billy to be very human. That's what comes to mind first and foremost. We were two human beings encountering each other around a set of experiences that lie at the root of the human experience. Billy did not explore his own mortality so much as other clients might as a reaction to their father's death, but he did encounter a great deal and as a result has come to know himself more clearly than before, and is now moving on in his life with a new-found sensitivity and perhaps appreciation of life, and certainly of those closest to him.

I also want to add something to that. It wasn't just a very human experience. I want to also highlight the man-to-man nature of our relationship. That felt enormously important. I haven't checked out with Billy what he thinks about that, maybe he'll have something to say on the topic in his reflection of the process so far. But for me it was important. I think my being a man was probably significant. Some of the moments of eye contact were profound. I felt at times that Billy was searching deeply for something, sometimes within me, and most certainly within himself.

For a man to cry in the presence of another man within a culture where that is not the norm, is a huge thing. I have a lot of respect for Billy, for the work *he* has done within therapy. And I do want to make that emphasis. He could have chosen not to engage in the process, but he did. I like to think that the relational attitude I offered helped him in this. I also know that where a client is in themselves, the stage they are at in coming to terms with something can also be an important factor.

Let me say something more about that. It links to the notion that incongruence in the client is a condition for constructive personality change. People can get something productive from therapy because they are incongruent, and perhaps more so as they become aware that they are incongruent. Not that someone wakes up and declares themselves incongruent, but rather they start to experience the effects of the internal mismatching of experience, awareness and what they communicate to the outside world. Somehow, somewhere inside themselves, is perhaps a knowing that something has to change. I think this is an important condition – or maybe some might describe it as a pre-condition – for therapeutic change.

I was and am touched by Billy's openness. Yes, the first session had lots of silences, but that's not unusual. Why should someone pour their heart out to a stranger about something so painful to them? Equally, for others the very fact that you are a stranger is the reason why they feel they can tell you their innermost thoughts and feelings, anxieties and hurts.

Key moments in the sessions? There were many. Some of the silences were profound, and the eye contact. Contact, we don't often talk much about that. The focus is often on congruence, empathy, unconditional positive regard. But the experience of contact, the actual therapeutic impact of contact is, for me, really important. And I sensed that this was the case for Billy. We did make contact, and profoundly so on a number of occasions. We were both affected by what emerged within Billy and into our relationship. And, yes, I was affected too, and my affect was present and I am sure was something Billy also recognised. I hope so. I want to be present to him and for all my clients. It's important.

What more can I say? It feels as though Billy is moving to how he wants and needs to be. He is moving on in himself, and in his life. He may not have many more counselling sessions, or he may choose to have more. I am quite happy for him to decide.

And I am so glad that he is feeling what he is feeling for his family. It must have been so hard for them while he was struggling to come to terms with his dad's death and what that meant for him emotionally, and in terms of his memories and his hopes and expectations.

Were the sessions so far typical of counselling someone for a bereavement? I don't think there are typical sessions. I don't want to sit with expectations of how a client will be, or an expectation of how many sessions, or feel a need to decide at what stage somewhat might be in their grieving process. I don't work that way. I hope I can accept my client as he or she is with what they need to bring and how they need to be. Every client will be different and I am sure that my responses will be different. I do think that the therapeutic relationship emerges, develops in its own direction and my role is to respond. I am sure, well I know, that I contribute to the direction even though my approach is non-directive. That's always an interesting debate. But what is important is that I am not *seeking to impose* a specific direction, but what is likely to emerge is that the client will find a direction from within themselves. The actualising tendency, that lies so much at the heart of the constructive emphasis within the person-centred approach, constructive in the sense of urging the person towards what-ever will give them the fullest satisfaction. It was satisfying to Billy to dwell on what he had lost following his dad's death. It satisfied his need to feel what he was feeling. Now, however, he seeks satisfaction in other ways, from his relation-ship with Clare, and with his two daughters, his mother and no doubt from other areas of life that perhaps now have more meaning for him.

I have said enough, more than I intended. I wish Billy well, whether he chooses a couple more sessions, or to continue longer. I feel satisfied with the work I have done with him and what I have contributed to his process.

From the client

Well, where do I start? I've been up and down, turned inside out, wracked with emotions that I didn't think were possible to experience, or survive. I really have been on a rollercoaster. And, well, things are settled or at least settling now. I hope they stay that way. Whether they will, I don't know. I know I have the poten-tial to get too intense and to become quite insensitive to the effect I am having on others. That worries me, and, yes, I still feel guilty about it. Well, I think that's fair enough. I have to put my hand up. Yes, there were reasons, but, yes, I was out of order. I am so grateful they stuck by me. It could have been worse.

Actually, since the last session that's something that I have thought about. It was another conversation with Clare. I don't know quite how the topic came up, it was about how difficult it had been to cope with me. And I said that I was so glad they stuck by me, even though I was all over the place. She said that she wonders herself now, looking back, but is glad she did. That she still loved me even though it was hard at times, particularly the mood swings. The drinking came up again. I didn't react this time, tried to listen from her point of view. And it got me thinking. What would have happened if she hadn't coped, hadn't stuck with me? What would have happened if it had continued, and everything had got worse? It made me realise something that was, well, sobering, I can tell you. I mean, yes, I'd like to have thought that I'd have coped, if that had happened, say we had split up, I know that's extreme, but it can happen. Where would I have been, away from my daughters, still stuck with the loss of my dad, and drinking. I think I can understand now how things can go badly wrong for people. While I don't think it could have happened to me, you don't know, do you? And what if it had been Clare or one of the girls who had died, how would I cope with that? I don't even want to go there. I guess that's normal. We don't want to contemplate for the worse, it's too painful to contemplate.

So, I've learned a lot. I didn't talk as much about it in the last session as I thought I might, but I do feel I've been let back in to the family, or have I let myself in? Different emphasis. Hmm, maybe a bit of both, that's probably closest to the truth. And what of counselling? I didn't really know what to expect. Mum said that counsellors listen, give you space, don't tell you what to do. At least that had been her experience and it was certainly mine too. Strange, in a way, but thank goodness for people like Chris. And you know, and I don't know what difference it made, but I'm glad it was a man. I think if someone had told me how I was going to feel, and that I would have a male counsellor, I'd probably have said no, I'd rather see a woman. But actually, I don't know, but I think for me there was something important about going through what I did with Chris. I can't describe it or explain it, it's just how it was, and I'm sure other people will say or experience something different. All I can say is what it was like for me. Something in his eyes, something about how he was. I respected him as the sessions went on.

Hmm. So much emotion, so much hurt, but he was somehow reassuring. It wasn't that he kept saying things to reassure me, though he did once or twice I seem to remember, but it was his presence, something about how he was. It wasn't just what he said, it was something more than that. I can't quite put my finger on it. He was calm, didn't seem at all phased by how I was, and yet I saw a compassion, a caring, some kind of understanding – more than saw, I felt it. That was important. There was something about, yes, we sort of made contact in some way. And that's strange because I know so little about him and yet he knows so much about me! But that doesn't somehow seem to matter. We connected and in a way I do know a lot about him; not facts, not things someone says about themselves, but more about how he is. And maybe, in some strange way, that's actually more important.

I think for me the key moments were when I said things that were the hardest things to say, about how Clare and the girls still loved me. That still gets to me, it really does, and I am glad it does and I genuinely hope I always will be affected when I think of that. If I lose my reaction then I will have lost a precious part of myself. And something about the way Chris didn't interrupt me. Even when I was lost inside myself, he sort of let me know he was there, but he didn't sort of, I don't know, interrupt. Maybe I might have wanted that and yet actually, thinking back now, that was quite important, maybe really important. But only because I knew he was there. Back to that sort of reassurance, back to something about him, just being there, being . . . , being there for me.

I think I can live a better life now. Yes, I have my memories, and yes, they can be painful, but not like they were. And now I feel more grateful for them. I feel more able to appreciate the good times rather than just miss them, or feel I've lost them. I haven't. They happened. They are part of me. Dad is part of me. Yes, it makes me tearful, of course it does, but that's how I am these days. But it's a different kind of tearful and there isn't the same intense hurt. Dad was a good man and . . . , and I'm proud to be his son. I think the counselling has helped me realise this in a new way, in a way that doesn't tie me to the past, to what's gone, to what will be missing from the future. He won't be there and yes, that makes me sad. But life goes on, new experiences, and I want to be part of that. And Dad will be part of that in a way because he will still be in all our hearts.

Part 2

Counselling session 8: The client is tired, emotional and due to see the doctor for a check-up

Nicola sat in the counselling room at the doctor's surgery waiting for her client, Barbara, to arrive. This would be their eighth session. She had been seeing Barbara for a couple of months now, having been referred by her doctor for support and space to talk through difficulties she was having at home. The main issues had been related to Barbara's husband's lack of support for her, and her sons causing her stress as a result of their behaviour. One son was using drugs and had been in prison for acquisitive crimes, the other drank heavily and had been quite disruptive at times. Her husband had disowned both sons, seemingly uninterested in either of them, arguing with them and threatening to throw them both out of the house. Barbara, however, had felt unable to do this. They were her sons, and much as she disliked how they were, she felt she had to help, try and make them see things differently. She had felt, and still felt, so responsible. And while the counselling had helped her to recognise that logically she was not responsible for their choices, emotionally she couldn't help feeling responsible.

Barbara had been feeling tired of everything, generally run down. It all seemed an effort. In a sense, that was not new, but somehow the fatigue felt worse. She didn't know why. She knew she wasn't eating much, didn't feel hungry. She knew it wasn't like her to be off her food, but at the moment she couldn't explain it, she just didn't feel like she had much appetite.

In fact not just for food. While she felt the counselling had helped, the past week or two – maybe longer – things had begun to feel hopeless again. It saddened her. But, well, at least she was staying sober. She knew how, in the past, she had coped – well, it hadn't been coping, but it had sort of helped her escape – by drinking. Quite heavily at times. She'd had to be detoxed on more than one occasion, but that was in the past. Sometimes the thought was there, but not so much now. Anyway, it wasn't something she wanted to do now.

Barbara had been having some discomfort in her stomach, and back pain, though neither was particularly unusual. She had just made an appointment to see the doctor, in fact she was seeing him the next day. Even that had felt like an effort. She had mentioned the symptoms to Nicola but without saying much more, other than that they did not help, just added to her stress and feeling that no one really cared about her or appreciated her.

The phone rang in the counselling room, it was reception. 'Your client has arrived.'

'Thanks. I'll come out and meet her.'

Nicola left the counselling room and headed down the corridor to the waiting area. She saw Barbara sitting in the corner. She didn't look well.

'Hello, Barbara, come on through.' Barbara followed, still not saying anything. They entered the counselling room and Barbara sat down. She wasn't wearing a coat, it was a warm day.

Barbara just felt so tired and suddenly so very emotional. Her eyes began to water, her throat felt hot, constricted, burning, and she burst into tears. Still not speaking.

Nicola pushed the tissues along the table so they were closer to Barbara. 'Something's really upset you.' She didn't voice her words as a question, it was obvious something was upsetting Barbara. She waited to see if Barbara was going to respond, or whether she simply needed the time and the space to release or express what she was feeling through her tears.

Barbara was catching her breath, trying to regain control. She swallowed but it didn't seem to make any difference. It felt like the emotion was coming from so deep inside herself. Low down, pit of her stomach. A strange feeling. And her back felt uncomfortable, a painful kind of aching sensation, didn't seem to change much when she moved. She'd thought it was just stiffness, but it clearly wasn't just that. But that was a side issue. 'Every day's the same, and I just feel like I'm ..., I'm ...,' Barbara paused, hesitated, not sure how to express herself. It was difficult to find the words, particularly as the waves of emotion continued to affect her. She took a deep breath and sighed, burying her face in a tissue.

'So much ...'. Nicola sought to empathise with the intensity that she was experiencing from Barbara's emotional release. She knew from the past counselling sessions how difficult Barbara was finding it all, and she had been tearful before, but somehow today was different, more intense, yes, and somehow deeper. But that was her word and her interpretation. She waited, maintaining a sense of warm acceptance for Barbara. No, it was more than that, it was a compassion, a caring, the kind of feeling a person has towards another who is suffering.

'I just feel like nothing changes and nothing will ever change.'

'Stuck?'

Barbara nodded, and blew her nose, putting the tissue in the bin before taking another to dab at her eyes.

'It's not what I want. And, you know, some days it's OK, I can cope. I get on with what I need to do, sort of shut it all out.'

'Mhmm, shut it all out.' Nicola wondered if the 'it' referred to something within her, or to her family.

'And I felt better, what, a couple of weeks back, I really did. I was starting to make choices for me, you know, and it felt good. Not easy, but it felt like I was doing something for me.'

'Mhmm, I remember, and I remember how important that was for you.'

'And I still do, but somehow it's like it's all such an effort, too much of an effort, and I feel, I don't know . . . ,' she paused, 'I don't feel well.'

Nicola nodded and the words in her head were, 'You don't look well either', but she didn't voice them, wanting to stay with what Barbara was saying. 'Just not feeling well, everything's an effort.'

'It's different, not like it was. It's like, I don't know, I feel tired. I mean, I felt tired before, but it was different.' She shook her head. 'It's hard to explain, but it feels different, I feel different.'

'You feel different, it's a different kind of tiredness?'

Barbara was taking a deep breath again, it caused her to cough. She'd been coughing more just recently, she wasn't sure why, thought it was a chill, it was that time of year. It jarred her back. That pain was more present again.

'I'm seeing the doctor tomorrow. Maybe it's the time of year, maybe it's a chill or something. Anyway, I guess it'll be OK.' She forced a smile. 'And, well, then I can get myself back together again. I have to, don't I?'

'It's important to you, isn't it, to get back on track.'

'I'd been feeling better, bit more energy, but now . . . , well, anyway . . . ,' she winced, her lower back again.

The session continued with Barbara talking a little more about how it had been at home and how she was going to try and make more time for herself, and not try and keep expecting more from her family, which she was coming to accept she'd never get. The session ended early, Barbara felt tired and wanted to rest.

Nicola expressed concern for her health, she didn't look good. She was glad Barbara was seeing the doctor the next day. She felt sure that had she not been, she may well have felt concerned enough to ask if she had considered a check-up.

After Barbara had left, Nicola sat down to write her notes and to ponder on the session. Yes, Barbara had definitely moved on, and was much clearer in what she needed to do to give herself space and some, well, self-respect really at home. Clearly this was what she wanted and, well, maybe her feeling not too good at the moment was a kind of physical reaction to inner change. Maybe. She wasn't totally convinced. She believed in the interaction between mind, emotions and body, and knew that sometimes released inner tension could be expressed physically. Perhaps the back pain and tiredness were linked to that? She didn't know and there wasn't much point in speculating. She wrote her notes and went to make herself a cup of tea. She had time, a bit of extra time as the session had finished early. She remained concerned, though, Barbara just had not looked a good colour, a kind of yellowish tinge to her features, she was sure that hadn't been there before.

Counselling session 9: cancer diagnosed, so many thoughts and feelings

Barbara was sitting in the counselling room, but this week she was feeling very different. She'd left that last sessions tired, yes, and she knew she wasn't herself, but she'd had no idea. It all seemed a blur and yet it wasn't. She had felt numb, not wanting to believe what she had been told. It was a strange sensation, knowing something and yet . . . . It was like it was too big, too overwhelming to really know. It was as though she had thoughts but didn't know what to think, had feelings but didn't know what to feel. And she had carried on with doing the usual things in her life, routine things. Just carried on.

Nicola waited. She noted how Barbara was not looking back at her but down to her right. She looked as though she had lost more colour in her face. She wasn't going to push her into saying anything. She trusted her client to say what she needed to say, when and how she needed to say it. She sat, keeping her attention focused on her client and maintaining her openness to the inner experiencing that was coming into her awareness. She could feel a tension, a kind of anxiety, a sort of knot in her stomach. Yes, she could feel the tension. Physiologically there was a reaction within her, and she felt as though her sensitivity was increased, as if she was on full alert for something, though she did not know what it was. She trusted these reactions, they had happened before.

As she looked across at Barbara – now in her late fifties – she realised that her thoughts had momentarily wandered into speculation. Some kind of shock. Someone had died, perhaps? Her immediate thoughts then went to Barbara's two sons, Alec and Graham. Knowing the emotional connection Barbara felt towards them both, in spite of how they behaved and their attitude towards her, this was what was uppermost in her thinking. She pushed the thought aside. It wasn't for her to sit speculating. She had to be open to the reality as she knew it, which was that Barbara had come in looking pale, little or no facial expression, and that she, Nicola, was feeling a tension and heightened state of alert within herself.

Where a client has begun a session by not saying anything it can make it difficult for the counsellor to hold their focus and attention on the client. The client has not disclosed their inner world. The counsellor may then, as in this case, drift into speculation. They have to try and maintain control, to be open to what they sense from the client but without going beyond what is present. Silences of this nature can be difficult. The person-centred counsellor will want to ensure that they are maintaining a sensitive openness, an alertness to whatever the client may be communicating through body language and facial expression, and a readiness, an availability to hear whatever the client may say when they begin to speak. It is highly likely that

> when the client does speak, what they say will need to be heard with parti-
> cular warm acceptance and responded to accurately.

Barbara was not really seeing, although she was looking down at the carpet and the leg of the table that was against the wall on her right. She hadn't wanted anyone to know, at first. They'd told her at the hospital. It all happened so quickly. She hadn't slept much that night, or the next one. She hadn't told her parents, she had felt she didn't want to worry them. Derek knew, but she hadn't told her sons, she didn't know what to say. And she knew she was seeing Nicola, and somehow, well, somehow she felt she needed to ..., she didn't know what. She took a deep breath. 'I've got cancer.' Those were the words in her mind, the words she knew she had to say, but they stayed in her head. Words that she did not want to hear herself speak. The cancer was advanced, her pancreas badly damaged, they couldn't operate, and there were already indications of secondaries having spread both to her lungs and her liver. They couldn't operate, they could try and slow it down, buy time, but .... Maybe months, could be weeks. She continued to stare down, feeling still quite numb and yet also aware of a disbelief as well as a kind of knowing. And now, as she sat there, she didn't know what to say or how to say it.

She looked up and across to Nicola. Her face felt strangely numb, and she could feel a sensation of nausea building up in her stomach. Her throat seemed sud-denly constricted, as if it was stopping her from saying what she knew she had to say. She swallowed. She looked into Nicola's eyes. Nicola was looking back at her. There was a deep compassion in her eyes. Barbara looked away, taking another deep breath. She coughed, it had got worse. Somewhere deep in her lungs was a kind of irritation, it persisted most of the time.

Nicola watched Barbara look away. In that moment of eye contact there had been something powerful take place, though she could not describe it. It was not a normal look, but a knowing one, serious, she did not know what other words to use. She respected Barbara's choice not to speak, and she also felt a pressure within herself to say something. She needed to say something, but she also knew that it was her need to reduce the tension that she was feeling. Her need. That wasn't good enough a reason. When did facilitating a client to speak become pressure and direction to speak? Barbara was no doubt experien-cing something hugely significant and, at this moment, her nature was keeping her silent. She felt she had to empathise with that choice. She spoke softly, choosing her words carefully. 'Something you need to be silent about.'

The words resonated within Barbara, they did capture what was present for her. She was lifting her left hand, her fingers touching the corner of her mouth. Her hand was trembling. She looked up at Nicola once more. Again, the caring in her eyes. 'Cancer.'

Nicola felt her heart thumping. Her thoughts went back to the symptoms Barbara had complained of in previous sessions, the aches and pains, the fatigue and her altered colour, the feeling strange, which had seemed like a stress reaction, and yet. She was making an assumption Barbara was referring to herself. It was a spontaneous assumption.

'You...?'

Barbara nodded.

Nicola felt her own lips tighten. Barbara's expression had not changed. Shock, Nicola thought, she's in emotional shock. Her inner nature may be stopping her from feeling the full extent of the impact.

'I'm sorry.' It was a genuine expression. 'Bad?'

Barbara nodded again. 'Weeks, maybe months.'

'The tiredness, the pain?'

Again Barbara nodded.

Nicola was feeling herself take in a deep breath. She needed to empathise with whatever was present within Barbara. At the moment she could only empathise with what she was communicating.

'I haven't told my sons.'

She felt a reaction of wanting to say in a slightly surprised tone, 'They don't know?', but pushed it aside. That wasn't empathy, and if her tone of voice sounded surprised it could be heard as being quite judgemental. 'You haven't told them.' She kept eye contact with Barbara, she was speaking softly, and nodded slightly as she spoke. It was a sensitive time, a human moment, more than a moment. Sitting with another human being who has been given weeks to live, she knew that she had to offer total acceptance of all the thoughts, feelings and reactions that Barbara experienced and chose to communicate.

'I know I have to, but I didn't when I came back after ...'. Barbara lapsed into silence, memories of being rushed into hospital. The pain .... She was unaware she was shaking her head. The pain had been so intense, excruciating, felt like her insides were ..., it was hard to describe, but she was convinced she was going to die. She'd been sedated, they'd scanned her, taken blood and then operated, exploratory they said. Strong painkillers for a day or two and it had eased. She was still taking them but on a reduced dose. Barbara closed her eyes. She knew she hadn't fully accepted it, and didn't really know what to think or feel about what was happening to her.

Nicola nodded and reached over, gently touching Barbara on the forearm. 'Not easy to talk to anyone.'

'No, no ...'. Barbara lapsed into silence. She just hadn't known what to say or how to say it. She'd made her husband agree to not tell them, said that she wanted to. She was worried about the effect it would have on them, how they'd cope. She also didn't want to hear herself telling them either. It was like she knew, but she didn't believe, and yet she did as well. It wasn't exactly denial, she knew, but she couldn't accept, couldn't quite imagine it was happening to her. But it was. 'I guess I'm sort of still, well ...,' Barbara shook her head, 'letting it sink in I suppose. And I know that I have to, you know, well, I have to tell everyone, but ...'.

'But ...'.

'They are saying maybe just weeks. I'm sure I should be feeling something, feeling something more. I mean, I am, but I also feel sort of numb as well. It's like, I don't know, yes, it is sort of numb, numb on the inside, in my . . . , in my . . . , everywhere. Except for the pain.'

'Like before?'

'More intense. They say they will control it if it gets worse, increase the painkillers.' Barbara looked away. 'It's like you know it's happening but you can't believe it. It doesn't make sense, but it's happening and what do I do?'

Nicola nodded, 'Now that you know, as you say, what do you do?' Nicola felt herself experiencing a mixture of feelings as well. Sadness, sorry to hear what Barbara had told her, an urge, no, a determination to be very present, very focused and attentive. She had worked with others who had faced their own death, but she also knew that the experience was a unique one to each person. How would Barbara wish to use counselling, if indeed she wanted to? Not everyone did.

The counsellor has maintained her focus and sensitivity. A devastating situation has occurred for her client, who is still in emotional shock. She is being allowed to say what she needs to say, and at her own pace. The person-centred counsellor will be alert to the need to stay very much with the inner world of the client. They may be feeling many things themselves, but this is not a time to be expressing their own inner world. The client is disclosing that she is facing death. The counsellor is offering warmth, gently enabling the client to say what has happened. She is talking about the event, the diagnosis, what she hasn't done. She has yet to move into talking specifically about how she is feeling, what she is now thinking. The person-centred counsellor will not be seeking to direct the client towards this focus. She knows that the client must process what has happened in their own way, at their own pace. Her role is to be a warm and caring companion to her client in that process.

'I have to tell my sons but I'm afraid how they'll react. Derek has been good, though he's in shock as well. He wanted to blame Alec and Graham. I won't let him say that. I haven't told my parents either. It's like I don't want to hear myself telling them.' She shook her head.

Nicola noted the silence that had developed between them. It wasn't an awkward silence, though it was painful. Nicola realised that she should have responded, but she had been momentarily caught in her own thoughts and feelings in reaction to what Barbara had disclosed. She had slipped into her own inner world. She needed to regain her focus and emphasis on what was happening for her client, while remaining open to herself as well.

'Yes, not something you want to hear yourself saying, and particularly not to them.'

Barbara shook her head slowly. 'So many thoughts rush through my head, it's like I think them but they're somehow separate from me. It's weird, hard to describe. Maybe the painkillers are affecting me as well, I don't know, it's like it's happening, I know it, but . . .'. She shook her head again. 'What do you do?'

'That's really troubling you, that question of what do you do given what you know.'

'I don't know, I just don't know. And so many people will be so upset, and I don't want them upset. I'd rather they didn't know in a way. But they will, won't they?'

'You'd prefer them not to know, but . . .'.

Barbara sighed, 'But they will, they have to. They have to face it as well.'

Nicola nodded, 'They have to come to terms with it as well.'

Barbara was lost in her own thoughts about her two sons. Yes, they had their problems, everyone did, but, well, she could just see how Alec would cope, he'd drink, she was sure of it. Bit like she would have done once. But that was then. Strangely that wasn't something she felt any need for at the moment. She didn't react the way she used to. But Alec would. And it would only make things worse for him, and between him and his father. And then there was Graham, she just wasn't sure how he'd be. Sometimes he could be fairly OK, if only he could stick to the methadone he got from the clinic for his heroin addiction, but she knew that he didn't. At least he wasn't injecting any more, having that regular prescription was helping, but he was still caught up in that world, she could only imagine him . . . . She shook her head.

Nicola noticed Barbara shaking her head and responded to it. 'Leaves you shaking your head thinking about it?'

'Yes, yes it does. I can see them both struggling, I really can. Derek can't cope with either of them. Not really. He doesn't want to know. Without me . . .'. She felt raw emotion rising up inside herself. Yes, without me . . . . She couldn't imagine a happy time for any of them. She closed her eyes and felt the tears trickling over her eyelids and spilling down her cheeks. 'I've tried, Nicola, I've tried so hard, but . . .'. She shook her head, wondering about how much she had contributed to how her sons were today.

'Tried so hard . . .'. Nicola spoke softly, not wanting her response to in any way disrupt the flow of experiencing that was clearly occurring for Barbara.

'And now this.' Barbara paused. 'Now this.' It was mainly sadness but there was concern, more than concern, real worry about how her sons were going to be.

The client has been focusing on other people and their reaction, or anticipated reaction. The counsellor has remained calm and quietly present. There is a tone to the therapeutic interaction that is expressive of the seriousness of what has occurred, and is occurring. The counsellor's empathy is sensitive and responsive to her client and what she is saying. It is a time that demands discipline of the counsellor, a firm but gentle self-discipline to ensure that the client is offered the space and the freedom to be as she needs to be.

'You know I drift into thinking about what's happening inside me.' Barbara paused, collecting her thoughts, which was not easy amidst the emotions she was feeling. But she wanted to finish what she had started to say. 'The, you know, knowing that something is happening, that my body is, well, sort of . . . , I don't know, like it's growing inside me, taking over. And the pain, I'm so scared of the pain. They say they can help me with that, but what I've experienced was so excruciating, so intense.' Barbara went quiet, outwardly, but inside that fear was so very present.

Nicola was very aware of how many different areas Barbara had moved through in the past five minutes, so much happening for her, so much to contain, come to terms with, try and make sense of. Concern for others but also fear for what was going to happen to her in terms of pain and, no doubt, the progression of the cancer. 'You've experienced the pain, and that's so, so scary to have to face.'

'It's not that I haven't known pain – what woman, mother, hasn't?'

Nicola nodded.

'But it is this knowing that it's growing inside me, and they've started me on treatment to try and slow it down, but I guess that, well, may just prolong the pain, maybe. They say they can control that.' Barbara stopped again, thinking about how it was going to be, the next few weeks and months. She was home, able to function, but she had been told that she would probably have to go into hospital, or maybe a hospice at some point when things got worse. She didn't want to think about that.

Barbara continued. 'They told me that what I have can be hard to detect early on, cancer in the pancreas. There aren't the symptoms, at least not ones to make you feel you have to be checked out. That's why it's so advanced, and spreading.' Barbara talked a little about the treatment options. Nicola listened. She knew most of them from what she had heard from other clients, and from her own mother's battle with breast cancer which, fortunately, had gone into remission and seemed to have been diagnosed and treated early enough to stop it spreading. 'I have to be positive, somehow, but I don't feel like it. I really don't, Nicola, I just . . . , I'm not some hero, just me . . .'. She shook her head and closed her eyes as the tears welled up once again.

'Feels like it's just you.'

Barbara nodded, fighting back the tears and the emotions, and then giving up. You-you never think it'll happen to you, not really. You d-d-don't, d-do you?'

'No.'

'You're not really sort of prepared for it. I mean . . .'. The words she had intended to say were, 'We've all got to die', but they were words she couldn't bring herself to say. She didn't want to die. Yes, life wasn't brilliant, but it was life. And she'd been feeling better about things before all this had happened. Somehow it didn't seem fair. It just didn't seem fair.

'Not something you think about happening to you.'

'You sort of know it can happen, but you don't really think about it, imagine it happening. Too busy coping with everything, I suppose.'

Nicola nodded, 'Busy coping with the everyday, this is not something you really think about.'

'I mean you do, sometimes, when someone close to you . . . , you know?'

Nicola nodded, aware that Barbara was finding it difficult to speak directly of death. She respected that. She imagined how she needed to try and contain the emotions associated with it at the moment.

Each person will have their own unique reaction. That uniqueness has to be appreciated by the counsellor. The person-centred counsellor will be seeking to accept how the client needs to be, not pushing them towards anything. The client here is struggling to use words like 'death' and 'die'. Perhaps the counsellor could point this out, but in this instance is choosing not to. A person-centred counsellor would be unlikely to focus the client on this, but would rather accept that the client needs to speak as they are doing. The client knows what they are struggling to say, and may not need the counsellor to tell them this. But there could be times when they will want to know that the counsellor appreciates the difficulty they are having with hearing themselves say particular words. It is for the counsellor to seek to ascertain the situation, and a professional (and personal) judgement as to what is the most appropriate response.

'Someone close, when it happens to them, then you think about it.'

'I mean, you know, what happens. But, well, that's the afterwards. I can't think about that at the moment. It's what's happening now, how it's going to upset the people I love, and . . . ,' she took a deeper breath, carefully, so as not to cough, '. . . and . . .', Barbara shook her head again, looking down. She couldn't find the words, but she was thinking about how it was all going to be, how it would end, what pain would she have to face, would she keep her dignity. She felt fear in the pit of her stomach, raw, naked fear. She swallowed, 'I'm so afraid.' She sobbed, wiping the tears from her eyes with her fingers. He breathing coming in short, shallow breaths.

'So much fear.' Nicola was again speaking softly. She could see Barbara sitting in front of her, head bowed, her shoulders jolting upwards with each sob. She felt her caring, her warmth for her. It was a mix of her own personal feeling towards her as someone she had got to know quite well, and something other, which she thought of as being to do with some kind of very deep human reaction to another person in pain and distress. She felt her own pain in response to what Barbara was saying and experiencing. And she was suddenly struck by the loneliness of it all. Her husband also in shock, two sons who didn't know but who may well struggle to cope without more alcohol and drugs, and she hadn't mentioned other family and friends. It could help to feel it as a shared battle even though, of course, the reality was that it was a very personal and individual reality. Yes, she thought, so much fear.

'I'm no hero, these people that, you know . . .'.

Nicola nodded, she thought of celebrities who had faced cancer, and the people who had found that their cancer had sort of spurred them into lifestyle changes and fundraising. But it wasn't right to compare, not really, though she could appreciate how easy that was to do. 'I'm sure everyone has their difficult times, we don't necessarily see it, though. And you don't feel like a hero.'

Hearing what Nicola had said helped. It was easy to forget that others would have their difficult times. 'I'm not there, just still coming to terms with it. It's like I don't know how to react. I feel like I sort of haven't, in a way. I mean, I have, but I haven't. It's like I can't stay feeling like this. I can't just sit and wait, though it feels like that, like just waiting. But I can't, I have to get on, do what I can. I have to.'

'Mhmm, have to not just wait, but get on, do what you can. That sounds important, the way you say it.'

The emotions had subsided. 'I'm not a hero though.'

Nicola was struck by a sense of how important it was for Barbara to say that and for it to be heard. 'You really don't feel very heroic in all of this.' Nicola was aware of her own thought that facing and coming to terms with your own death was a pretty damned heroic act. But it was not how Barbara was feeling and she didn't want to say something from her frame of reference that clearly differed from Barbara's. What Barbara felt and experienced was what mattered, her inner world was what needed to be heard, respected and warmly accepted. It was so easy to rush in with an alternative view, to try and, well, often with a motive to help the client feel better – often driven by a need in the therapist to feel better. But the reality was, facing death, whatever one's beliefs about what came next, wasn't necessarily easy. She put her thoughts aside, they were for later, or supervision, but not for now.

'I'm no hero, just a woman with cancer . . .'.

'Mhmm, just a woman with cancer.' Nicola felt herself to be very connected to Barbara as she responded. The words, and the emotions associated with them, perhaps attached to them was more accurate, seemed so very present. That was how it felt; what Barbara had said clearly reflected what was so present within her inner world, her awareness, a sense of her situation, and it was this that Nicola needed to convey that she had heard. She spoke softly, very much aware of the words and the meaning, and the emphasis as she spoke them, seeking to reflect back accurately the same emphasis that Barbara had given as she had spoken.

The person-centred approach values the inner world of the client. The responses made by the counsellor are warmly and humanly empathic. There is no attempt to present an alternative view, no comment, for instance in response to what has been said by the client here, along the lines of 'you're more than that'. The person-centred counsellor has no intent to create or encourage a different experience or perspective for the client. Yes, that may emerge as a result of the client feeling heard and warmly accepted, but there is no specific intention on the part of the person-centred counsellor to encourage a particular experience within the client. The client feels what she feels; the role of the person-centred counsellor is to warmly accept this without judgement, and to convey what they have heard, what they have understood to be the client's experience.

It is this disciplined response, the person-centred counsellor unwavering in their focus on the client's experiencing, that lies at the core of the person-centred approach, and is an example of how it differs from other approaches that embrace the introduction of alternative perspectives by the counsellor. From the person-centred theoretical stance, it is the very human quality of feeling heard, feeling that your inner world, the essential experiencing that is present in a person's awareness, is appreciated, accepted and to some degree understood, that is so powerful.

While a client may feel terribly alone within their inner world, in the moment of sharing that inner world with another, of feeling heard and accepted, something powerful occurs. It seems that there is a kind of healing power in these genuine person-to-person moments of connection that the science of psychology has yet to fully understand. It lies at the heart, and literally so, of person-centred practice.

Just a woman with cancer. The words stayed with Barbara, and hearing them spoken back to her made them sound not exactly different, they were still the same words, but they left her with a moment of reflection, a questioning of what she meant. It felt as though for a moment she stepped aside from herself. Yes, she was just another woman with cancer; and yet .... Somehow, no, it didn't capture the full extent of her experience. It was *her* cancer. And she was Barbara, not 'just another woman'. It seemed subtle and yet it was profound. What she had said she had meant, but now, no, now she felt that she wouldn't want to say the same words again.

'I'm more than that.' She looked up at Nicola who was looking back at her. To Barbara she seemed so caring, so supportive, so steady, so available – that was a funny word to come to mind. She glanced away as her thoughts returned to what she had been thinking. Yes, she was just another woman with cancer, well in one sense anyway, but she wasn't just that, no, she was *herself*, with *her* cancer.

'Mhmm, more than just another woman ...'.

'Much more.' Barbara looked back at Nicola again. She felt her lips tighten. She thought back to how she had come to counselling to resolve stresses in her family life. Nicola had really helped by listening, giving her space, letting her ..., she wasn't sure how to describe it to herself. It was something about having a sense of her being there, her presence. Something like that. Whatever it was, she was grateful for it, for how Nicola was and had been. She had grown to trust her and to feel good that she was there. But now it was serious. This was different. This was life and .... She found herself taking a deep breath. Nicola seemed steady, still very much with her. She didn't seem as though she had retreated from her in any way when she had disclosed about the cancer. She was grateful for that.

Nicola sensed the searching behind Barbara's eye contact. She maintained it, allowing the moment of connection to remain undisturbed by words. For Nicola there was a sense of Barbara claiming her unique womanhood, more than just a woman, more than her cancer, perhaps? She hadn't said the latter. Nicola let the thought go and maintained her focus and connection with her warmth for Barbara.

Barbara was slowly taking a deeper breath, careful not to inflame the irritation that might cause her to cough. 'I just can't sit and wait.' She continued to look into Nicola's eyes as she spoke. Nicola heard Barbara's words, they sounded very affirming. She nodded slowly in response, maintaining eye contact. To Nicola it felt as though the atmosphere had been turned up a notch in intensity. It seemed a vitally important moment, not simply because of the words Barbara had said, but because of what was within Barbara that had urged her to say those words. The person themselves, their experience, the emotional texture of the moment, the emergence into awareness of fresh insight – all these factors were significant. For Nicola, these moments of contact (could they be called therapeutic contact? She wasn't sure, she knew they didn't only happen in the therapy room) were key, and she knew her response must be, in effect, a response that took her through Barbara's words to the experience behind them, and to the tone of experiencing that was present within Barbara. In a sense her slow nod and maintained eye contact was an important element of her response.

'Sitting waiting isn't an acceptable option.' They weren't the exact words Barbara had used, yet in the context of feeling so connected with Barbara, and her own openness to her own inner prompting, they seemed to be the words that needed to be said. They felt right, not by some clever design or intention, they just simply felt right.

Empathy from a person-centred perspective is so much more than reflecting the words of a client. Empathy, perhaps we might clarify and define it in this context as 'therapeutic empathy', is a response that emerges out of connection, relationship, a genuine entering of the inner world of the client, of seeing, glimpsing, the client's reality as they see it, that the words they have used may only in part have captured. It is not telling the client what they must be feeling or thinking, and it is not a response rooted in some intellectual appraisal of what the client is saying and therefore must be thinking or feeling. Therapeutic empathy is a genuine, *heartfelt* response to a sensed presence within the client that is conveyed through the texture and tone of the therapeutic relationship into the awareness of the therapist. It impacts on the therapist's awareness as a result of their being openly present and available to the client and to themselves. It is a level of relatedness that takes place beneath the words. Whether it is psychological depth or a matter of the degree of psychological contact is a matter for further reflection. But in these special moments there is a mutual reaching out and connecting. And in these moments it seems a healing energy becomes present, made possible by the presence of the therapeutic conditions.

Barbara heard Nicola's response. Not acceptable. No, it wasn't acceptable. That was exactly it. It wasn't good enough to just wait, to be passive. 'No, no, it isn't. OK, so maybe it doesn't look good, but I've got to carry on, face it.' As she spoke, Barbara felt doubt arising, like a reaction to what she was saying to herself, the wanting to not think about it, to try and carry on in a way as if nothing had happened, nothing had changed, except that it had. She had to carry on, but in a different way. And she felt, knew, instinctively that just waiting wasn't good enough. She heard Nicola responding.

'Carry on and . . .', the words 'ultimate challenge' came into Nicola's mind, though she didn't voice them. Seemed a bit dramatic, and yet . . . . She had hesitated in adding those words and the moment passed. Barbara was responding.

'. . . the reality is that cancer is in my body, and giving up is not what I want. It's just, I mean.' She paused and shook her head. 'How do I tell people? I don't know what to say. Derek was with me at the hospital when they told me, us, you know? But *I* have to tell them, and I have to give them time to come to terms with it as well, haven't I? I've told Derek not to say anything, it wouldn't be right to now tell him to do it. No, and anyway he'd struggle, maybe more than me. No, it's what I have to do this week. I have to.' She lapsed into silence thinking of her parents, who she knew would be shocked. But she also knew they would be supportive, and that felt positive. But her sons . . . , they were a different matter.

'Sounds like you are giving yourself that task during this week.'

'I have to sit down with Graham and Alec, tell them together. Then tell my parents. That feels right. They'll be supportive and I think I'll need that. I know I will.' It felt much easier to think of it that way around, neither would be easy, she knew that, and she knew her parents would be upset, but felt that they would be able to cope with that and be there for her. Her sons she really wasn't sure about.

'Knowing your parents will be supportive – it's important to have that after telling your sons.'

Barbara nodded, thinking about her sons, how might they react. 'I sort of think that Alec will be OK, he's more sensitive somehow. What I mean is that he is good at listening, although the drinking messes his head up and gets him into trouble. But Graham I'm not so sure about. He doesn't show his feelings much, I suppose that's part of his reason for using drugs. The medication he gets sort of takes the shine off him, so to speak. I don't know, it seems to go back to a relationship break up – he had a girlfriend at school, well, he'd known her for most of his secondary school, at least through teenage years. He thought the world of her, but she went off to university, and he didn't and, well, she moved with a different group and, well, I genuinely think he was heartbroken over it. It really affected him. He'd dabbled before with drugs, smoked cannabis and of course drank, but it was then that it got out of control. I guess talking like this makes me realise that he is sensitive too, but doesn't show it, maybe can't. Can't let himself feel, you know?'

Nicola nodded.

Barbara continued. 'They're good boys, well, not boys really, not any more, you know, but they'll always be my boys. It's going to be a shock for them.' She could feel her own emotions welling up again and tears filled her eyes. She took a tissue, blinked and dabbed at the tears that trickled down her cheeks. 'They're going to need me, need me to be strong.' Barbara paused again. What she had just said had only really just begun to dawn on her. Another reason to not give in or give up and just wait. Life had to go on. Her life had to go on. Their lives had to go on. Life, she thought . . . . Still, while she was breathing she was still living and she had an example to set and a family to prepare for a future none of them had anticipated or planned for. A strange thought struck Barbara, it was linked to what she had just said about breathing. It was about what it would be like to not breathe? She felt anxious. It didn't feel right, it was unnerving. She didn't know, couldn't answer it and pushed the question aside. It went away, but not completely. She didn't want to dwell on it.

Nicola hadn't responded immediately to what Barbara had been saying about her sons, she sensed that Barbara was very much in her own thoughts. The silence that had emerged was not an awkward, not-knowing-what-to-say silence. It was very much a working silence, as it were. She did not want to disturb Barbara's thoughts.

Barbara looked up. 'It's good to be able to just sit and think a bit. It wouldn't be the same on my own. It's different having someone listening. It helps. I don't understand how or why, but it helps. Thank you.'

'I'm glad it is helping, Barbara, and I hope that I can continue to be with you in a way that is helpful.'

Barbara smiled, and Nicola smiled back. Both were wondering for how long. Barbara had a feeling that Nicola was thinking what she was thinking, and Nicola was thinking the same about Barbara. It was Nicola who voiced her experience. 'I'm aware of wondering how long, and want to say that I'll be here for you for as long as . . .'.

Barbara smiled, taking a deeper breath and nodding. 'Thank you.' The words stuck a little in her throat, which she cleared. 'Thank you.' The words felt so genuine and they meant a lot to Nicola to hear.

Barbara nodded again to herself and glanced over to the clock. 'Time's nearly up.' That, she thought, was an understatement if ever there was one. Strange, although she had the thought she didn't feel the upset she almost expected. 'That says it all, doesn't it?'

Nicola nodded. 'Nothing I can add to that.' Both women appreciated the injection of humour at the end of what had been an intense and emotional session.

'So, next week, same time, and I'll tell you how I've got on. It won't be an easy week. But, it has to be done.'

Nicola nodded. She didn't say 'It'll be OK', that wasn't a therapeutic response, and she didn't know if it would be OK anyway. It could turn out to be an awful week for Barbara, with people reacting worse than she expected. She chose to convey her perception of Barbara. 'Yes, as you say, has to be done, and it does seem to me that you are clearer now as to what you have to do.'

'It's not the *what* but the *how* that's bothering me.'

'Yeah.'

'I hope it goes as you would want it to, Barbara, and I'll see you next week.'

'Thanks, thanks a lot. I think coming here and seeing you is going to be really important for me.'

'I hope I can be what you want, what you need.'

Nicola's response felt very reassuring to Barbara. 'Thanks.'

After Barbara had left, Nicola found herself aware of how emotionally drained she was. It had been an intense session and she had had to be very concentrated throughout. The issues that Barbara was facing were, to say the least, challenging. She thought back to those words that had come to her mind but which she had not said, 'ultimate challenge'. Was it? Was that how she would have felt faced with what Barbara was facing? Probably. But it was her stuff. Whether that would be Barbara's view, in truth she did not know. She was glad she had hesitated and the moment had passed.

It left her thinking, though. What was more challenging than facing your own death? Was it harder to face the impending death of a loved one, and the anticipation of loss that would follow? Who could say for sure. Everyone is different. She sensed that Barbara was more concerned for those around her. It was her way. Perhaps it would help her through, though that might depend on how others reacted. And what she needed to focus on this week may change next week. Nicola felt the tiredness in her eyes once more and she knew she needed to wash her face with some cool water and get some fresh air. She went outside, it was cool and refreshing. She appreciated it. She appreciated it more; the fragility of life brought home to her by her client left her with a greater sense of being glad to be alive, and of not taking it for granted. She took a couple of deep breaths before going back inside. She knew that how she felt was probably something Barbara might now never feel, and that made her feel sad.

Points for discussion

- How has the session left you feeling? Can you trace why those particular feelings have emerged for you?
- How effective was the counsellor in conveying the therapeutic attitudes and values of the person-centred approach in these sessions?
- How might you have responded differently to what the client was saying had you been the counsellor, and why?

- What, for you, were the key responses or moments in this session, from a therapeutic perspective?
- What would you take to supervision from this session, why, and what would you hope to achieve?
- Write notes for this session.

CHAPTER 9

Supervision session 2: Exploring the process from a person-centred perspective

Nicola had already been talking about another client to her supervisor, Mark. But she wanted to talk about Barbara and her reactions to what was happening for her client. She knew how important it was to use supervision to ensure that she was being authentically present, that she was able to genuinely offer empathic responses that were clear and focused on what the client was saying, experiencing and communicating. For her, this lay at the core of supervision. Yes, it could be an opportunity to discuss theory, to speculate on the therapeutic process, but essentially she wanted to leave supervision with a sense of having identified and resolved anything within herself that might be blocking her from seeing clearly and responding accurately to her clients. And, yes, another important feature was support, and she didn't want to overlook that aspect as well. She had been grateful for that at times, when working with clients who were presenting with very traumatic experiences that impacted on her own sense of humanity.

'I need a little time to reflect on my work with Barbara, my client who has been seeing me for stress that is related to coping with her family.'

'Yes, yes, I remember. She had been doing well, taking some power and control back in her life if I remember correctly.' Mark had felt good about the work Nicola had been doing with Barbara. He had worked with clients with similar difficulties and he knew, from his own experience, how rewarding it could be to see someone in situations like that, in a sense reclaiming their own needs and wishes in the face of incessant demands from those around them, or from a seeming inability to let go and allow others to take responsibility for their own lives. And he knew how hard that was for a parent and, it seemed to him, particularly so for many mothers. But he had also worked with fathers who seemed to need to live out their dreams and hopes through their children to a degree that they couldn't move on in their own lives as their children grew up.

'Well, she's been diagnosed with cancer.'

'Oh, and in the context of her doing so well.' Mark felt pained at what Nicola had said. It felt like a sudden intrusion into what had felt like a really positive therapeutic process. His thoughts went to Nicola, feeling his supervisory responsibility to ensuring her wellbeing. 'How are you with what's happened?'

'That's what I want to explore. In the session, when she told me, yes, it was a shock but it didn't feel like a shock. I felt very connected to her, and there were some powerful moments in that session, usually in silence with really significant eye contact. I really felt we "met" on a number of occasions.'

'Mhmm, so a shock, but one that are you saying you don't think you fully felt, for yourself, that is?'

'Yes, it was like I was so focused on Barbara and what she was presenting to me that, well, effectively I didn't really have time to focus on what was happening for me. I mean, I did, I was present, but I suppose since the session, and in a way it hit me first just after the session when I was outside taking some fresh air, it left me thinking about, you know, feeling glad to be alive and then I felt quite sad for Barbara. It sounds as though the prognosis isn't good. She hasn't said much about it, but it's in the pancreas, and was a late diagnosis, and they're talking weeks, maybe months. I guess it all depends on how much it has spread, and whether any treatment can slow it down. She's getting treatment but hasn't said anything much about it. More concerned about how to tell her sons and her parents – they don't know yet. Her husband knows, he was there at the hospital. She was rushed in suffering acute pain. That's what led them to discover it.' Nicola paused. 'And she was doing so well. And now this.'

Mark nodded. He wanted to highlight what Nicola had been saying. 'I'm struck by the sense of connection you experienced with Barbara, that must have been important for her, and maybe for you too. And that sadness. And seems like things are happening fast. And she wants to continue with the counselling?'

'She does. I feel strangely privileged that she wants to do that. I can imagine some people wanting to spend their time in other ways, but, well, clearly she feels it will help her. I don't think she's really out of the shock, not really.'

'Very likely. It can be a shattering experience to a person's structure of self.' The thought crossed Mark's mind as to what awareness there was within the person in situations like this. The organism has a disease and it knows that disease is there. So, arguably, the organismic self may know that something is different, but it hasn't reached consciousness, it hasn't entered into the person's everyday awareness, as it were. Symptoms could be felt yet minimised or interpreted differently by the person experiencing them as a way of containing the experience and of denying to awareness the possibility that something serious was happening. He let the thought go, he would ponder on it further after the session, unless it felt pressing and appropriate to voice it within the session. Nicola was responding to what he had just said.

'We know we all have to die some time, but it's when it is unexpected, when it cuts across your plans for the future and your sense of existence, well, your sense of relative permanence, so to speak. I mean, you can't imagine yourself not existing, can you?'

'No. The moment you try and imagine it, and even if you succeed, there is still the you that is doing the imagining continuing to exist.' He wondered whether the Buddhists or others who engaged in deep forms of meditation could reach a point of non-being in awareness, but he didn't know.

'And so much is connected to personal belief about death and what comes after. If you are absolutely convinced that you continue in some other form, then you don't have to worry about your non-existence. And I know some would argue that is simply a way of facing existential death, but that in turn is also based on a premise that is unproven, that consciousness is no more than an experiential by-product of having a physical body and brain. That's a gross simplification, but that's my take on it.' Nicola had her beliefs, and she was comfortable with how she had made sense of life and the meaning and purpose of human existence. She didn't feel like saying any more.

'It sounds like a pretty clear differentiation to me, and no doubt there are other positions along the continuum of whether consciousness can exist independent of body, or whether it is a by-product of complex physical processes.' Mark paused. 'We can discuss this at length, of course, but is this what you need at this time? You were talking about shock and what your client may be going through.'

'Yes, yes, thanks for bringing the focus back, I do need to take time to reflect on what is happening within myself and with Barbara.' She thought for a moment. 'It's, hmm, I mean, I really can't say how it will be over the coming weeks, months – I sort of think months, but maybe because I can't imagine anything happening faster. I know it does, of course, but, well, Barbara doesn't look well, but she doesn't look like she is dying, if you know what I mean. But I don't know how it will be, and of course Barbara won't, either. It's day to day, hour to hour, isn't it?'

'And at times probably minute to minute, as powerful feelings can arise at any time as her inner processing takes its course. And there will be physical pain as well, most likely.' He paused for a moment, acknowledging to himself what he had just said. It felt important to make this clear within the supervisory relationship.

'Yeah.' Nicola had nothing to add. It had served to sharpen her own focus as well.

Mark's thoughts turned back to Nicola. 'What do you need? It's going to be a psychologically demanding process – not that you need me to tell you that.'

Nicola thought, tight-lipped and nodding her head slightly. It would be demanding emotionally and mentally, and as she had already experienced, intense sessions could be so physically draining as well. 'I need to look after myself, but I'm good at that. I take plenty of exercise and eat healthily. But I'm going to need to unload where feelings, thoughts build up, so I will need this time for that. And, well, it's all linked, but perhaps more importantly check out my own congruence, be sure that I am genuinely present and available for Barbara. I have to watch my own agenda. I don't feel like I am going to try and rescue her from painful experiencing, I know I cannot. I need to stand beside her, with her, be a true companion for her. But I may be tempted at times to say something from my own frame of reference that may simply not be appropriate.'

Mark looked questioningly towards her, inviting further elaboration.

'In the last session, for instance, I thought about saying in response to something Barbara had said, about what she faced being the ultimate challenge, in the sense of facing your own impending death. I hesitated. It didn't get said. And I'm glad, on reflection. It was my stuff, as it were, and I want to reflect on this. I was assuming, perhaps, that Barbara would see it like that, but would she? Does she? I don't know. Maybe, at some point, and maybe not. But it was not where she seemed to be at that moment. Her focus, her concern seems to be largely towards her family, towards telling them and how they will cope, how they will react.'

'And you need to stay with her on this.'

'I know. But I have to be aware that, well, so much is written about stages people go through in relation to bereavement and facing death, and I am sure they all play a part, but not, well, I don't know, it seems to me that what is important is not to have expectations, but rather to be open to accepting what emerges for her, and that what she experiences will emerge in its own time and at the right time.' Nicola paused, collecting her thoughts.

Mark did not respond. He nodded, holding eye contact as Nicola continued. 'It really is about trusting her, isn't it, trusting her psychological process, trusting that her actualising tendency will enable her to achieve what she needs; that she finds a way to be that is right for her. And I am aware in saying all of this that there may not be much time.' She paused. 'And in saying all that it sounds like I'm thinking of some way of being that she has to achieve, like some culmination, or something like that. Is that what I mean?' Nicola wasn't sure. She didn't want to feel Barbara had to work towards some predestined goal, no, predestined wasn't the right word, but that there was some definable and achievable way of being she needed to reach. Yet there was a sense within her that at the end of a life there did need to be some kind of experience, a time when the threads of experience were drawn together in some way and, hopefully . . . . Hmm. She wasn't sure, she knew that wasn't always possible. But when it was, wasn't that a good way to end?

Mark was frowning and had begun to respond, checking out that he was hearing what Nicola was trying to say. 'You mean like you bring into the therapy room the notion that Barbara has to find some, I don't know, particular way of being – a kind of culmination of her life – am I catching your meaning?'

Nicola nodded. 'Mhmm. Hadn't expected this to emerge, but it has. Do I have an expectation, aim, goal? I don't know that I have a specific goal as such but, yes, I do have a hope that Barbara will die in a place in herself that, I don't know, I suppose where she can feel at peace. That's what I want for her. And maybe that's not possible, and I know not everyone achieves this or necessarily tries to achieve it. But yes, I have to own that being my hope.'

'A hope is not necessarily a goal.'

'No, but either way I don't want to find myself wittingly, or unwittingly, trying to direct Barbara towards . . . , whether we call it a goal or a hope, it doesn't matter to me. I don't want to direct her, but I do need to own that hope.'

'And I suspect that it is a hope that perhaps most people carry. But, as you appreciate, we can't start trying to push our clients towards it in some way.

It is good when it happens, it must be satisfying to the person themselves and probably to those who are close to them. And maybe it is all a bit of a value judgement on my part. Some people may want to die feeling angry about something, or perhaps die during some act of perceived revenge for something. But there's still something about being at peace with yourself, or maybe feeling true to yourself, and that takes me to wondering about congruence and the process of death and dying. Perhaps, and this is my speculation, and it's getting us away from Barbara again, the more congruent the person at death, the more at peace they are with themselves. Maybe. I don't know. I'd need to give that more thought. Having said it, I want to think about it some more.'

Nicola was listening to what Mark was saying, but also very much in her own thoughts as well. 'I suppose the danger is seeking this, I mean, wanting this for my client so that it affects my responding, or of wanting it so as to avoid being with someone still having heightened levels of psychological and emotional stress right up to the end. I mean, I do want my client to be congruent; as person-centred therapists we all must own wanting that because we are, I guess, defining constructive personality change as being a change towards greater congruence. But it is about not seeking specifics, a particular way of being congruent, as it were. And, hmm, being congruent could mean someone being rightly anxious and stressed as they approach death because of the circumstances. I'm not so sure, hmm, I was going to say I'm not sure about equating congruence at death with peace. Someone may be in absolute turmoil. I guess my hope is that their circumstances will allow them to be at peace with themselves, and, yes, congruence will be a factor in achieving that being at peace with themselves.'

Nicola lapsed into silence. She had said a lot and wasn't too sure how much she was sure about. It all felt something of an exploration. What was the theoretical standpoint of person-centred theory in the context of working with someone near to death, or preparing to die? Was constructive personality change still a goal? It might occur, but were a set of relational conditions that were linked to this possibility what were most needed? Yet she knew that instinctively she felt that they were. They were the core features of a healing relationship, and if ever a person's structure needed healing then the shattering effect of knowing you were going to die, and probably in pain, surely required a relational experience that could in some way have a constructive effect on what could become a somewhat broken structure of self. And she also knew that not everyone reacted like that. For some people, the closeness of death seemed to draw something stronger out of them, almost as though it liberated them in some way from the structure of self that had previously conditioned their sense of self.

'You know, so much is going to depend on how her sons react. That's what it hinges on in many ways. If Barbara is to find peace with herself she may well need to feel that either her sons have responded in such a way that she can feel secure that they will be OK, or reach a point when she can genuinely let go of feeling responsible for them and their choices. She has been working on the latter, as you know, in previous sessions. What will now emerge, well, only time will tell.' Nicola could imagine a state of unresolved anxiety, and yet, that anxiety could be utterly realistic to what was happening around her, and congruence was about realistic reactions to experience.

'Mhmm, as you say, a lot hinges on their reaction to her, but also her reaction to their reaction.'

'And how much will be resolved ahead of a time when Barbara may be on high levels of painkillers, probably morphine, that in itself may suppress anxieties. How congruent may she have the capacity to be once the more powerful drugs kick in? But then, if it brings her some peace of mind and eases the transition . . . ?'

'We can only speculate, but perhaps our exploration has extended our awareness of the implications of the therapist's thoughts, hopes, beliefs on their ability to respond empathically in a non-directive manner. An, yes, you may be working with a client with a somewhat shattered structure of self and what will emerge we do not know. We just do not know. But we do know that therapeutic relationship has a healing effect. Barbara will be stronger for having you as a therapeutic companion, I want to say as a human companion. It is up to her how she feels she needs to use it, and for how long.'

'I know, and another thought has come to mind, and it's to do with just how much my thinking is coloured by the doctors' expectations. And I know they are often right in these kinds of situations, but there has to be some uncertainty. Treatment may help to delay the cancer developing and spreading. And by treatment I don't just mean chemotherapy or radiotherapy – I'm not sure what Barbara is going to receive – but some of the more holistic ideas around diet and attitude that many people turn to. And as I say that, it reminds me of Barbara saying in the session that it wasn't acceptable for her to just wait, she needed to live. Something like that, I'm not sure now that she expressed it quite that way, but she had to, what was it she said, something about it not being acceptable, yes, yes,' Nicola recalled Barbara's words, 'she said at one point that "I'm just another woman with cancer", but then, hearing herself say those words, or maybe hearing me saying them back to her in my empathic response, she questioned it, and quite strongly. She wanted to affirm herself, that it was her cancer, and she had to face it. It was very self-affirming, a powerful moment in the session.'

Mark was struck by the two distinctive ways Barbara had expressed herself. 'That sounds as though one part of her said one thing, and when she heard it, another part emerged carrying a different set of thoughts and feelings – we could think of this in terms of "configurations within self".'

As mentioned in the introduction, configurations within self is a theoretical stance or model for understanding, within the person-centred system, the phenomenon of people having different parts within their nature, each having associated thoughts, feeling and behaviours. The number and range of these 'parts', and their nature and presence, will vary from person to person. Working with clients who are facing significant events in the lives – such as coming to terms with their own death – is likely to draw con-figurational states powerfully to the surface. Each part may have its own reaction to what has occurred, and may need to express this. But again, this will vary from person to person. And, of course, new configurational states may develop in response. The person-centred counsellor will seek to be open to this process, seeking to offer each part the same quality of empathy and warm acceptance.

'A part of her that almost devalues herself, and another part that carries a real affirmation of herself as Barbara the woman, individual and unique in her own right.' Nicola was nodding as she spoke. What Mark had said made a lot of sense to her and what she now added helped it to become clearer still. 'And I've got to offer equal warm acceptance to both, to all of Barbara. She's probably going to express different thoughts and feelings, and yes, I have to feel accepting of both. It's more than conveying acceptance, I have to actually be accepting, don't I? That's the challenge of unconditional positive regard. She's going to feel strong sometimes, and at other times, as she said, just feel like another woman with cancer. Quite what she feels beneath those words, I don't know, she didn't say, but it felt like a real devaluing of herself to the point of feeling like just another statistic. That's hard to hear. But I have to hear it when it is present and communicated to me. And thinking back to the session, it really felt like she did not want to hold that particular focus. Like she acknowledged it, it was there, but by so doing she was then able to affirm something else, something other.'
'She processed it in the session, you mean?'
Nicola nodded. 'There was a lot of that. That's why I think it felt so intense. And there was a lot of contact and connection. I don't imagine she fully processed what was happening, I don't know, but there was a shift occurring for her. It really does reinforce for me the therapeutic power of empathy, real empathy, not some vacuous repetition of what clients say, but a real getting beyond or behind the words, the tone, the emotional texture present with and being pre-sented by the client, you know? I'm sure there's a case for thinking in terms of "therapeutic empathy" as much as "empathic understanding". Yet they are probably very similar, two ways of approaching a similar reality, of really con-veying a sense of what is happening for the client.' Nicola felt good about what she had just said. It felt important. Yes, it was in part something that she wanted to believe, she genuinely felt there was a healing power in feeling heard and understood, really heard and understood at a visceral level, and par-ticularly those deeper personal feelings and thoughts.
Mark was struck by a sensed difference in tone in Nicola as she now talked. 'Maybe a shift in you, too, a different tone to your experience as Barbara shifted from her "just another woman with cancer" to a more self-affirming sense of self.' Mark had not responded to all that Nicola had said, the shift he referred to had struck him and it had persisted as Nicola had continued to speak.

'Yes, and that's interesting. I mean, it's natural, the client draws out different responses within the therapist. Hmm. There's something about trusting myself to be how Barbara needs me to be. And that feels so important. It's back to being non-directive, or client-led. Can I be how my client needs me to be, and maybe that's more than what she consciously is aware of feeling she needs, it is also to do with what her actualising tendency needs from me, needs to maybe draw from me.' Nicola paused, aware that what she had said opened up another whole area of debate. Could one person's actualising tendency directly interact with another person? What did such a notion mean? What mechanism might be involved? 'And all of this in the context of facing death and very likely in the not too distant future.' Another pause. 'This is time-limited therapy in its fullest sense.'

Is the actualising tendency localised within the person? Rogers wrote of the actualising tendency as being an aspect of a wider, greater, all-embracing formative tendency at work throughout creation. He wrote:

> I hypothesise that there is a formative directional tendency in the universe, which can be traced and observed in stellar space, in crystals, in micro-organisms, in more complex organic life, and in human beings. There is an evolutionary tendency towards greater order, greater complexity, greater inter relatedness. In humankind, this tendency exhibits itself as the individual moves from a single cell origin to complex organic functioning, to knowing and sensing below the level of consciousness, to a conscious awareness of the organism and the external world to a transcendent awareness of the harmony and unity of the cosmic system, including mankind. (Roger, 1980, p. 133)

But does this formative tendency, described as the actualising tendency when applied to persons, work in isolation within each form, or is there cross-connection, a kind of universal process within which each individual process is embedded? And does the actualising process within the client connect to that within the counsellor in some way, allowing the counsellor to be, if you like, inspired to be as the client needs them to be?

The person-centred counsellor will want to be able to be present in such a way that they are able to respond therapeutically to their client. Sometimes there is a sense of knowing the response that is needed, at other times it is utterly spontaneous, unformulated within a conscious process, and yet therapeutically helpful. Rogers wrote that:

> When I am at my best, as a group facilitator or as a therapist, I discover another characteristic. I find that when I am closest to my inner, intuitive self, when I am somehow in touch with the unknown in me, when perhaps I am in a slightly altered state of consciousness, then whatever I do

seems to be full of healing. Then, simply my *presence* is releasing and help-ful to the other. There is nothing I can do to force this experience, but when I can relax and be close to the transcendent core of me, then I may behave in strange and impulsive ways in the relationship, ways which I cannot justify rationally, which have nothing to do with my thought pro-cesses. But these strange behaviours turn out to be *right*, in some odd way: it seems that my inner spirit has reached out and touched the inner spirit of the other. Our relationship transcends itself and becomes a part of something larger. Profound growth and healing and energy are present. (Rogers, 1980, p. 129)

Mark nodded. 'That goes to the heart of the matter, "can I be how my client needs me to be?" and, as you say, there is then the matter of is what a client needs always what they think they need? We often don't know. Our safeguard is our accurate empathy and our warm acceptance of our clients and those aspects of the client that emerge into the therapeutic relationship. The way we try to be is in line with the therapeutic attitudes and values of the approach. In that we place our trust. And yes, counselling in preparation for dying is time-limited therapy of a different order.' Mark appreciated the discussion, but he wanted to check out the implications for his supervisee. 'Where does all this leave you as you prepare to see Barbara again?' How was it affecting her?

'It just seems to open it all up, and in one sense it can seem so very complex and yet at the same time it feels as though there is a simplicity in all of this, the sim-plicity of two people in a therapeutic relationship. Yes, I can think about all of this and think myself into a headache. That won't help. What it does, though, is bring me back again to the reality that we have, myself and Barbara, sitting together in a room as she contemplates her own death and works through all that arises or emerges in relation to this. That's what matters. And that's what I have to be focused on. And if I can be congruently present, if I can offer the therapeutic conditions and they can be received by Barbara, then I believe that what will emerge from her, and from me, will be therapeutically helpful. What form that therapeutic helpfulness will take, and to what effect, I cannot say. I don't know.'

'I can't add to that, Nicola, that is exactly it, and I am glad you said it. I needed to bring the focus back and what's great is that the complexity of the con-cepts we have been discussing have informed your thinking, but not dis-tracted you from the essence of what is being asked of you as a person-centred counsellor.'

Nicola smiled. 'I think PCA is embedded somewhere in my heart these days. You can't switch it on and off. It's a set of values that you try to live by. That doesn't mean being everyone's therapist, but you're mindful of them, you carry them with you.'

'I appreciate what you are saying. There's a transition somewhere from "doing person-centred" to "being person-centred", and I don't know that you can train people in that; it happens for some people, but I'm not sure it happens for everyone. And I think some people are naturally person-centred who have never been anywhere near a person-centred training course, or therapy. They just have it, are it, the values are part of who they are. Rogers didn't have copyright on them, they're fundamental elements of the human experience.'

'We're all on a journey, aren't we?' Nicola paused, an image had come into her mind. She was back with Barbara once more. 'The idea of sharing a train journey with someone comes to mind, like being with someone who got on the train expecting to go the full distance to the end of the line, to the train's final destination. She has sat down next to you, and you both have the same expectation, and then she is told she has to get off, but she's not told when or exactly how long she has on the train. But she will be getting off and she won't be reaching the final destination. And I am there, here, with her, sharing her journey, but I know I will continue beyond the point when she has to get off.' As she spoke it felt as though the image became more real. It just felt incredibly present, there was a kind of knowing, a quality of knowing was a better way of describing it. It just felt right to be describing it in these terms.

'And I guess you also have an expectation of sharing a longer part of the journey with her, and now you have uncertainty over how long you will journey together, and maybe too will be left wondering whether you will be asked to get off at some point as well?' Mark had a sense of where Nicola was heading with her imagery. Life, a journey, assumptions that we will go the distance, seeing fellow travellers having to get off, maybe some to take another train, but for others it was journey's end, no more trains, no more travelling, no more life.

Nicola nodded. It did make you think about your own journey, but she wanted to focus on Barbara. 'Mhmm, share the journey with her, share her journey and all that she feels she wants to share with me. She shares with me; I may share my experiences with her at times, and somehow you're on the journey too – bit like a conductor who comes along from time to time . . . , maybe that's taking the analogy too far.'

'Maybe, but does it make sense, does it have meaning for you?'

'Yes it does. I can see my role more clearly. It's another angle on what I said just now. I'm glad it has come to mind as a result of what we have been exploring. It feels enough, though. We are on a journey, there is uncertainty, but there is time together and during that time therapeutic work can be done. And we will go as far as we can with the time that we have. And I hope that there is time to prepare for the end of the journey, that it won't be too abrupt, but it may be and I'll have to deal with how I feel about that if it happens that way. No, somehow the image feels right and I feel strangely calm thinking about it in this way. It feels, I don't know, like it runs deep, very deep. I think I need to move on, I know I'll talk more about Barbara in future supervision sessions, but this feels like the place to stop today, and give myself time for a couple of my other clients.'

Points for discussion

- What images and impressions has the supervision session left you with?
- Do you feel that Nicola used the supervision session as fully as she needed? Were there other issues that might usefully have been addressed?
- What do you feel was resolved during the supervision session, and how did this occur?
- How were the principles of the person-centred approach applied by the supervisor?
- Would you have found the supervisor's responses helpful, or would you have wanted more or something different, and if so, what and why?
- What notes would you write for this session if you were the supervisee?
- If you were the supervisor, what might you be considering taking from this session to your own supervision?

CHAPTER 10

Counselling session 10: Pain and anguish, and relationships with her sons

Barbara began the session telling Nicola more about her treatment and how it was leaving her feeling. She also described what else she was doing to try and help herself. She had checked out some websites offering advice from the angle of holistic and complementary therapies, and she had started to change her diet. 'I need to try and give myself time', was what she had said to Nicola, 'I need to give everyone time to get used to what is going to happen'. She had then gone on to talk about how her sons had reacted to the news.

'I was right to tell them first, and then my parents. We told them together, but I did the actual, you know, but I was glad Derek was there. Funny, this week he's been different. It's like, yes, he's struggling with it, I know he is, but he's been far more attentive and, well, he's just around more, a kind of presence, you know? In the past he'd be out doing something, but now he just seems to be staying around more. I'm grateful for that. I guess not everyone's like that, wasn't really expecting him to be, but I'm glad that he is. I think he'll need to talk to someone as well sometime, he doesn't say a lot, just quietly there.' She felt herself becoming emotional. 'More like he used to be, somehow. Strange that.'

'Feels strange him being like he used to be, but clearly it means a lot to you as well.' Nicola sought to respond to both Barbara's words and the tears in her eyes.

Barbara nodded. 'He's been good. He's self-employed, builder, he's got jobs on but he's making time to be at home. I guess some men would just lose themselves in their work. I suppose I had half expected Derek to do that, but he hasn't, thank goodness, and hopefully he won't . . .'. The words 'while I'm here' came into her mind but remained unspoken. She couldn't bring herself to say them. She didn't want to think about how it would be afterwards. 'Anyway, he's being great but I know it's not easy for him, for any of us.' She tightened her lips as she thought back to the evening they'd spoken to her sons. 'I was right, I mean Alec went quiet, really quiet. Actually they both did, but, well, he's, I don't know, he's struggling, he's hurting, and, yes, he's drinking, but he's being

129

sort of controlled about it. He's spent time with me, we've talked. But he's hurting and shocked and is struggling to come to terms with what's happening, will happen.' Barbara took a careful deep breath and shook her head. 'He's tried to reassure me as well, saying that everything would be OK. Said that doctors get it wrong sometimes and that I needed to not accept what they were saying, but fight it. He doesn't want to lose me, and I can't blame him for that. And I, well, you know . . .'.
'Don't want to lose him?'

The counsellor is describing the client's inner world as she senses it to be. By putting into words, albeit with a questioning tone, what the counsellor thinks the client is trying to say enables the client's emotions to become more fully present in her awareness, finding expression and release. The client's feeling of the unfairness of it all in particular is voiced.

'I can't . . .'. The emotions got the better of her. 'I-I c-can't . . . ,' she let out a long breath and burst into tears. They were hot and stinging to her eyes. Her throat burned, her chest felt like it had a weight on it. Her breath came in short bursts and, reaching for a tissue, she buried her face in her hands. She felt fear, sadness, anxiety, loneliness, so many feelings and all of them left her feeling wretched and helpless. 'I-I-It wasn't m-meant to b-b-be like this.' She swallowed, the sobs continued, her breaths getting shorter. 'Why me? Why? I-I d-don't deserve this, I r-really d-d-don't.' Her breathing had become very shallow and rapid.
'No, no, it's so awful and so unfair.' Nicola's response was in part empathy, but also in line with the feelings that were present within her.

Another short, empathic response, spoken with warmth and unconditional positive regard for the client. In a sense it is a summary, letting the client know that the awfulness and unfairness is heard, but more than that. It is a response that is also coming from the counsellor's own experiencing as well. Hence it is authentic and genuine, more than a letting know that the client has been heard. Such responses can be hugely validating for the client. It becomes a kind of shared experience, both client and counsellor holding similar feelings. Empathy becomes a sympathetic response. This can be most powerful. It is not a 'you poor thing' kind of sympathy, it is more of a moment of shared feeling, an affirmation, if you like, of this is how it is, we both know it, we both feel it in our own ways.

Barbara shook her head. She had lifted her face from the tissue but she still had her eyes closed, her breathing remained the same. Somehow she felt calmer.

Yes, awful and unfair, and hearing Nicola's response somehow seemed . . . . She couldn't put it into words, it simply felt helpful. It felt so caring, like she was really in touch with what she, Barbara, was feeling. She swallowed and felt irritation deep in her lungs, she swallowed again. It was a painful, burning sensation and she couldn't stop herself coughing. It jarred her body and made it feel worse. She winced and took a sharp intake of breath, which triggered more coughing. She tried to swallow again to regain control. She felt the phlegm in her mouth, she took a tissue, she wanted to spit it out. There were traces of blood. That wasn't new. It wasn't fair. Yes, she had smoked, but the doctors didn't think it had originated in her lungs, but they were weakened. Her smoking and drinking in the past, neither had helped; her lungs and liver, the doctor said, had both been compromised. She'd been stupid, but she didn't deserve this, she really didn't.

She felt herself calming down a little, the irritation had eased. She reached for the glass of water, it felt cool and refreshing in her mouth as she sipped it slowly. 'I'm supposed to rest, I try to, but, well, it doesn't come easy. I've always been active and, well, like I said last week, I can't just give up. I feel like it sometimes, but I can't, I won't, I mustn't.'

Nicola looked at her and felt for her. Battling against the odds. 'No, you feel like it but you have to keep going, you want to keep going.'

'I have to. I have to.' Her voice trailed off as her thoughts went back to her sons, how they'd reacted. 'Alec will struggle, I know he will, but at least he's talking to me. Maybe he'll get through OK without drinking like I know that he can. He gets quite selfish when he's drunk, it really changes him. It's all about himself. I think in a way though it seems to help him release his feelings. He is concerned about how he will cope without me, how he will cope with his feelings. When he's sober he worries about me, tells me he'll be there for me, and I know he means it, he really does, but after a few drinks, he just, I don't know, he changes, he listens but he doesn't, not really, too full of what he's feeling. I think alcohol opens him up in a way. It used to close me down, used to stop me feeling. Thank God I'm not still drinking. I won't go back to it now, been too long away from it. Funny, I used to go to AA [Alcoholics Anonymous], long time ago, but I kept the literature, been reading the book, you know, thinking about the steps. Funny that. Keep thinking about that 'Higher Power' they talk about. Always meant something to me, that. I know it wasn't for everyone, but it meant a lot to me. Give yourself over to a Higher Power. Yes, I sort of feel like that now, and I know that I need to do my bit as well. That's what I learned then and that's what I need now.' Barbara paused. 'And accepting the things I can't change, you know, from the serenity prayer?[1] I'm not there with this. I haven't really accepted it, not really, and in a way I have. I'm probably not making much sense.' Barbara looked up at Nicola, who looked back, holding

---

[1] God grant me the serenity
to accept the things I cannot change;
courage to change the things I can;
and wisdom to know the difference.

the eye contact. She looked so serious, Barbara thought. She felt a wave of emotion, a warm feeling.

'Well, I'm hearing you say that some aspects of the AA programme have found new meaning for you, and it's hard to feel you've fully accepted things, you're not sure that you have.'

'I have and then I haven't. It's not consistent. It changes, I change. Sometimes I feel quite calm, almost like I understand what serenity means, and then at other times I feel angry, sad, confused, terrified. I want to shout at God. At other time I want to plead with Him. And then I just feel tired of it all, of everything, I just want it all to go away.' The tears welled up, 'But I know what that means, and I don't want that either, I really don't.' She closed her eyes and tears trickled over her eyelids and down her cheeks once more. She wiped them with the back of her hand and sniffed. 'No, no, I can't keep crying. I know I have to, but I also have to have control as well.' She felt suddenly very hot. 'Is it me or is it hot in here?'

'It is warm.'

'I need to take my jacket off.' Nicola reached over and helped her, as Barbara was finding it hard to flex her shoulders back to take it off.

'Thanks, thanks. Silly things are suddenly difficult.'

'That's OK. Are you comfortable in the chair.'

Barbara nodded. 'Yes, it's really very supportive. Better than the one I have at home, actually.' She paused. 'I still haven't finished talking about Alec, and then there's Graham, and my parents. As I say, at least Alec is talking, I think actually he'll be OK. I know myself the dangers of drinking heavily, and, well, I don't like to see him drinking, but that's how he is and I know people cannot change until they are ready. We've talked a bit about all of that and, well, actually I think that what's happened is making him think. But he's torn, he wants something to take his pain away, but he knows he has to find some other way.' Barbara paused for a moment, full of her memories of the chats they had had over the past few days. 'I think the fact that the doctor has said that the drinking in the past damaged my liver, which has reduced any resistance to the spread of the cancer, has made him think a bit. He's started to look at some of my AA books, he's not done that before. I think he can see that it's helping me, and that's drawn him to it. I feel more reassured because of that.'

Nicola had listened attentively. She was struck by the way Barbara was speaking about Alec. There seemed to be a greater calmness in her voice. She voiced what she felt. 'It seems that Alec has become closer to you, or you closer to him. And you're feeling more reassured because of how he's responded.'

'He's a good lad, but he needs to change, settle down, make a more settled life for himself. And he's going to have to do that for himself. I can only do what I can do, and then it will be up to him.' Barbara sighed. 'I hope things turn out well for him and, well, I wish I could be part of his future, but that's not going to happen. And that's . . . ,' Barbara closed her eyes as she felt her sadness rise up inside her and the tears well up once more, '. . . and that's so hard to accept.' She was shaking her head now, slowly opening her eyes as she looked down. Her hands felt strangely tingly, and her stomach, chest felt sort of cold, hollow,

it was hard to put into words. Like a mild shock reaction. 'Yeah, not being part
of their lives. I know they give me grief, that's their way, but I love them just the
same, you know?'
Nicola nodded. She spoke softly in response. 'I know. They're your boys, you're
their mum.'

The loss of her future has become very present for Barbara. Loss is such a
significant element of the bereavement experience for many people, particularly when they have either a vision of their future which will not now come
to pass, or a sense of responsibility and duty that they will not be able to dis-
charge as fully as they had hoped. The counsellor's response is particularly
powerful. Often saying 'I know' is unhelpful. How can a counsellor know?
They are not the client. Saying 'I know' is not empathy. What do they know?
Why should the client accept that the counsellor knows? But in this case, it
has been spoken and then followed up with words that do convey an understanding of how it is and why Barbara is feeling the way that she is.

'You never think that, you know, you won't be there for them. Don't think you
ever stop being a mum, not really.' She swallowed. Thoughts were crowding in
on her and the sensations she had felt just before had intensified. A question,
one that had come to her over the recent two weeks, was back with her again.
She felt the sadness, anxiety – it was more than anxiety, but not as strong as
terror – building up inside herself once more. 'What's going to become of me?'
It was the question she couldn't answer. She didn't know. She couldn't know.
She knew what she believed but she couldn't imagine it.
'That's a powerful question you need to try and answer, "what's going to become
of me?".' Nicola responded with Barbara's words, holding the question before
them both.

No clever attempt to try and answer the question. Rather there is pure,
simple and direct empathy for the question that is so present for the client.
The question is acknowledged. The client does not know. She wants an
answer but for the moment what is needed is to allow the question to be,
allow the client the time and the space to process that question as they
need to without disruption or interference from the counsellor. It enables
the client to develop their own train of thought, which lasts for a while,
during which the counsellor seeks to maintain her focus, her feelings of
warmth and acceptance towards her client.

Barbara sat, staring ahead, unable to grasp an answer. She didn't know. She
hoped that, well, there'd be something more. And that wherever she was

she'd be able to look down on her family and maybe, perhaps, somehow still be a kind of unseen presence in their lives. She did believe that you lived on in some way. At least, that was what she hoped for. She wasn't religious, but most religions in her view seemed to agree that there was a part of her that would carry on, but what that would be like, what would she be like, she could only imagine herself as she was. She took a deep breath.

Nicola watched Barbara as she sat in her own thoughts. The question she had asked was a profound one. She believed people had to make their own minds up about what they wanted to believe, based on what felt right to them. She wasn't going to introduce any answers. Barbara would know within herself what she thought, hoped for, how reliable her conclusions felt for her. And Nicola was also aware that as well as thoughts being in her head, there were powerful feelings present. Facing that question, a challenge to a person's sense of continuity, and of their own existence. She found herself taking a deep breath as well.

Her mind momentarily went to something she had read about Zen koans, statements that to be answered required you to think differently, or not think at all, that took you beyond the logical and the rational in some way. What happens when you are faced with a question that you need an answer to but there is no answer? She took her thoughts back to Barbara, who was continuing to sit, looking anxious and thoughtful, still staring down, her hands clenched on her thighs. She did not look relaxed, but how can you feel relaxed when you are facing questions of your own mortality?

Barbara found her thoughts ranging across different topics. Here she was, sitting in a counselling room, contemplating her own death, or at least what would it be like? But it wasn't the after death that concerned her, it was the dying, the pain, the loss of dignity. How long would it take? She had asked the doctors these questions and they had sought to reassure her. But she ... the thought that was present for her was, well, not so much a thought, more a feeling, the actual moment. And she didn't want to think about it. Her sons came back into her mind. She'd talked a bit about Alec. She hadn't said anything about Graham. And she really had to try and make sense of what was going on, she really needed to help him, somehow. She didn't know how. So many thoughts, so much, so little time. She looked up at Nicola. 'I feel like my head is going to explode.'

'So many things to think about, you mean? Feels like it wants to explode with it all.'

Barbara nodded. 'It's like there's so much I could talk about, and things I want to talk about, and things I need time to get on with and, well, I want to have this time, and then I wonder if I'd be better off doing all the other things.'

'You question whether being here is good use of your time?' Nicola could understand that. Some people needed the time for support, or to be able to reflect on or make sense of what was happening, or to release feelings they were keeping from their family and loved ones. Others didn't want that, maybe they had enough support and people giving them time, or were in a family situation where they felt that how they needed to be was more fully and openly accepted.

> The client's wonder about whether counselling is the best use of her time is accepted, not questioned, and no attempt is made to persuade her to think a particular way. Having voiced her concern, the client is then able to realise, for herself, that she has a topic that she needs to explore and use the time for. The client is trusted to make the choices she needs to make.

'I have to talk about Graham. I can't seem to, I don't know. He's withdrawn, goes out, he's just, I don't know, I don't know if it's him, if it's the drugs, what it is. He's my son and yet sometimes he seems like a stranger to me.' Sadness welled up in Barbara as images of her son came to mind along with the feelings of being so alienated from him.

'You feel like Graham's become a stranger to you.' Nicola spoke slowly, very aware of the emotional atmosphere that had arisen in the room, or perhaps more accurately in the relationship between them. 'That can't be an easy experience for you.' Nicola had felt a strong reaction as Barbara had spoken, a real feeling of sadness for Barbara, a sense of what it means for a mother to not feel connected to a son, but this was more than that, of not feeling maybe important to him, maybe invisible to him in some way. She waited to see how Barbara wanted to continue.

'He ..., I don't know, it's like I can't relate to him. He's moody. He's out a lot. Well, he is and he isn't. He's either out or in his room at home. But when he's out, I don't know where he goes, who he's with. He's been out more lately. When he's home he seems to sleep a lot. And since I told him, I mean, I don't know, it's worse. I mean, don't get me wrong, he's had good times. He's got a good job. People think because you take drugs you can't hold down a job, but that's not true. Since he's been on the methadone script that's really helped, really made him more stable. But he can still be moody. But, well, I don't know, I think he's using more, or something. I told him, he needs to talk about what he's going through. He's got a keyworker at the clinic, but I don't know if he talks to her like I think he needs to.'

'Sounds from what you are saying as if you're really concerned about him.' Nicola did not seek to empathise with the content of what Barbara had said, more with the tone and her sense of the underlying feeling and emotions.

'I need to feel he's coming to terms with what's happening. But, well, I guess it's too soon, he's only just, you know, been made aware, but I need him to change. Alec's going to try and talk to him. Sometimes he listens. No good asking Derek, Graham and him just argue ...'. Barbara was shaking her head, looking down as she spoke. How she wished it could have all been different. And yet, somehow she couldn't imagine it being other than how it was. That was how it had been for too long now.

'That's so important for you to feel that to some degree he has come to terms with what's happening to you.' Nicola felt for Barbara, and for Graham. She knew how people using drugs were often misrepresented, seen as just another 'addict', but they were people, with thoughts, feelings, hopes, dreams, but affected by a need to use substances to feel different, or to use substances to simply stave off physical withdrawal.

'He's a good lad, he is. I know he's got problems, we all have, but, well, he just can't seem to cope without drugs. I think he was hurt too much when he broke up with Ros.' Another pause as Barbara felt her own feelings emerge more into her awareness. 'He's not how I hoped he'd be, but he's settled down a lot in the last couple of years. It's just, I think he's going to lose it and I don't know what I can do, Nicola,' her eyes filled with tears, 'I don't know what I can do, and now all of this is happening and . . . ,' the emotions cut across her attempt to speak. She broke down in heart-rending sobs. It felt to Barbara as though she was suddenly dropped into a great lake of pain, hurt, anguish, everywhere, like it was all there was. The tears continued to flow, her sobs became wails, horrible sounds and yet clearly so expressive of the pain and anguish that she was experiencing.

> The client has been enabled to engage with, make visible and release feelings, emotions associated with her younger son and her knowing she will not be there to help and support him in the future. The person-centred counsellor will need to have the emotional strength to sit with the depth of feeling that is brought into the therapeutic relationship. Yes, it can be shocking in the sense that it can emerge unexpectedly and powerfully. The depth of pain and anguish that human beings have the capacity to experience may be known to the counsellor, from their work or their own experience. For the novice counsellor who may be new to such intensity of feeling, it can be a challenge to be open to the feelings and emotions that it induces within them. But they have to maintain their focus, continue to offer the therapeutic conditions while maintaining their authentic presence as a human companion sharing in the painful process of engaging with distressing feelings, emotions and thoughts.

The intensity rocked Nicola. The pain, the sounds of hurt and anguish were all too plain to see, and to hear. They tore into her own heart.

'Everything, just everything.' Nicola felt no need to try and reflect any of the pain in words. She felt sure that what she was experiencing was being expressed in her tone of voice.

Barbara nodded through her tears. The pain was still very present, she felt lost in it, sort of, it was as though it was more than her simply feeling the pain, more that she *was* the pain, and the pain *was* her. It felt blinding, utterly blinding. She couldn't see through it, beyond it. It was all there was. 'I-I c-can't s-see a way out.' Her breathing came in short, sharp breaths. Her chest felt tight, so tight, the muscles in her ribs ached, they felt so painful. Her head was throbbing, her throat burned. Her arms and legs felt heavy but somehow strangely distant, as if she was her pain first and her body second.

Nicola had moved closer to Barbara and had reached out to her. Barbara had her face in her hands, her shoulders shuddering now and then as she caught her breath. She took a gentle but firm hold of Barbara's right shoulder. She felt it was the right thing to do. She knew it might take the client away from her focus, perhaps, but she felt clear in herself that that was not her intention. She wanted to communicate her presence, her support, her heartfelt caring and compassion.

Barbara felt the contact, and she was grateful for it although it also felt strangely distant. 'I-I . . . , I-I'm . . . ,' she sniffed, 'oh God'. She shook her head, still holding it in her hands. 'Oh God, oh God,' her breath still in short, shallow breaths, 'I-I've nev-ver f-felt an-anyth-th-thing l-l-l-l-like th-this.' Another breath, 'Oohh'. She blew out the air through her mouth. 'Oh God.' Pain all around her, everywhere, and fear. 'I-I-I'm so afraid,' the breaths still short and shallow, 'I-I d-don't know what t-t-to d-do.' Barbara tried to regain control, but it was useless, she felt utterly lost to the surge of pain and fear that seemed to envelop her. 'Wh-what do I d-do? I don't kn-know w-what to d-do.'

Nicola pressed and rubbed Barbara's shoulder. She had momentarily closed her own eyes as she felt her own anguish rising and tears welling up in her own eyes. 'You so wish you knew what you could do.' She wasn't sure about her response and yet she didn't know what else to say.

Empathic responses are spoken with warmth and a quality of tenderness. A note of compassion is present within the counsellor and is conveyed in the tone of her response, facial expression and physical response. The counsellor knows she cannot make it easier for her client, that it is not her role even if she could. What Barbara is feeling is utterly appropriate. There are so many questions that cannot be answered, the answer must emerge from within the client as they become aware of what they have to do. The counsellor's feeling as she responded may be linked to a sense of helplessness on her part. What can she do either? She can't take the pain and anguish away, however much that very human urge is present within her. The simple empathic response can feel not enough, but this is because the humanity of the counsellor wants her to do more. But she is doing all that she can in this therapeutic context. She is offering the relational experience, which contains the possibility of healing.

Barbara swallowed, it was painful. She lapsed into silence. There was nothing more to say. She did so wish she knew what to do, and could do it, but she didn't, she couldn't. She was exhausted. So tired of it all, of everything. Her breathing began to ease a little, she felt physically weak. Her head throbbed. Her eyes still burned. And the ache in her chest, her heart. She took a slow breath, her eyes clenched, and breathed out through her mouth. 'I don't know what to do. There is nothing I can do. I can't, I've got to cope with me. I can't, I haven't the energy. I can't . . .'. She paused. 'Oohh,' she blew the air out as she spoke, 'I can't.' She began to wipe her eyes with her hands, her finger tips pressed against them for a moment. She blew out another breath and dropped her hands into her lap. Her head bowed a little lower as she did so.

Nicola responded with a little more pressure as she gently squeezed her shoulder. Barbara reached up with her left hand and pressed down on Nicola's hand. 'Thank you.' She blew out another breath. 'Thank you.' She nodded her head and looked across at Nicola. Their eyes made contact. Nicola nodded, tight-lipped, her eyes themselves looking quite watery. Barbara noticed them. Somehow it seemed reassuring. She didn't know why and wasn't trying to think about it anyway. There was just something reassuring about the fact that Nicola's eyes looked watery and her face looked so serious. And caring. Barbara nodded again. 'Thanks. I'm OK.'

Nicola took that as an indication that Barbara wanted her to remove her hand, which she did, and moved back into her seat. Meanwhile, Barbara had reached for another tissue and was drying her face, her eyes, and blowing her nose. 'I can't, I'll try and help him, but I can't . . . , I can't be responsible for him. He's got to rely on others and, well, on himself. He does get support. He goes to a clinic. Maybe I must talk to them. Yes, maybe he hasn't told them. Maybe they need to be aware. I hadn't thought of that, but I can do that. Yes, that would be something. He's got to get support from them. I'll . . . , I'll be there for him as much as I can but . . . , but I can't keep giving, can I? I mean I know that, we talked about that before, having to let him take responsibility for his own choices, it's just that, it all feels like my responsibility. It's because of me that he's struggling.'

'You make it sound as though you are responsible not just for him but for being unwell.'

'Maybe I am. Haven't had the most healthy lifestyle, but, well, a lot of that was in the past. I don't know. But I have to try and be there for him, for them. I just have to.' Barbara felt so strongly about this, she couldn't imagine it any different. She felt so responsible, she had to be there for them, had to try and make things OK. She felt her anxiety rising as she thought about them, about herself, about how it would be without her there.

Nicola sat with her own reactions, so aware of Barbara's focus on her 'boys' – how they were so clearly a major concern, and yet aware that beneath her concern was her own fear of what was to become of her, with all the uncertainty that that brought.

'That's so important for you, Barbara, you feel so much that you have to be there for them.' Nicola had noticed the time, there were only a few minutes of the session left. She didn't want to disrupt the focus, it felt important, but she also recognised the importance of ensuring her client was aware of the time frame she was working within. 'And I'm aware we only have a few minutes left.'

'Never enough time when you want it.' I've got to use my time, all of my time. She didn't voice the last sentence, it remained as a thought. 'But I haven't said anything about my parents, I'll have to leave that. They're being very good. Upset, but supportive.' Barbara felt her own upset as she spoke.

Nicola, noticing Barbara's eyes welling up, responded empathically to what she sensed to be happening. 'It upsets them, and their upset is affecting you.'

'They don't need this, not at their age. They're both in their eighties now.' Barbara felt more of her emotion welling up, a sadness that they had to feel what they were feeling, and that they .... She swallowed. The thought of them having to attend her funeral. That wasn't something she had somehow really thought about, but there it was. She didn't want them to have to go through that. And she had been expecting to be there for them in their latter years as well.

'So much for them to come to terms with, and for you. So much sadness'. Nicola's response was general, it felt to her that there was just so much sadness in the atmosphere, no doubt affecting everyone.

Barbara was taking a deeper breath. And she knew that she had to get on in spite of it all. She could cope with her own sadness, that was how she felt, but she didn't want to cause others hurt, and she found that so hard to accept. But she didn't mention it. It was time to go. She would have liked to have stayed and said more, but she was tired. It had been a long session, it felt like it. 'I have to head off. Thank you. I do need this, it is helping. It's not easy, nothing is, not now. It's not going to be an easy week, more hospital appointments. They're very good, very supportive, but this is different. I can be me, here. Even at home, I mean, well, I try to make things normal, sort of. But it's not, is it? I really need to just come here and be me, and then try and put myself together again to face the next week. That's how it feels.'

'I'm glad this is helpful, and, what can I say? I really do hear what you are saying, that image of having to put yourself back together to try and make a normal week at home. Doing what you have to do.'

Barbara nodded. Yes, she thought, yes, that's exactly it, doing what she had to do. There was no choice, not really. She had to try and make things normal, however much she felt anything but normal. She got up to leave and immediately felt quite dizzy. 'Till next week.'

'Yes. You OK?' Nicola noticed Barbara's unsteadiness.

'Bit dizzy. Treatment can leave me feeling like that, and I do feel tired, and the pain, of course. It's not been easy, today. I do feel tired.'

'Are you OK for getting home? Can we call anyone, arrange a cab?'

'No, no, I'll be OK. Just get my balance and take it carefully. I've not that far to go.'

'OK, but if you change your mind, mention it at reception and they can arrange a cab for you.'

'Thanks, I do appreciate your concern.' Somehow it meant a lot to Barbara, she felt quite emotional. People didn't often really think of her, not like that. It just touched her, quite deeply. She felt good and sad at the same time. It was nice, but it made her aware of how rare it was. Nicola had opened the door for her. Barbara looked over at her, a moment of eye contact. Something in the way Nicola was looking, again that caring and concern. 'Thanks, you're a godsend, you really are.'

Nicola smiled back. 'Sure you are OK?'

'Yes, I'll be fine. Thanks again.' Barbara left, but those few moments stayed with her. She couldn't explain why, she didn't try. They just did. Yes, she felt good about Nicola as her counsellor, and she felt sad as well. She felt the support of her presence, and she felt the loneliness of her life.

She got outside and appreciated the warmth of the sun on her face. But the tiredness was still very present. She knew she needed to just get home and lie down for a while, get her energy back. She was going to keep coming to the counselling, it really was important. She didn't have to explain herself. She liked the way Nicola listened. She didn't say a lot. But she listened, and that felt so good somehow. She didn't really understand it, it was how it was. Yes, I can just be as I need to be. She helps me get the pain out. It's not nice, but I know I have to. She was very much in her own thoughts as she walked slowly along the pavement.

Such a relief not to have to pretend, to be strong for other people. At home it felt like she had to keep up a pretence. But here she could let go – she didn't feel she had much choice when the feelings really ran high. But it was time to go back. She was aware of feeling breathless. Everything just seemed so much more of an effort.

Nicola was very much in contact with her own feelings after the session. Something about Barbara's situation. It was complex. Yes, she knew how families could react in different ways to these kinds of situation, and maybe there was a case to have someone work with the whole family, a kind of family therapy service specialising in bereavement, in preparing the family for what was to happen and how to move on and through the death of a loved one. Her thoughts switched to Barbara's parents. What must they be feeling? It was one thing to lose a parent, but for a parent who loses a child, at any age, that was often so hard to bear. At the end of your life, having to face the death of your own daughter, or son .... Yes, it happened, but somehow it was something that went against natural, psychological conditioning. Another attack on a person's expectations and on the assumptions that contribute to a person's sense, or structure, of self.

As she sat and thought about it she realised that she wasn't surprised that the counselling was important for Barbara, and it left her with mixed feelings: glad that she could offer something that was being received and experienced as helpful, and sad that Barbara needed to turn to a counsellor in her time of need, that her husband and sons couldn't quite be there for her in a way that might have made everything very different and, of course, may have meant she may never have needed to come to counselling in the first place. She realised, as she had these thoughts, that she was being simplistic, that Barbara would have had a part to play in how the family system developed. Not that she was seeking to blame anyone; what had developed had developed and everyone contributed. But parents did play a significant part, though often what they brought into the family system came from their own familial experiences. Patterns could repeat themselves so easily. Still, Alex seems supportive and understanding, and she has found strength through her AA books and philosophy. Yes, Nicola felt comforted by that. Barbara had turned to something that had obviously given her strength and meaning before, and now, well, now it was offering her something else. Everyone had to find what they needed, and no one could prescribe for another where it should come from.

Points for discussion

- Critically evaluate Nicola's offering of the therapeutic conditions in this session. Was she as effective as a person-centred counsellor as she could or should have been?
- What are the key issues for Barbara as she faces perhaps the last few weeks or months of her life? What thoughts, feelings does this leave you with and how would you deal with them if you were her counsellor?
- What key elements of the person-centred approach are important when working with a client facing up to the reality of their own death? Do you think that a client facing death needs a counsellor to evidence particular therapeutic qualities and, if so, what are they?
- What should Nicola consider taking to supervision from this session, and why?
- Write notes for this session.

CHAPTER 11

Counselling session 11: Reflections on the past

Barbara had not had a good week. The tiredness had persisted, and she had felt nauseous much of the time. Her mood seemed to fluctuate a lot, although generally it was low. She had bouts of feeling angry, feeling responsible, feeling sad, feeling alone, anxious, afraid. And then there were other moments, strange moments in many ways, when she seemed suddenly quite calm. She wanted to talk about it, and she wanted to talk through some of the things she wanted to do for herself in the weeks ahead. The prognosis remained poor; the doctors were particularly concerned about her liver. She didn't feel she had much time to do what she wanted, and somehow she was feeling she wouldn't be able to do everything. She didn't want to lose hope, but she knew she also had to prepare herself, and everyone else, for what was probably inevitable – her death. Yet it still seemed impossible to think about, to imagine. And it was too painful . . . .

The session had started. Barbara had said a little about her week and the treatment she was receiving. But she didn't want to dwell on that. 'I know I have to accept that I will die, Nicola, I know it. I still can't really accept it though, but I have to. And part of me doesn't want to believe it, wants me to just carry on as if nothing is happening. But it is. I feel like crap most of the time. I look in the mirror and I don't see myself, I mean I do, but I look awful. That depresses me. I'm losing weight. But . . . . There are things I want to do, need to do. Places I want to visit one last time, if I can. I want to go back to where I spent my early childhood. I haven't been back to Norfolk for a few years now, and we moved away when I was 12. I just want to see places again, it still feels like home.' She smiled and Nicola smiled back.

'Important place for you, to feel like home.'

Barbara nodded. 'Very. I didn't appreciate it so much then. I was young, it was a long time ago but, well, I like the fresh air . . . and the big sky – people often don't know what I mean, but it's the relative flatness, you see the horizon further away and it sort of gives you a sense of a bigger sky. No hills to reduce the horizon, if you know the right places!'

'That big sky seems to really make you smile.'

'It does, it really does. Nothing like it on a cold winter's morning, with the frost on the fields and the sun overhead, or on a sunny summer day.' She took a deep breath, forgetting she needed to be careful, and started coughing. She took a tissue, as usual there was a little blood in the phlegm. 'Sorry about that.'

Nicola nodded, not wanting to focus on it as it had cut across what Barbara had been saying and she felt she wanted to hold open the option for Barbara to continue with what she was saying rather than be drawn into an interaction about her coughing.

'It feels like a place to expand and I need that. And I just want to see places again, you know, places that had special meaning for me all those years ago, and since.' She paused.

Nicola did not respond, respecting the silence, as it seemed to her that Barbara had thought of something and was engaging with the thought, whatever it was.

Barbara looked up. She seemed to be reaching out somehow, or so it felt to Nicola. She responded. 'A place of special meaning . . .'.

'Places I want to see, and probably for the last time.' She tightened her lips. Those few words really had brought it home. It was one thing knowing something, but hearing the words, hearing yourself say it and knowing it as well. 'Yes, that's how it has to be.'

Nicola felt a quietness in herself. She also felt a sudden strong sense of respect for Barbara, for what she was saying, what she was contemplating doing. How would it be for her? Yes, important to see places again, but how would it be as she left?

For Barbara, though, it was something of a kind of pilgrimage. Not religious, nothing like that, but there was something about wanting to go home. She couldn't really understand the strength of the feeling, but she knew she had to.

For some people, knowing their time is limited, there can be an urge to revisit important places or people, sometimes very much from the past. However, it can also happen for people who are not aware that death is close, who just suddenly experience such an urge. And they may not be aware of why they are doing it; the person finds themselves contacting people they haven't been in touch with for a while, having a last conversation in some way, though not necessarily with that consciously in mind. It is as though they know, at some level, that the end is close at hand. On the face of it this may seem strange, how do people know? But perhaps there are deeper levels of knowing, and where a progressive disease is present then the knowing that death may be close at hand may be known at some organismic level, although not present in the person's awareness.

For others it can be much more of a conscious process. They are fully aware of what they are doing, and why. Either way, the person-centred therapist will be honouring the client's needs, warmly accepting how they need to be and what they need to do.

Nicola was responding, 'That's how it has to be – special places, places to experience again and, as you say, knowing it will probably be for the last time.' Nicola felt her own jaw become tight. It was a very emotional moment. She felt a lump in her own throat and swallowed. This could not be easy for Barbara to talk about.

'And you know, yes, as I say all this, yes, I am sad, and yet . . . I don't know, I get these moments, well, they're longer than moments, but I feel calm, almost as though, I don't know, I can't describe it.'

'You can't put into words something about this sense of calm.'

Barbara thought for a moment. 'It's not like a dream, but it sort of is, like I'm watching myself, sort of. Strange . . .'.

'Like you're watching yourself in some way?' Nicola didn't feel she was really grasping what Barbara was saying. Yes, she was responding to the words, but she did not feel sufficiently connected to the sense of what Barbara was trying to describe. 'I'm not sure I'm really getting a sense of what you are saying, and I want to.'

An extremely authentic response. The counsellor is sufficiently self-aware to know that her response was to the words, but in fact she wants to empathise with her client, not offer a classic reflection of the counselling skills kind. She is a therapeutic counsellor, she wants to understand what her clients means, what she is experiencing and seeking to communicate. She therefore responds openly and authentically, allowing the client opportunity to explain further – if the client wishes to do this.

Barbara sat silently again for a moment or two. Her thoughts had moved on. 'I'm still reading the serenity prayer, that line about accepting the things you cannot change. I can't do it all, can I?' Barbara looked at Nicola as she spoke. 'I can't, and it's hard to accept that. I always thought I could accept things not changing, but this is different. It means accepting that I can't make those changes to other people. I can only really be responsible for me. And I thought, well, I know that about my drinking, and I dealt with it, but now it seems different somehow. It is different. I want my sons to change, but I can't change them, can I?' Barbara looked away, shaking her head as she did so. 'It's now about me, how I am, the example I show, meeting my needs. I have to do the things I want to do now.'

Nicola again responded to the last comment from her client, seeking to enable her to feel heard but to minimise any interruption to the flow of experiencing that Barbara was putting into words. 'The things you want to do.'

'I've been thinking about that.' Barbara went on to describe how there were two places that she wanted to visit: Norfolk, because that was where she spent her early childhood before her parents moved to the Midlands; and Llandudno, where she and Derek had had their honeymoon. 'You may think I'm silly, but I want to see them both again.'

Nicola did not feel in any way that Barbara was being silly. 'I don't think you're silly at all. I think that both places and what they mean are really important to you. Places for you, places with memories, places you need to experience again.'

'Opposite directions, of course, and, well, I somehow feel like I need to just breathe the air, take in the scenery, hear the sounds, smell, yes, smell the salt water. Do you know Norfolk?'

Nicola nodded, she had spent time there. 'I know the north Norfolk coast.' It seemed appropriate for Nicola to say this, although she wondered whether by so doing she might in effect be robbing Barbara of the opportunity to describe the place in her own words. It was never an easy situation, she felt. But she had said what she had said now.

It is an interesting dilemma. A client talks about a place and asks if the counsellor knows it. The counsellor could say something along the lines of, 'It's important for you to know if I know of the place?' But is that really therapeutically helpful. A client asks a direct question. Why? Usually, because they want an answer. But it opens up the debate as to how much self-disclosure is therapeutically helpful, but who is the counsellor to judge that? The person-centred counsellor seeks to be transparent. That does not mean that they will initiate endless self-disclosure. But there are times when a client does need to know something about the counsellor. Perhaps it might be reassuring. Perhaps it will inform their decision as to what to say about something or somewhere. What may be unhelpful is getting into a conversation about a place. The counsellor is not there to offer conversation as such, but to help the client explore their inner world. Having said that, there are times in therapy where the communication does become quite conversational. This can certainly be the case as therapy draws to a close, but not uniquely so. There is a place for more 'conversational counselling', but where it occurs the counsellor needs to be clear on their motivation in engaging with the client in this way. The focus is, after all, on the client's experience and the counsellor's attempt to understand and accept what is present for and within the client. Conversation should not detract from this primary emphasis.

'Well, I want to stand and look down at the pier at Cromer. We used to live nearby and I used to play on the sands. And go along the coast, Walcott, Mundesley, Yarmouth, Lowestoft. The model boat ponds at Lowestoft. The things that come back to you. And the piers at Yarmouth, and the snails, there were big snails that you rode on, and a Noah's Ark you went in and everything moved inside.' She stopped and shook her head again, thinking back to those times. 'I expect it's all changed now. Maybe I don't want to go to some places, but Cromer won't have changed much.'

'You want to see the places that you think won't have changed too much?'

Barbara nodded. 'The Norfolk Broads, the windmills, and the reeds at Filby Broad, funny but that's stuck in my mind. I can't tell you why.'

'Important place for you, something about how it looked?'

'I remember we had a rowing boat out. We used to go back after we had moved, holidays, visit friends. My grandparents were there. Strange. Something about a sense of home, of needing to go home, something about "home".'

'Something about going home.' Nicola put only a slightly questioning intonation in her empathic response. It felt very much in tune with what Barbara was saying and the way she was questioning herself as to what it was all about.

> For some people 'going home' can be like a metaphor, and sometimes more than that, for returning to some pre-birth state of consciousness, or it may reflect a religious belief, or thoughts of rejoining family members who have died. Sometimes the outer urge, while having its own meaning, might also be a symbolic expression of some inner process.

Barbara was nodding. 'Going home. Finding some peace. I liked it there. I hated moving away. I just remember it being quiet, peaceful, open space. My problems were all later, well, you know the story, I told you when I started seeing you.'

Nicola felt a strong sense of how much Barbara looked back to those early years, how important they must have been to her, and be to her now in her memory. 'Feels like you lost something when you moved away.'

Barbara's thoughts went back to the years after the move, and the problems she'd begun to have. She always wanted her independence but she had fallen in with what she could now see were the 'wrong crowd'. She'd smoked cannabis, experimented a bit with LSD, experienced her 'summer of love'. 'I had a good time, but, well, it did get out of control and, well, I got into drinking too much as well, as you know. That was a big part of the problem. It all feels a long time ago now. I just . . . , I don't know, am I being silly wanting to go back?'

'That seems a really important question you're needing an answer to, "Am I being silly wanting to go back?".'

'In a way I think I am, but it's what I want to do. Feels more than a want, something I need to do. I feel like I'm always there for everyone else, and, well, it's like this one's for me.'

Nicola nodded, struck by the tone of Barbara's voice. 'A real statement – I'm going to Norfolk for me.'

'I'm sure people would think there are better places to want to go to. Why go back, why somewhere you already know. But maybe that's it. Maybe . . .'.

'Something about going to a place you know?'

'It's about memories, but it's about knowing a place, something certain, something you can imagine.'

'Something sort of predictable, or have I got that wrong?' The word had come into Nicola's mind immediately as Barbara was speaking, but she wasn't sure, she may be giving undue emphasis by what she had said.

'Mhmm, I think you're right. And it's home. It'll always be home. I need . . .'. She swallowed. Emotions arose in her and her eyes watered. She was caught by the suddenness of it. 'Oh dear.'

'Painful thought?' Nicola spoke gently. She sensed immediately that something had emerged for Barbara.

Counsellors need to be sensitive to material, thoughts, feelings suddenly emerging into a client's awareness. It can be extremely powerful, intense and momentarily overwhelming. It can also be extremely disorientating, particularly when the material is of a nature such that it threatens a person's view of themselves. This is not the case here, but where it is, then either the new material has to be absorbed into an adjusted structure of self – and that may take time to happen – or the suddenness and intensity can, in extreme cases, lead to psychotic breakdown, the person's self-concept is shattered.

In terms of facing death, one area that can be quite profound is the sudden realisation in an immediate and personal way of one's own mortality. People can create a strong structure of self around a belief in their own seeming immortality and invincibility. Yes, as we grow older we all know at some level that we will die, though many people will push the thought aside, not wishing to dwell on it. But when the reality of death arises earlier in life, or to the person who still feels full of life with no expectation of death on the horizon, the impact on the person's self-concept and structure of self can be devastating. The counsellor needs to be sensitive to this, to the far-reaching psychological consequences of facing death in such circumstances.

Barbara had closed her eyes, trying to regain control of her emotions. She nodded her head and held her breath. She knew what it was, but it felt so difficult to say.

'I need . . . ,', she paused again, the lump in her throat made it difficult. 'I have to say this, it wouldn't be making me feel like this if it wasn't important.'

'Take your time, Barbara. Take your time.' Nicola spoke softly and waited, not wanting to pressure Barbara in any way. Barbara knew what she was feeling, she didn't need her to interrupt or try and push her in some way. She had said she had to say it.

The words finally came out in a rush. 'I need to say goodbye.' Barbara was blinking, she could feel the tears trickling over her eyelids. She took a short breath, breathed out and swallowed.

'Mhmm.' Nicola felt herself taking a deep breath, it was instinctive. 'Needing to say goodbye.' She nodded as she spoke, acutely aware of the emotions that were present. It felt like a defining moment in some way. Barbara was sharing her innermost sense of what was motivating her. In voicing and acknowledging it she is helping herself to integrate it into her awareness, and at a more visceral level.

There is a difference between a thought of saying goodbye and the feeling that it *is* goodbye. The client here is connecting with a knowing that is not just in her head, but in her being, her heart, her feelings. She has moved from the earlier recognition that that was what she was doing, to a deeper engagement with the reality, the implications, the actual sense of the good-bye experience. It has become a reality at some more personal and profound level. Is 'level' the right word? Possibly not. It is a deeper knowing that is beyond the logical, thinking mind. The realisation and the utter knowing, with all the feelings associated with it, that a person is now in the process of saying goodbye.

Barbara nodded. She felt the raw emotion in her body, her chest, heart, head. The way Nicola had spoken told Barbara that she had an understanding of what Barbara was saying, really saying. Places passed through her mind, places and people. She opened her eyes and looked over to Nicola. 'Derek says I don't need to put myself through it, that I have my memories, that should be enough. Maybe he's right, I don't know, but he's wrong as well. I need to do this, for me. It will not be easy in so many ways and for so many reasons, but something is calling me home. I know it will be painful, but . . .'.

'Painful, but something you have to do.'

Barbara felt herself nodding again in response. She didn't really understand why it was so important. She did, in a sense, in her head, but it felt more than that somehow. Was it an escape, an attempt to recapture the past? Maybe, but she didn't know. In a sense, making sense of it didn't matter. She didn't want to say anything more, she didn't feel she needed to. She knew what she had to do and she felt that Nicola was hearing that need, and accepting it, and that felt good. Like she didn't have to explain herself.

Nicola did have a sensed appreciation of Barbara's need.

And Barbara could also think logically about it, how it would very likely take a lot of energy and bring pain of all kinds, and perhaps her condition might worsen. But dying wasn't just about physical condition. It was also about head and heart, about the inner person, inner needs. If you don't do what you need to do at a time when time was running out, then when would you do it? She had things she had to do. 'Alex understands. He wants to come with me.' She sniffed. 'He thinks I should go straightaway, not hesitate. He can be really sensitive. He's right. I don't know if he'll come or not. In a way I want time on my own, but that's not really practical. Not how I am feeling at the moment. But I need time to be with my thoughts. I spend a lot of time with them anyway, but I want to be in that space, feeling the cool wind off the North Sea, hearing the waves on the shore.'

'Time to be with your thoughts, and in the place that is home in so many ways. And the wind . . . and the waves . . .'. Nicola sought to both capture in her empathic response what Barbara had said and the context in which she was speaking.

Barbara sat for a little while in a place in herself where she could relive something of how that felt. Her thoughts moved to different memories and she talked a little more about her past. Her focus had brought back a lot of memories and she wanted to share them, hear herself retell how it was and feel listened to. It made her, them, feel important, real, valued in some way.

For Nicola, as she listened, it felt that there was a kind of reverence in how she was feeling towards Barbara. It wasn't a confessional kind of interaction, but there was something about bearing witness. And the way Barbara was speaking about her past, there was something so meaningful. Like an inner pilgrimage, and she wasn't sure what she meant by that as the thought crossed her mind, but it somehow seemed to make sense.

Barbara also talked about the cinema, how her parents had been great cinema goers. She talked of the queues at the local cinema she remembered as a child. 'You really looked forward to it – it was a treat.' She paused as a thought struck her. 'You know, in those days you were prepared to wait. We're not like that now. Everyone wants things immediately. Like buying things, you used to save up, now you use the credit card and pay later. Something's changed in society, in people, or maybe it's just me? We did used to wait and it was OK. It's not like that now.'

'You feel that in the past there was a greater readiness to wait?'

'Like I say, you saved up, you waited, you anticipated. Now there is no time for that. Someone wants something, they go and get it, a feeling that they have a right to what they want somehow. I don't know, something precious has been lost.'

The client clearly needs Nicola to hear about her past. She is telling her story. She is having her experiences validated, perhaps in the process saying goodbye to them. She might be thought of as drawing together threads from her own experience, gathering herself into herself. It may not only take place in the therapy room. What she is saying is, 'This is me, this is what I have experienced. These are the changes I've seen.' There is also a reflection on these changes, space for some personal wisdom.

The person-centred counsellor will listen, honouring the client's need to have their experiences and conclusions heard and appreciated. It is important for the client's perspectives to feel valued. She is summing up aspects of her life and how she sees things, what she has learned, maybe; perhaps she might even touch on what she might do differently if she had her time again. This process can be short, or may take many sessions, it will vary from person to person and, of course, may be limited by the time available.

What can be particularly challenging for the counsellor is where the client looks back and feels that their life was unfulfilling, that they perhaps made the wrong choices, that they are left with unresolved and unresolvable regrets. The counsellor has to remain the client's companion, warmly accepting the difficult and painful feelings and the realisation that are emerging within their client. This can be particularly difficult. The client's summary of their life is how they see it and experience it. The person-centred counsellor will not just accept their view, but warmly accept it, being open to how it touches and affects them. It is hard to die with a heart full of regret for what might have been, or for what was. The counsellor who stays with their client's inner world where this is the case may feel emotionally shredded, and is likely to need the restorative experience of extremely supportive supervision. And, of course, such experiences may well impact on how the therapist begins to view their own life, and can be a catalyst for them to question themselves and to make changes.

Nicola listened to what Barbara was saying. She sensed that she was very much speaking from the heart about something that was very present and real for her, this contrast in attitude and behaviour between the past that she had known and the present. 'You can see a change, and there's a loss, it feels to you like, as you say, something precious has been lost along the way.'

Barbara nodded. 'Maybe my situation makes me more reflective. Yes, I'm all over the place sometimes, I know, but these moments of calm that I have, I don't know, they really leave me thinking. Talking to you now, it's really good, remembering about how things were. They were good times. Yes, bad times as well, but I do have good memories. I wonder what people feel if they are in my situation and don't have good memories?' She shook her head.

'Hard for you to imagine what that must be like, no good memories . . .'.

'It's strange, but sometimes I can feel quite fortunate. At other times, well, things haven't worked out how I'd hoped, but lots of families have problems, you know?'

Nicola nodded.

'But it's like I'm sort of more aware of the things that are important to me, things I appreciate somehow.' She paused to take a deep breath. The emotions were close to the surface. 'I suppose it's knowing you'll lose them, but I'll have my memories.' She forced a smile. 'You see, I don't think you die, not really. I know we don't really know, but I can't imagine not being me. I know people talk about going to sleep, you know, and not waking up. But even in sleep you dream, you have a sense of yourself. No, I'm happy to think it's not the end. I guess I've come to think like this more and more.'

'A sense of continuity, of you continuing to be you, of having a sense of you in some other state?'

'Of being me. Maybe I'm fooling myself, but I don't think so, I don't think I'm wrong. And if I am, well, I won't know, will I, and it won't matter anyway.' She smiled at what she had said.

'It sounds like you have found a philosophy, a way of making sense of it, for yourself, and it sounds really positive.'

Barbara found herself aware of her doubts as well. 'I know I have my doubts too. And, well, I forget and become anxious and sad, and that's at the thought of not being here, not being able to share a future ...'. Her voiced waivered as she spoke. 'Sorry.'

'No need to feel sorry, take your time. "Not being able to share a future ..." '.

'It's that loss that hurts most.' Barbara's eyes filled with tears. It was that thought of not being there to share her family's future. So life hadn't been easy, but .... She closed her eyes, there was another pain within her that had come to the surface. She swallowed, her mouth had become very dry. But she knew she needed to say what was in her head. 'And not being a grandmother.' She felt the surge of emotion and lifted her hand to her mouth and then across her eyes as she bowed her head, crying gently.

'That really hurts.'

Barbara nodded through the tears, unable to speak, her throat suddenly feeling hot and raw, and an emptiness in the pit of her stomach.

Nicola sat and did not make any further comment. Painful feelings were emerging and needed time to be released. She maintained her own feelings of warmth and compassion towards Barbara, allowing herself to be affected by what she was saying and feeling, feeling perhaps robbed of an experience that she so wanted for herself.

Slowly, the emotions began to settle. It wasn't to be. Even if she hadn't got cancer, it may still not have happened. She thought of her sons, wondering how they would be in the future. Would they settle down and make good fathers? She thought so, if they got their problems sorted out. She could have helped, she'd have wanted to help. She found herself voicing her thoughts out loud. 'I could have made a difference, not solved all their problems, but I could have helped them to see things differently.'

'Maybe you are.' Nicola hadn't really thought through her response, the words just formed and in a sense demanded to be voiced. The thought that was present for her was that their facing up to their mother's condition, and likely death, could make a difference, could make them think differently, perhaps, though it might depend on how they handled their own pain and loss.

Barbara smiled. 'Maybe.' She sounded quite reflective. 'Maybe ...'. She looked up at the clock, 'It's a nice thought to end on, anyway.'

The counsellor might be accused of rescuing the client from their painful feelings by putting a positive spin on the situation. Maybe. But maybe she was simply being authentic, expressing a feeling that had emerged strongly within her at a time when she felt a particularly strong connection with her client, and trusting that it was appropriate and helpful to voice. Who can say what the effect was or would be. Barbara has a different perspective. She may reflect on it. May reject it. That will be her choice. Sometimes a comment such as this can be incredibly helpful. But, it has to be empathic to the reality. What does this mean? That it is a response that is true, even though the client has not seen it that way. And of course the counsellor does not know if what she said is true, is empathic to the reality of what is happening for her client's family in response to her condition. But clearly the counsellor here will be thinking or feeling that it is true. A person-centred counsellor would not say it unless this was sensed.

The session drew to a close. Nicola was left pondering her own thoughts. Was a world in which there was one chance of life and then judgement, the creation of a wise and loving God? Or would such a world be tempered by a God of Mercy such that all was taken into account and therefore there was a genuine wise justice? Or was there a succession of lives, justice being the result of the working out of a law of cause and effect, or karma? Or perhaps there was no God, simply a creative process, and we are in truth simply a chemically driven biological process that has culminated in the emergence of consciousness, intelligence, love and will, and the many other higher human qualities. Or maybe, and this thought appealed to her, maybe we had only just begun, and there are deeper human qualities, capacities and potential to yet discover that will take us, well, the words that came to mind were 'God knows where', as we explore the heights and depths of inner space. Inner space, hmm, perhaps that's the true 'final frontier'. She put her thoughts aside and attended to her notes for the session.

Points for discussion

- How has the session left you feeling? How does this contrast with other sessions?
- When clients move between different emotional states within a session, what enables you to be open to the changing impressions made on your own awareness?
- In terms of person-centred theory, describe Barbara's psychological processes as she finds ways to come to terms with her anticipated death.
- Pick out any significant responses by Nicola during the session that seemed to have particular therapeutic value.
- What were your thoughts in response to what Barbara was saying about living on after death? Was this easy for you to accept, and if she were your client would you be able to convey your acceptance of her view? What would you do if she had a view that was hard for you to accept?
- What would you take to supervision from this session?
- Write notes for this session.

CHAPTER 12

Counselling session 12: Telephone contact – a difficult decision

When Nicola arrived on the following Monday there was a message for her. Barbara had phoned to cancel the session, but had asked if she could call her at the time when she would have seen her.

Nicola had two other clients to see first that morning, and she was aware that Barbara wasn't too far from her thoughts at times, but she felt she managed to keep her focus. It was not knowing why, but at least she had left her home number, so she was at home, maybe not feeling well enough to come out.

After the second session Nicola wrote up her notes and then sat down to contemplate her call to Barbara. She was aware of feeling a little anxious. It was concern for Barbara's wellbeing. She was glad she had called and had asked to be called back. It couldn't be that serious, just enough to stop her getting to the surgery. She thought about visiting her at home. She spent a few moments thinking it through. She could switch to counselling at home if necessary. She had done that before. It changed things, but that didn't mean it wasn't helpful.

Oh well, she thought, no point in me sitting here speculating about what may have happened, and what I can offer, I won't know until I've spoken to her. She closed her eyes for a moment, she found telephone work could be quite demanding, no physical signals to add to the vocal communication. And she wasn't sure whether Barbara would want a telephone counselling session, or a chat to convey some news, or to simply arrange the next appointment. She lifted the receiver and tapped out the number. She heard the phone ringing.

'Hello?' It was a man's voice.

'Oh, hello. I'm Nicola, from the surgery. Can I speak to Barbara please?'

'Yes, yes. I'll get her to pick up the phone.' She heard the phone being put down, and Barbara's name being called in the background. She heard the phone being picked up.

'Hello.'

'Hello, is that Barbara?'

'Yes.'

'It's Nicola.'

155

'Hello, thanks for calling. I'm so sorry but I'm not feeling well at all.' She coughed before she could add anything further, and winced with the sudden pain that it brought. 'I couldn't face coming up to the surgery, but I do want to talk to you.'

'That's OK. I'm sorry you are not feeling well, but we can talk. Are you in a place where you can talk?'

'Yes, I'm in the bedroom. Derek's at home, but I'm on my own in here. So, yes, I can talk.' She coughed, 'Sorry, it feels worse at the moment.' Barbara paused, before continuing with something she had very much on her mind. 'What we talked about last week, we booked up to go away at the weekend, this coming weekend, like I'd talked about, but I'm not so sure now. I've got a few days to try and feel a bit better, I felt good when we organised it early last week. Now I'm really not sure.' She paused again, getting her breath. 'Just talking is tiring at the moment.'

'Talking is making you tired, that must be so wearing.'

Barbara felt tired, and the pain was intense at times, although the medication helped some of the time. And she felt anxious, but almost too tired to feel anxious. 'They want me to go into hospital. They said they would stabilise me, control the pain. This was on Friday. I wasn't sure, I just thought that I'd feel a bit better if I took it easy over the weekend. I didn't want to go in, they might not have let me out to go away. So I said no.'

'It's important for you to go away, and hospital seemed like it might stop that.'

'I really thought I'd be OK, but I'm not. I may have to accept what they are saying. So I don't know, I don't know what will happen.' Barbara was feeling anxious as she spoke.

Nicola could hear the anxiety in Barbara's voice. 'Makes it all very uncertain and must cause you anxiety.'

Barbara found herself nodding as she held the phone. 'I'm scared, Nicola, scared of what's happening. I don't want to go to hospital, I won't have any control then, I won't be able to make my own choices, and I want to be here, with Derek, Alec and Graham – Graham seems to have settled a bit this week. Seems to be a bit more steady again. I just want to be here for them. I don't want to go in, and if I do, I won't see you either, and it's really important to me. Really important.'

'Going into hospital feels like you'll lose control and not be there for your family, or be able to get to counselling.'

Barbara went silent. Nicola stayed with the silence, aware that her own thinking was along the lines of how flexible the surgery was and that she could go and see clients elsewhere. She had undertaken home visits for counselling sessions. Visiting Barbara at home or in hospital was possible. She wondered whether to say anything at this point. Would it take Barbara away from what she was feeling and thinking? Was she trying to rescue Barbara, or by mentioning that she could see her in hospital would it sound as though she was encouraging her to go in? 'I could visit you in hospital if you go in, or at home if it is difficult for you to get here.'

'Could you? That would be lovely, oh that really would be good of you. You're sure that's not a problem?'

'No, no, not a problem.'

'If I go in, I don't know how long it will be for.' Barbara paused. 'How can I let you know?'

'Leave a message for me here at the surgery.' Nicola paused for a moment. 'Is it OK if I talk to Dr Adams to let her know and so she can keep me up to date?'

'Can you? That would be good.' Barbara knew that she still didn't want to go into hospital. What she was not voicing was her fear of not coming out. It was very much in her thoughts as she lay in bed, holding the phone to her ear. What would happen? Would that be it? The doctor had encouraged her to think about it as a few days to get her cancer more under control and to ease some of the symptoms. She wished she could be at the counselling session. It felt easier to talk there, somehow. It was good to be talking on the phone but it wasn't the same. She wanted to tell Nicola how she was feeling, but it seemed to her that that was all it would be. And she might just feel worse. But she knew she needed to say something. It seemed to her that Nicola was someone she could trust with her fears. That was important.

Nicola had responded, acknowledging that it was possible. Barbara began to express her fears. 'I'm so afraid, really afraid. It's all become too real. Only last week I was planning what I wanted to do and now, well, now . . .'. She stopped speaking.

Nicola could hear Barbara crying. Her heart went out to her. She felt like she wanted to rush round and comfort her. At least she wasn't alone, her husband was there. 'Happening too fast, so afraid . . .'.

Barbara felt awful. It wasn't what she had expected. Not now. Not before she had done what she wanted to do. 'I just feel awful, I can't begin to tell you. I'm in more pain, but I just feel like I have no energy. I'm not me, Nicola, I'm just not me. I hate it.' She paused, taking a deeper breath and closing her eyes. She felt so tired lying there. 'So tired, so scared.'

Nicola felt her own lips tightening, pressing together. 'Tired and scared of what's happening.'

'It just feels hopeless. I don't know. I can't get comfortable. I can't keep my eyes open. I don't want to eat, I don't want to die, Nicola.' The crying had begun again, 'I d-d-don't want t-to die . . .'. Barbara's voice trailed off into a fit of coughing. It felt like a violent spasm, she could only imagine the pain it was causing for Barbara, who was suffering enough distress anyway, without that.

Nicola felt herself react. She closed her eyes.

'No, no, you don't . . .'. What more could she say?

'I hadn't thought it would be like this. I mean, oh, I don't know, maybe things'll improve again, they do, don't they, sometimes?'

'Yes, things can improve.'

Barbara knew it happened, but would it happen to her? She usually felt more posi-tive. She knew things were bad, serious. She accepted that. But . . . but now it felt like it was too real, too close, and she just felt too awful and weak. She felt that she needed something to hang on to. 'Can I see you again?'

'Sure, I can book you time and, as I say, see you at home, hospital, I can make the time for that. If I make the time at the end of the morning then I can be a little more flexible, gives me time to get to you, particularly if you are in hospital.'

Barbara felt glad about that. 'Thanks, yes, I really appreciate that. You've been so much help. When will it be, next Monday?'

Nicola had been leafing through her diary, it would have to be next Monday.

'That's good. Give me time, give them time to do what they have to do. Try and control the pain. That's what they have to do. It's been bad. It comes and goes, like it was when it all first happened. And worse. I think I have to go in. I know it, I just don't want to, but I know I can't go on like this. The pain just wears you down. If they can control it then I'm sure I'll feel a bit better.'

'Pain can drain you so much, and can be so excruciating. As you say, if they can control that, probably on a pump.'

'That's what they have said. It would be more consistent pain control, maintain levels of a stronger painkiller in my system. I have to accept it. You've been so good, Nicola, I really do appreciate you being there for me, listening, helping me. You really have been such a help, you really have.'

Nicola was struck by a profound sense that Barbara was saying goodbye. It was the way Barbara was speaking, not just the past tense that she was using. Her own emotions were welling up and she felt a constriction in her own throat, she felt tearful.

'I'm so glad that I have been, Barbara, being a part of your struggle and getting to know you, it's been a privilege, it really has.' Nicola realised her response was also in the past tense. She hadn't intended that, it was how the words came out.

Barbara hoped that she would improve, but she knew she did need treatment, it was that fear of going into hospital. She knew things were not good. The doctor had wanted her to go in but she had resisted, saying she wanted to be at home and that she hoped that things would ease a little. He had increased her pain-killers but had made it clear that was the limit, any more and she had to go in to have the pain controlled. The palliative care nurses were visiting her, they seemed very nice and Barbara told Nicola about them. She wanted Nicola to know that she was being looked after. She could hear the emotion in Nicola's voice. She was sort of glad to hear it. It felt right. And she could imagine that Nicola would maintain that professional attitude, yet with that personal touch. She was probably sitting there and her face would be a mixture of calm, serious and concern.

'Anyway, I'll get myself sorted out in a few days and see you on Monday. You take care of yourself. I just need them to reduce the pain, and build me up a bit.' She paused. 'And it would be so much easier if someone would tell me what to do. And I suppose they have, I don't want to do it, but I have to, don't I?'

'Feels like you have been told, and that it's what you have to do?'

'I guess I know I do. I worry everyone being here. I don't want to be a burden. I have to, don't I?'

'You don't like the effect it's having on your family, makes you feel you have to go to hospital?' Nicola heard the intake of breath at the end of the phone.

'I have to. I have to. Just got to get myself stronger, more comfortable.' A pause. 'I'm feeling tired. I think I have to go now.'

'Sure, you rest, you'll make the right choice.'

'Yes. Thank you.'

Nicola was aware of a voice in the background on the phone.

'My parents have arrived. I'll go now and I'll make sure the Surgery knows where I am.' She wanted to say 'See you next week', but the words stayed in her head. 'You look after yourself.'

'You too.' Nicola heard the phone being put down. She sat, the phone still in her own hand for a few seconds, aware of the emotions that were present within her and which suddenly seemed quite overwhelming. She blinked and felt tears on her cheeks, her throat was raw and a little constricted. She decided to stay with her feelings, let them be present, let them find the expression they needed.

Supervision session 3: Exploring the effect of belief on empathy and warm acceptance

'Barbara's in a bad way, she didn't attend this week. We spoke on the phone. She may be back in hospital by now, she probably is, I don't know. She left a message for me to call her at home on Monday as she wasn't going to get to the counselling session. She's taken a turn for the worse. All happened quite suddenly.' Nicola went quiet as she thought back to the session at the beginning of the week, and the feelings it had left her with, and which were still present.

'Sudden worsening, sounds like it wasn't expected.' Mark was struck by what he was hearing concerning the suddenness of it.

Nicola nodded. She told him how Barbara had been planning a trip back to where she'd spent her early childhood. How it had been hard for her to say that she was planning it to 'say goodbye', and how in a sense it had felt very positive. 'And now it has all changed.'

'One week it sounds as though you were feeling positive, and the next week everything has changed for the worse.' Mark was aware that he had brought the focus on to his supervisee and what she was feeling. He realised that she may need to retell what she had heard from her client, but he was also aware that painful feelings would have been present too. How had his supervisee been affected? Was he trusting her, truly trusting her, by responding as he had? His supervisee would know what she needed to talk about. Was this his issue, his agenda? As a supervisor, he knew he had a responsibility to his supervisees and through them to their clients. But he was person-centred, seeking to maintain non-directivity.

Mark could have kept the focus on Nicola's client in his response, but he has chosen not to. In his thoughts he believes this to be in line with his responsibility to enable his supervisee to deal with the impact on her of her work with her client, particularly where that impact risks affecting her ability to offer a genuinely therapeutic relational experience. In this instance the supervisor has probably come in with his focus on his supervisee too soon. There is time for the supervisee to 'tell the story' of her work with her client. During that process, and when the time is right for her, the feelings that need to be addressed will become present.

'It's the suddenness. I mean, in my head I know things can change fast when people have a life-threatening condition like cancer, particularly when it is advanced and affecting major organs. And yet, while she was tired and yes she doesn't look well and is clearly in a lot of discomfort, there was also something so alive in her when we met last time. Yes, that was it, *so alive*. Yes, she was sad, but she was talking about a place, about experiences from her past that were important to her. They were alive to her, and she to them. Yes, it brought something alive in her – not in a lively sense but in terms of her presence.' Nicola paused. 'Hmm.' She found herself reflecting on what she had just said. What did she mean by 'presence'?

'Presence, something about her presence struck you as being so alive.'

Nicola nodded, remaining with her thoughts 'There was a calmness, she's been working on acceptance. She talked about Alcoholic Anonymous's serenity prayer – I'm not sure if that's what it's officially called – that it had fresh meaning for her. She talked about believing she wouldn't die in the sense of ceasing to exist. She felt sure something of her lived on.'

'Mhmm, something in her lives on.'

'And I know there are different takes on it, but I respect her way of making sense of what is happening for her. I know some will say she's avoiding facing up to the reality of existential death, but that is based on a hypothesis. And most of humanity believes something else, some kind of continuity of consciousness, I know I do.'

'And I'm not so sure, but I am open to suggestions. It is one the fundamental elements of human life and yet, well, we don't know, that's the bottom line. But your client clearly believes in something of her living on.'

'She does. And I'm OK with that, I can accept that. Maybe if I believed something different that would be more difficult, but that's OK for me. And I do wonder about the emphasis on existential death. I mean, do we really want to spend our lives working through feelings about not existing at the end of it? I don't know. I mean, if there truly is existential death at the end of life, then that's it, there's nothing to worry about. What we have to deal with is the question of mortality and the loss of those experiences, or of our sense of being alive while we are still alive. But surely if existential death is your belief then that's ever more reason to live to the full. Wasn't it Nelson Mandela who said something about our greatest fear not being of death, but of life? I may have misquoted, I don't think so.'

'Something for you about becoming overabsorbed in worrying about death when actually once it happens there's no you to worry or to be aware of what has been lost?'

'Maybe it's simplistic, and I suppose I'd feel different if I had a different belief. But isn't it often how we die that is the major concern – pain, loss of dignity, loss of control, being a burden to others, being helpless perhaps, being alone? These are so big, such causes for fear and anxiety.' Nicola felt strongly about what she was saying and it showed in her tone of voice.

'So what you are saying is that for you, it is not the what does, or does not, come next that is the issue, but what is experienced in the process leading up to the moment of death?'

> The role of the supervisor can be to help the supervisee clarify their thoughts, feelings, behaviours and experiences. Sometimes such clarification might be in the form of theoretical exploration, but at other times it will be very much centred on restoring congruence and enhancing the supervisee's psychological and emotional availability to their clients.

Nicola thought for a moment, 'Yes, yes, that's right. I feel comfortable in my belief, but the thought of what I might die from, how I might die, yes, that becomes a concern if I allow myself to dwell on it. And I don't think dwelling on it or trying to work it through makes much difference, because you can only know how you will react, truly react, when you are genuinely faced with it. And of course we all are, but it's ahead of us, that is until it isn't, until, as with Barbara, it is suddenly there. Then there is no choice about focusing on it. I just wonder if we really can address our feelings about death until we are faced with it. And what's important for me, as a therapist, is whether I can offer Barbara, or any other client who is facing death, the quality of empathy that they have a right to expect from me as a client coming to me for therapy.'

'Mhmm, can you offer the empathy that you would expect, hope to offer, to a client facing death?' Mark kept his response focused and to the point. He recognised that Nicola was flowing, he didn't want to disrupt the flow, but he did want to acknowledge the point she had made in relation to her expectations of herself.

'In so many ways, my beliefs, my fears, while obviously real and important to me, are very much centred within my frame of reference. I do not want them intruding to the degree that they influence my ability to experience and communicate acceptance of my client's perspectives and the thoughts and feelings that arise within them.' She paused taking a deep breath. 'But does this present a fundamental problem?'

Mark responded, inviting Nicola to continue. 'Can you say more?'

'Well, my beliefs sustain me, but I've not been tested, so to speak, by truly facing my own imminent death. And in a way, perhaps my belief sustains me in being with clients like Barbara. But I suppose any belief would sustain me because you develop beliefs for that purpose. Anyway, that aside, the question in my mind is when dealing with something so fundamental to the human experience, can I be genuinely congruent and acceptant of a client's view of death if it is not my own?'

'Let me check out that I am hearing this as you intend. If your client's experiences as they face death are rooted in a belief or a perception that does not match your own, does that mean your acceptance is somehow less genuine?'

'I'm not sure, I mean, I believe I can accept the feelings that are present which will be linked to the client's beliefs, and I can accept their right, need, to believe what they believe. But if it is not my belief, can I accept their belief? I can accept that it is their belief, but do I need to accept the belief, be open to it in some way? And can I do that when I genuinely think differently, and about something that is so fundamental?' Nicola paused. Yes, that was what was troubling her. 'And I am still wondering, as I speak, what my view is of all of this. I'm not sure. Barbara has brought the question into focus, although she is not an example of what I am talking about.'

'Your view doesn't differ from hers?'

'We haven't gone into detail, but at the level it has been mentioned, no, not really. She feels something of her lives on, and I agree with that.' Nicola thought for a moment.

Mark did not interrupt, he could see that Nicola was wrestling with something from the expression on her face.

'No, I think it's easy to think we can't empathise when there is a difference when we are thinking about it, like this, but not actually in the room with the client, actually in the therapeutic relationship. I think that within that connection, when it exists, there is a very human quality present, at a genuine person-to-person level. And it's OK, you do empathise. You connect to thoughts and feelings. You sort of go through and beyond the cause of those thoughts and feelings. You're not empathising so much with the cause, though you will let the client know that you are hearing and understanding it, but the true empathy – that may not be quite the right way of putting it – maybe I should say the focus of therapeutic empathy is more on the thoughts and feelings that flow as a result of the cause.' She paused. 'To empathise with a client's fear I may not agree with what it is that is causing the fear, but I can feel their fear, and empathise with that and feel unconditional positive regard for my client in her anguish.'

'Mhmm, OK, so empathy, your empathy, is focused on what the client is experiencing, the visceral reality, if you like. Yes, in terms of death, their fear may be because of what they believe, but when that fear is present within the therapeutic relationship, then your sense is that your empathic sensitivity is soundly focused on it?'

Nicola smiled, 'That's an interesting word.'

'What?'

'Soundly.'

Mark looked taken aback. 'What do you mean?'

One exciting aspect of supervision is how something can emerge that turns out to be extremely apposite to a theme being explored. This is such an example. A word voiced without thinking of a secondary meaning is immediately seen in the other light by the supervisee. Supervision can be such a creative process, at times it can feel almost magical in the sense that something emerges seemingly out of nothing. It can feel quite awe-inspiring as a train of thought in one person becomes present for both supervisor and supervisee, each seemingly building on the joint insights that are emerging. There is often a wonderful energy present at these times. Co-professionals seeing something new for the first time, pushing their boundaries of understanding. It is an important element of super-vision as a living, collaborative process

'It is like hearing a sound, isn't it? Maybe it was a figure of speech, but it is like being able to distinguish a sound, isn't it – the sound of fear, in this context. The client sounds fearful, literally, and I hear it and respond to it. I don't know why, what you said has meaning for me. But it also leaves me with another question which is about what happens with a very dogmatic client with beliefs that are not your own. And then, the sound of their dogmatism may, if you like, yes, this makes sense, the sound of their dogmatism may, to my hearing, my empathic sensitivity, drown the sound of the fear, or pain, anguish, whatever is present.' Nicola felt a sense of satisfaction in what she had said. It somehow made so much sense. Yes, the more dogmatic the client if their beliefs were dif-ferent, then perhaps, maybe, it would get in the way, become a distraction, something difficult to keep hearing and yet loudly present.

Mark nodded thoughtfully, the conversation had taken him into an area of thought that he hadn't addressed before. 'So, a different belief, vociferously and dogmatically held, could negatively impact on the quality of empathy from the therapist holding a different belief.'

'And maybe even more so if they are dogmatic in their belief too, of course.'

'Mhmm, that makes sense. OK, this is all very interesting, and it is certainly some-thing to think about, and I am mindful of Barbara. This is not what you experi-ence with her?'

Nicola shook her head. 'No. No her belief is close to mine, close enough anyway from what has been disclosed. Hmm. And then there's the issue of how one person may find another's belief threatening to their own. If Barbara, for instance, strongly believed that there was no existence beyond physical death, therefore accentuating her thoughts and feelings associating death with being a huge experience of loss, and therefore she wanted to cling to life at all costs, I wonder, would my belief make me want to reassure her, or would I be able to stay with her on that edge of desperation? Or would my belief make me some-how convey reassurance, a sense of OKness that would be clearly out of sync with what the client would be experiencing?'

'You mean your empathy, the quality or tone of it, would be modified by your different belief?'

Nicola nodded.

'And it might convey motivations that would not otherwise be present?'

Nicola nodded again. 'Which could affect the quality or tone of my empathy, or my acceptance of what she was feeling, and could I be congruent? What would it mean to be congruent?'

'How do you mean?'

'Well, congruently holding my own beliefs in awareness could cause such modification, so I have to, maybe, hold them out of awareness. Is that compromising congruence, or is that simply what we have to do as part of the process of attending to the inner world of the client, focusing on their frame of reference even though we exist within our own?'

'And that's the challenge, particularly working with clients facing death, for instance.'

Nicola was nodding again. The supervision session felt so alive, it was sharp, like she was breaking into new ways of thinking about theory, practice, herself, what happens in therapy. 'Hmm.' The word 'alive' in her mind took her thoughts back to Barbara, and then to her work with her, and with clients facing death. 'And in so many ways it all comes back down to helping people – when they want this – to come to terms with what they are leaving behind, and the actual leaving behind of loved ones, unresolved issues and relationships, hopes, plans. And, as well as that, again where this is the client's focus, helping them to prepare themselves for the after-death experience that they believe in, or for uncertainty where that is what is most present for them.'

'So we work to, or within, our client's beliefs and expectations.'

'But I think the issue remains about what happens when beliefs differ, and people can feel, well, quite fanatical in their beliefs, and I'm thinking of some religious elements, although not exclusively so.'

'For some people there can be a fanatical edge to their religious belief.'

'And yet it is also such an individual thing. Broad statements don't really help. I come back to it being a matter for the two people in the therapy room, working towards some mutual understanding, some way of being together, therapeutically, in the face of death, with all that that brings out in a person. And it happens, you listen. Of course you listen. My client's pain, anguish, doubt, whatever is present for them is likely to be powerfully present. Yet my sense is that for me, and I haven't had this experience, if I had a client holding a particular belief that was different to my own, and who was quite vociferous and dogmatic about it, I might find it really difficult to empathise with and warm to them. I sense that as a real possibility, but I could be wrong. An ex-client who was a hunter comes to mind. I abhor hunting, but I could empathise with his suicidal ideation and the difficulties he was having in his life. It didn't matter, it wasn't in the way. His emotional state was much more present in my awareness as we sat together.'

Mark had been listening, appreciating what Nicola was saying and the way she was working towards her own clarification of the issues that had become present for her. 'So, for you, there is something about being able to relate to the feelings of the client, like you bypass the context, it doesn't, and I'll use the metaphor from earlier that I used by accident, it doesn't "sound" so loud, but dogmatic views differing to your own about death and what happens beyond could become a barrier to hearing the client's feelings, concerns, anxieties, whatever is happening for him or her as they face death.'

'It's about getting to know the person, really getting to know them, what they think, feel, what's really them, what's present in their experience as you sit with them.' Nicola paused as she thought of Barbara, of the last session and the telephone conversation. 'Barbara is out there now; she may be at home, in hospital, she may even have died, I don't know. I will know. I don't need to know at this moment. Maybe I don't want to hear that she has died. Hmm.' Another pause.

Mark sought to convey his understanding of what Nicola was saying, and feeling beneath the words. 'That sounds very present for you as you say that, not sure if you want to know, not sure because it may mean knowing she has died.' He spoke quietly and the room felt suddenly very quiet. Very quiet. It was Nicola who spoke first.

'I want her to be able to do the things she planned. They felt so important to her, the things that made her come alive as she thought about them. I want to hope that if she dies, well, no, that's not right. She may have to realise she is not going to be able to do them, but I hope that if that is the case she is able to accept that, and her memories are strong enough for her to feel good about that part of her life.' Nicola lapsed back into silence. It was strange, she felt sad and yet she felt somehow calm as well.

'Mhmm, you would want that for her.'

Nicola nodded. She felt the sadness growing inside her. She shook her head. 'Right from the start, from coming to counselling, it was all about her realising that she not only had needs, but that she had a right to try and meet those needs. How to find her own life, get her needs met within a family context that placed so many demands on her and within which she placed such demands on herself. It's like she was claiming her authority, no, I mean autonomy, well, maybe I mean both.'

'Authority and autonomy.'

Nicola nodded. 'She was striving to grow beyond being a mother, if that makes sense, beyond feeling so responsible for two adult children who could so easily draw her into co-dependence, and did so. And that was where she had allowed herself to be, and, yes, contributed to keeping herself there as well. She was attempting to break free, and she was achieving this. And then the cancer, and yes, something about that doesn't seem fair. That's what it is. That's what saddens me.' Nicola felt more animated. 'Just as she begins to move on, life deals her another blow, as it were.'

'And it's that which seems so unfair, and which saddens you.'

'So much struggle, and for what?'

'Precisely. And immediately I say that I think of how, you know, maybe there is a purpose to it, somehow. I know some people see life as a journey, some a journey over many lives, a sort of "evolution of consciousness" approach. Personally, I'm not sure, but it does seem unfair for this to happen to her just as she was beginning to assert her needs, to turn that corner, to begin to start that process of breaking free from, well, from herself really.' Nicola was struck by a thought. She looked up at Mark, quite intently. 'Except . . .'.

'Except?'

'Except she didn't just get it, did she? She already had it, but was unaware of it.' Nicola paused again. The implications of what she was thinking and saying were making a strong impression on her. 'I wonder whether at some level, organismically I suppose, there would have been a kind of knowing that the cancer was present even though it was not something present in her consciousness. Could the urge to change have come from that organismic level where there was a knowing that the cancer was present?'

Mark nodded, not wishing to disturb Nicola's train of thought.

'Hmm, well, of course there is, it's the actualising tendency, isn't it! I just hadn't come at it from this sort of angle. OK, so what am I saying here? The actualising tendency, operating from a level where the presence of cancer is known, the organism knows it is under threat but this information isn't present in the conscious awareness of the person.' Nicola paused again, the implications of where her thoughts were taking her were becoming clearer. 'It's all linked! Realising she needed counselling, starting to change. At some deeper level the actualising tendency could have been urging her to change and maybe prepare herself to cope. Maybe that's not the best way of putting it, but something like that.'

Mark responded, seeking to help to clarify what Nicola was saying. It felt extremely important, a real sense of the livingness of the actualising tendency and its actual presence and influence. 'Listening to what you have been saying, I am left with a strong sense that for some people, that urge to make changes could be an outer expression of an inner knowing, though a knowing that is not in the person's awareness, that the organism is under serious threat. An inner experiencing of the threat is present that is beyond the edge of their awareness. And the urge to change, yes, as you say, maybe is part of the process preparing someone to cope. Or something like that.'

'Something like that.'

'It would make a fascinating study which could, in a sense, bring the notion of an actualising tendency more into the open. If it was shown that people tend to initiate a process of psychological, emotional or other kind of change when their body is affected by a life-threatening condition, but before they are aware of it.' Mark could see the implications. 'It would make so much sense.'

'As though, while we may not be aware of physiological processes, they nevertheless may trigger psychological processes and behaviour change even though the person remains unaware of the real, inner cause.'

Such a study of pre-death behaviour change would be extremely interesting. We are not consciously aware of everything that is occurring within our bodies, or indeed within our structure of self. We can communicate experiences without being aware of them – for instance body language that reflects anxiety when we are not experiencing anxiety in awareness. If we have a life-threatening disease then our bodies know this. The body will be trying to combat it at a physiological level. It will only be when some visible or experiential indicator enters awareness that we may be alerted that something is wrong – pain often being the first sign, though tiredness can be another factor and, as in this case pallor due to the impact of the cancer on the liver.

Both Mark and Nicola paused. It was Nicola who broke the silence. 'So it brings me back even more to trusting the client's process, and the timing of that process, and to my role as a person centred-counsellor to be a companion to them as that process works out. The inner wisdom, so to speak.'

Mark nodded. 'Put like that, yes, it feels quite awesome.'

The discussion and exploration had reached a high point. For Nicola there was a sense that whatever happened for Barbara, it would be OK. She still hoped that she would see her again and that she would get to do the things that she wanted, but she felt clearer in herself. It felt as though her sensitivity had been restored, she felt more open to herself. That was how she thought of it anyway.

The session drew to a close, and as Nicola left she was still very much affected by the thoughts and ideas that had come alive to her. And she thought of Monday, of Barbara. Yes, she did feel more open and accepting towards the situation, more trusting. Not trusting that something in particular would happen, but that what was happening was a trustworthy process. She knew she would dwell on it from time to time over the weekend, and wonder how Barbara was. But somehow she felt that she would be OK. She felt goose bumps up the back of her neck as she had that thought.

Monday morning

Nicola arrived early at the surgery. She was feeling anxious. There was a note from Barbara's doctor asking her to see her when she came in. She went round to the doctor's room; morning surgery had not yet begun.

'Ah, hello Nicola.' Doctor Adams had swivelled in her chair to face her.

Nicola nodded. She knew. She could see the expression on Dr Adams' face, but it had been her tone of voice more than anything. Her own eyes were watering and she could feel the lump forming in her throat.

'Barbara?'

Dr Adams nodded.

'When?'

'Friday afternoon, about 4 o'clock.'

At the end of my supervision session, Nicola thought.

'What happened?'

'Massive liver failure. She was in the right place, in hospital, but they couldn't save her. She'd become progressively more unwell and jaundiced.'
'She hadn't been a good colour for a while.'
'It worsened, and she was in so much pain. She had to go in. They probably got the pain more under control, but . . .'.
Nicola nodded, taking a deep breath as she did so.
'Well . . .,' Nicola realised she was smiling at the thought passing through her head, which was 'she knows now'. She explained to Dr Adams. 'She'd been talking about what happens after death and I just had the thought "she knows now", if there is anything to know.'
Dr Adams smiled back. 'Nice way to think about it.'
'Thanks for letting me know.' They exchanged a few more words before Nicola left for the counselling room. She stopped for a cup of water on the way and then went in and sat down. She wanted to dedicate a few moments to Barbara and collect her thoughts ahead of her first client. And she wanted to honour the time when she would have seen Barbara later that morning by thinking about her, and by appreciating that she had been part of Barbara's journey at the end of her life.

Points for discussion

- How are you left feeling? How would you prepare yourself for your next client in this situation? What issues might arise?
- Evaluate the counsellor's responding to her client during the telephone contact. Was it therapy, support, a conversation? Would you have responded differently?
- What effect might your thoughts/beliefs about death and what follows have on your work with clients facing death – their own, or of a loved one?
- What might make it difficult for you to warmly accept or empathise with a client in these circumstances?
- What was not addressed in the supervision session? Was the theoretical exploration a diversion, an avoidance or a timely process for both counsellor and supervisor?
- What would you now expect Nicola to take to supervision following the news of Barbara's death? Should she contact him soon, or leave it until their next booked appointment?
- Write notes for the telephone contact, and the supervision session from the perspective of Nicola.

Author's epilogue

It seems somehow appropriate that the theme of this book, death and dying, is addressed in what is expected to be the last of the 17 books in the English language *Living Therapy* series. And I am left wondering how much of my own beliefs have become entangled in the therapeutic processes described in this book. I guess it is inevitable. And, as with all the books, I am left wondering about Billy and Barbara, what happens to them, in life and in death.

It seems to me that working with people who are facing death or who have suffered bereavement, is to work with people who have been affected by not only the process of death, but the process of life. Death is the contrast that can make life seem more precious. Opposites, perhaps, and maybe that is the essence of the human story, coming to terms with opposites: pleasure and pain, loss and gain, life and death, happy and sad. They are all around us and within us.

What is the secret to coping with this reality? Perhaps to find a middle way, to neither run desperately towards one, nor to desperately avoid the other. For if opposites are inevitable and are a part of life, and, to quote from Kipling's 'If':

> If you can meet with Triumph and Disaster
> And treat those two impostors just the same;

then we may have a clue to a way forward. Yet it is easy to say 'find a middle way'. The reality is that death brings life into sharp relief, and life does the same to death. We want life, if it is a good experience for us, and to avoid death. Of course, for some, death is a welcome relief from the pain of life.

Faced with death, our own, or that of someone dear to us, we are affected. We do not know the truth of death. People have their own experiences, which shape what they believe to be the reality. Others follow what is given in spiritual or religious texts. Still others prefer to accept what science tells them. Are we brainbound beings, or is there more to the human being? Do we have one chance in this world, or is there more to it than that? For me, I try to imagine what an all-knowing, all-loving creator would do in creating a world and watching it develop. For such a God, all things would be possible, however difficult they may be for science to grasp. If there is a God, we can be sure his creation is greater than human thoughts, feeling and behaviour. What else is there for us still to discover, and what light may that cast on life and death, birth and dying?

Enough of speculation. When faced with a person, a fellow human being facing death or coming to terms with the death of a loved one, suffering fear, anxiety, depression, perhaps feeling very alone, the counsellor is called to listen very seriously and attend very sensitively to what their client is experiencing and communicating. It is the raw, human edge of life. We do have to have resolved our own issues, as best we can, about loss, death and dying – and we may never really appreciate how we feel about death until we face it for ourselves. The death of a loved one may not bring us to the place in ourselves where we look over that edge and discover in that moment what emerges within us. And clients may tug on it as they look over their edge. The counsellor needs supportive supervision both to enable them to release their own emotions, and also to explore their own thinking and reactions. The counsellor needs to be able to return to the therapy room openly available once more to their client, able to peer over the edge of life (or rather the edge of death) with their perhaps terrified client and be their companion as they try to come to terms with what they perceive, what they experience, what they may feel themselves instinctively shrinking back from.

For some, death is to be feared; for others, it is another step on a path; and for a few, it may be regarded as a great adventure. However our clients view death, as counsellors we are required to see it through their eyes and to share in whatever emerges for them as they seek to come to terms with what it arouses in them.

Some may say that death and dying are perhaps the hardest of issues to deal with. Perhaps. When I wrote *Counselling Victims of Warfare*, it was not so much the death but the manner of it that marked it as atrocity, the impact that one human being can have on another. That was a painful book to write. As was this one. And yet looking back, most of the *Living Therapy* series has dealt with pain of one kind or another. And in many of them that pain has been the result of the actions of others, of the impact of destructive and damaging human relationships.

The fact is that relationships can damage and relationships can heal. The person-centred counsellor strives to offer a healing relationship, not to take the pain away. Pain can be a symptom of the healing process, and certainly a sign that something is wrong and needs attention.

Reading this book may have caused you pain. It may have contributed to your encountering feelings and thoughts that are uncomfortable. I hope that this book and the effect that it has does bring self-insight and greater understanding of the role of the person-centred counsellor or therapist when working with clients who are addressing the issues of death and dying. I am sure I have not touched on all of the issues. I have not tried to write the definitive person-centred perspective on death and dying, or on working with clients affected by the death of others or their own process of dying. But I hope this has been an experiential read, a book to be read not just from the head but also from the heart. It seems to me that for many people, the empathic counsellor offering warm acceptance and unconditional positive regard, and providing a genuinely authentic and congruence presence, is offering qualities of the heart. Perhaps heartfelt listening and understanding are as precious as life itself.

I wish to end with some references to Carl Rogers' ideas about death and dying. These are his personal views and I have left them to the end because these views are not to be considered as the person-centred view of death and dying. They remain controversial within the person-centred movement. However, they show us his changing thoughts in the light of his own experiences.

Writing in a section entitled 'Growing old: or older and growing' published in *A Way of Being* (Rogers 1980, pp. 87–8) within the last decade of his life, Rogers wrote:

And then there is the ending of life. It may surprise you that at my age I think very little about death. The current popular interest in it surprises me.

Ten or fifteen years ago I felt quite certain that death was the total end of the person. I still regard that as the most likely prospect; however, it does not seem to me a tragic or awful prospect. I have been able to *live* my life – not to the full, certainly, but with a satisfying degree of fullness – and it seems natural that my life should come to an end. I already have a degree of immortality in other persons. I have sometimes said that, psychologically, I have strong sons and daughters all over the world. Also, I believe that the ideas and the ways of being that I and others have helped to develop will continue, for some time at least. So if I, as an individual, come to a complete and final end, aspects of me will still live on in a variety of growing ways, and that is a pleasant thought.

I think that no one can know whether he or she fears death until it arrives. Certainly, death is the ultimate leap in the dark, and I think it is highly probable that the apprehension I feel when going under an anaesthetic will be duplicated or increased when I face death. Yet I don't experience a really deep fear of this process. So far as I am aware, my fears concerning death relate to its circumstances. I have a dread of any long and painful illness leading to death. I dread the thought of senility or of partial brain damage due to a stroke. My preference would be to die quickly, before it is too late to die with dignity . . .

My belief that death is the end has, however, been modified by some of my learnings of the past decade. I am impressed with the accounts of Raymond Moody (1975) of the experience of persons who have been so near death as to be declared dead, but who have come back to life. I am impressed by some of the reports of reincarnation, although reincarnation seems a very dubious blessing indeed. I am interested in the work of Elisabeth Kübler-Ross and the conclusions she has reached about life after death. I find definitely appealing the views of Arthur Koestler that individual consciousness is but a fragment of a cosmic consciousness, the fragment being reabsorbed into the whole upon the death of the individual. I like his analogy of the individual river eventually flowing into the tidal waters of the ocean, dropping its muddy silt as it enters the boundless sea.

So I consider death with, I believe, an openness to the experience. It will be what it will be, and I trust I can accept it as either an end to, or a continuation of life.

Although published in 1980, the above was written in 1977, and Rogers updated his thoughts in 1979. This followed the death of his wife and particular experiences that he had at the time which led him to state the following. Again, I wish to emphasise that this is his personal view:

> All these experiences, so briefly suggested rather than described, have made me more open to the possibility of the continuation of the individual human spirit, something I had never before believed possible. These experiences have left me very much interested in all types of paranormal phenomena. They have quite changed my understanding of the process of dying. I now consider it possible that each of us is a continuing spiritual essence lasting over time, and occasionally incarnated in a human body. (Rogers, 1980, pp. 92–3)

If he is right, then his words provide us with the basis for a revolution in our Western, science-based psychological understanding of the structure of self, the nature of consciousness and, of course, the purpose of, and context for, counselling for death and dying.

References

Anderson C and Wilkie P (1992) *Reflective Helping in HIV and AIDS*. Oxford University Press, Buckingham.

Bozarth J (1998) *Person-Centred Therapy: a revolutionary paradigm*. PCCS Books, Ross-on-Wye.

Bozarth J and Wilkins P (eds) (2001) *Rogers' Therapeutic Conditions: evolution, theory and practice. Volume 3: Unconditional Positive Regard*. PCCS Books, Ross-on-Wye.

Bryant-Jefferies R (2006) *A Little Book of Therapy*. Pen Press, Brighton.

Bryant-Jefferies R (2001) *Counselling the Person Beyond the Alcohol Problem*. Jessica Kingsley, London.

Bryant-Jefferies R (2003a) *Time Limited Therapy in Primary Care: a person-centred dialogue*. Radcliffe Publishing, Oxford.

Bryant-Jefferies R (2003b) *Problem Drinking: a person-centred dialogue*. Radcliffe Publishing, Oxford.

Bryant-Jefferies R (2005) *Counselling Victims of Warfare*. Radcliffe Publishing, Oxford.

Bryant-Jefferies R (2006) *Counselling Young Binge Drinkers: person-centred dialogues*. Radcliffe Publishing, Oxford.

Cooper M (2004) Towards a relationally-orientated approach to therapy: empirical support and analysis. *British Journal of Guidance and Counselling*. 32(4): 451–60.

Embleton Tudor L, Keemar K, Tudor K, Valentine J and Worrall M (2004) *The Person-Centered Approach: a contemporary introduction*. Palgrave MacMillan, Basingstoke.

Evans R (1975) *Carl Rogers: the man and his ideas*. Dutton and Co, New York.

Gaylin N (2001) *Family, Self and Psychotherapy: a person-centred perspective*. PCCS Books, Ross-on-Wye.

Green J and Sherr L (1989) Dying, bereavement and loss. In: Green J and McCreamer M (eds) *Counselling in HIV Infection and AIDS*, pp. 207–23. Blackwell Scientific Publications, Oxford.

Haugh S and Merry T (eds) (2001) *Rogers' Therapeutic Conditions: evolution, theory and practice. Volume 2: Empathy*. PCCS Books, Ross-on-Wye.

Kirschenbaum, H (2005) The current status of Carl Rogers and the person-centered approach. *Psychotherapy*. 42(1): 37–51.

Levitt BE (2005) *Embracing Non-Directivity: reassessing person-centred theory and practice for the 21st century*. PCCS Books, Ross-on-Wye.

Lynott P and Moore G (1979) Sarah. From the album *Black Rose*. Mercury Records, London.

Mearns D and Thorne B (1988) *Person-Centred Counselling in Action*. Sage, London.

Mearns D and Thorne B (1999) *Person-Centred Counselling in Action* (2e). Sage, London.

Mearns D and Thorne B (2000) *Person-Centred Therapy Today*. Sage, London.

Mearns D and Cooper M (2005) *Working at Relational Depth in Counselling and Psychotherapy*. Sage, London.

Merry T (2001) Congruence and the supervision of client-centred therapists. In: Wyatt G (ed.) *Rogers' Therapeutic Conditions: evolution theory and practice. Volume 1: Congruence*, pp. 174–83. PCCS Books, Ross-on-Wye.

Merry T (2002) *Learning and Being in Person-Centred Counselling* (2e). PCCS Books, Ross-on-Wye.

Moody RA (1975) *Life After Life*. Bantam Books, New York.

Moore G with Lynott P (1985) *Out in the Fields*. 10 Records. Exclusively licensed to Mercury Records, London.

Natiello P (2001) *The Person-centred Approach: A passionate presence*. PCCS Books, Ross-on-Wye.

Norcross JC (2002) Empirically supported therapy relationships. In: Norcross JC (ed.) *Psychotherapy Relationships that Work: therapist contributions and responsiveness to patients*. Oxford University Press, Oxford.

Patterson (2000) *Understanding Psychotherapy: fifty years of client-centred theory and practice*. PCCS Books, Ross-on-Wye.

Rogers CR (1942) *Counselling and Psychotherapy: newer concepts in practice*. Houghton Mifflin, Boston, MA.

Rogers CR (1951) *Client Centred Therapy*. Constable, London.

Rogers CR (1957) The necessary and sufficient conditions of therapeutic personality change. *Journal of Consulting Psychology*. **21**: 95–103.

Rogers CR (1959) A theory of therapy, personality and interpersonal relationships as developed in the client-centred framework. In: Koch S (ed) *Psychology: a study of a science. Volume 3: Formulations of the person and the social context*, pp. 185–246. McGraw-Hill, New York.

Rogers, CR (1967) *On Becoming a Person*. Constable, London. (Originally published in 1961)

Rogers CR (1980) *A Way of Being*. Houghton-Mifflin Company, Boston. MA.

Rogers CR (1986) A client-centered/person-centered approach to therapy. In: Kutash I and Wolfe A (eds) *Psychotherapists' Casebook*, pp. 236–57. Jossey Bass, New York.

Sanders P (2000) Mapping person-centred approaches to counselling and psychotherapy. *Person-Centred Practice*. **8**(2): 62–74.

Steering Committee (2002) Empirically supported therapy relationships: conclusions and recommendations on the Division 29 task force. In: Norcross JC (ed.) *Psychotherapy Relationships that Work: therapist contributions and responsiveness to patients*, pp. 441–3. Oxford University Press, Oxford.

Tudor K and Worrall M (2004) *Freedom to Practise: person-centred approaches to supervision*. PCCS Books, Ross-on-Wye.

Vincent S (2005) *Being Empathic*. Radcliffe Publishing, Oxford.

Warner MS (2000) Person-centred psychotherapy: One nation, many tribes. *The Person-Centred Journal.* 7(1): 28–39.

Warner MS (2002) Psychological contact, meaningful process and human nature. In: Wyatt G and Sanders P (eds) *Rogers' Therapeutic Conditions: evolution, theory and practice. Volume 4: Contact and perception*, pp. 76–95. PCCS Books, Ross-on-Wye.

Wilkins P (2003) *Person Centred Therapy in Focus*. Sage, London.

Wyatt G (ed.) (2001) *Rogers' Therapeutic Conditions: evolution, theory and practice. Volume 1: Congruence*. PCCS Books, Ross-on-Wye.

Wyatt G and Sanders P (eds) (2002) *Rogers' Therapeutic Conditions: evolution, theory and practice. Volume 4: Contact and perception*. PCCS Books, Ross-on-Wye.

Contacts

Bereavement

Cruse Bereavement Care

Cruse Bereavement Care exists to promote the well being of bereaved people and to enable anyone bereaved by death to understand their grief and cope with their loss. The organisation provides counselling and support. It offers information, advice, education and training services.

Day by Day Helpline 0870 167 1677
Young Person's Helpline freephone 0808 808 1677
Email: helpline@crusebereavementcare.org.uk
General Email: info@crusebereavementcare.org.uk
Website: www.crusebereavementcare.org.uk

Central Office:
Cruse Bereavement Care
Cruse House, 126 Sheen Road
Richmond, Surrey
TW9 1UR
Administration Tel: 020 8939 9530
Fax: 020 8940 7638

Northern Ireland Regional Office
Piney Ridge, Knockbracken Healthcare Park
Saintfield Road
Belfast BT8 8BH.
Tel: 028 90 792419
Email: northern.ireland@cruse.org.uk

Cruse Bereavement Care Cymru
Ty Energlyn, Heol Las
Caerphilly/Caerffili
CF83 2TT
Tel: 029 2088 6913
Email: cruse.cymru@care4free.net

Cruse Bereavement Care Scotland – National Office
Riverview House
Friarton Road
Perth, PH2 8DF
Tel: 01738 444178
Email: info@crusescotland.org.uk
Website: www.crusescotland.org.uk

Person-centred

Association for the Development of the Person-Centered Approach (ADPCA)
Email: adpca-web@signs.portents.com
Website: www.adpca.org

An international association, with members in 27 countries, for those interested in the development of client-centred therapy and the person-centred approach.

British Association for the Person-Centred Approach (BAPCA)
Bm-BAPCA
London WC1N 3XX
Tel: 01989 770948
Email: info@bapca.org.uk
Website: www.bapca.org.uk

National association promoting the person-centred approach. Publishes a regular magazine, *Person-Centred Quarterly*, and promotes awareness of person-centred events and issues in the UK.

Person Centred Therapy Scotland
Tel: 0870 7650871
Email: info@pctscotland.co.uk
Website: www.pctscotland.co.uk

An association of person-centred therapists in Scotland which offers training and networking opportunities to members with the aim of fostering high standards of professional practice.

World Association for Person-Centered and Experiential Psychotherapy and Counselling
Email: secretariat@pce-world.org
Website: www.pce-world.org

Aims to provide a worldwide forum for those professionals in science and practice who are committed to, and embody in their work, the theoretical principles of the person-centred approach first postulated by Carl Rogers. Publishes *Person Centred and Experiential Therapies,* an international journal which 'creates a dialogue among different parts of the person-centred/experiential therapy tradition, supporting, informing and challenging academics and practitioners with the aim of the development of these approaches in a broad professional, scientific and political context'.

Index

Ramses

The Temple of a Million Years

Ramses

The Temple of a Million Years

Christian Jacq

Translated by Mary Feeney

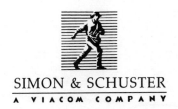

SIMON & SCHUSTER
A VIACOM COMPANY

First published in Great Britain by Simon & Schuster Ltd, 1998
A Viacom Company

Simon & Schuster Ltd
West Garden Place
Kendal Street
London W2 2AQ

Simon & Schuster Australia
Sydney

A CIP catalogue record for this book is available
from the British Library

ISBN 0-684-821-206

Typeset in Times 12/14pt by
Palimpsest Book Production Limited, Polmont, Stirlingshire
Printed and bound in Great Britain by
The Bath Press, Bath

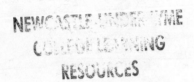

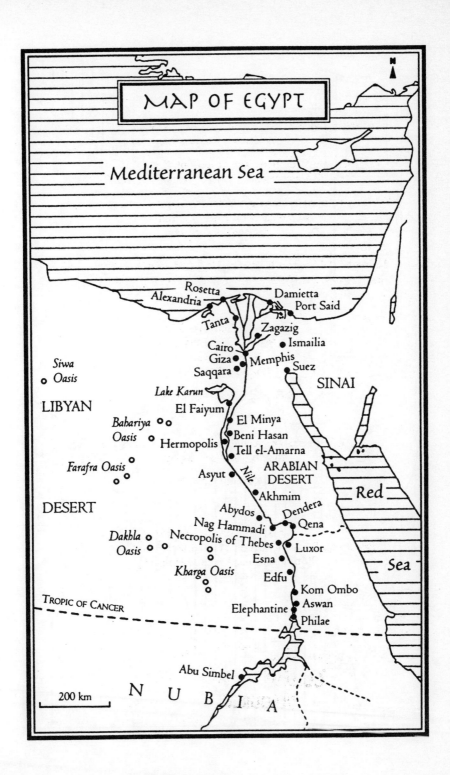

MAP OF EGYPT

Mediterranean Sea

Rosetta
Alexandria
Damietta
Port Said
Tanta
Zagazig
Cairo
Ismailia
Giza
Memphis
Saqqara
Suez
Siwa
Oasis
SINAI
Lake Karun
LIBYAN
El Faiyum
El Minya
Bahariya
Oasis
Beni Hasan
Hermopolis
Tell el-Amarna
Farafra Oasis
Asyut
Nile
ARABIAN
DESERT
Akhmim
Red
DESERT
Abydos
Dendera
Nag Hammadi
Qena
Dakhla
Necropolis of Thebes
Oasis
Luxor
Esna
Sea
Kharga Oasis
Edfu
Kom Ombo
TROPIC OF CANCER
Elephantine
Aswan
Philae

Abu Simbel
N U B I A
200 km

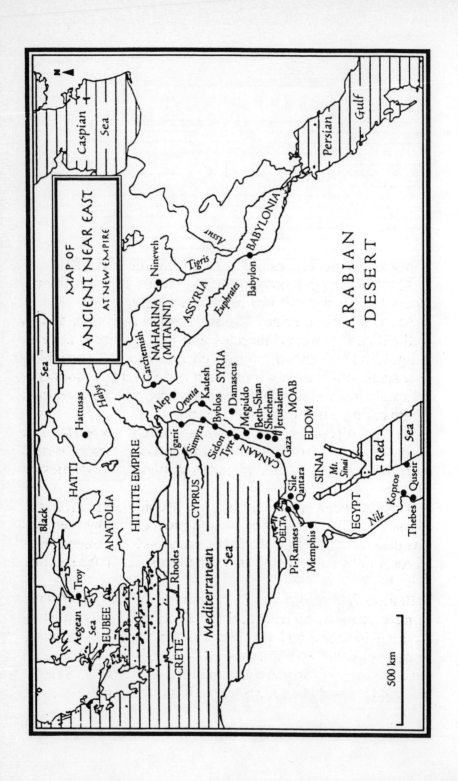

MAP OF
ANCIENT NEAR EAST
AT NEW EMPIRE

Caspian Sea

Black Sea

HATTI

ANATOLIA

HITTITE EMPIRE

Hattusas

Troy

Aegean Sea

EUBEE

Rhodes

CRETE

Mediterranean Sea

CYPRUS

Halys

Carchemish

NAHARINA
(MITANNI)

Nineveh

ASSYRIA

Assur

Tigris

Euphrates

Babylon

BABYLONIA

Persian Gulf

ARABIAN DESERT

Alep

Orontes

Kadesh

Byblos

Sidon

Tyre

Ugarit

Simyra

SYRIA

Damascus

Megiddo

Beth-Shan

Shechem

Jerusalem

MOAB

Gaza

CANAAN

EDOM

Sile

Qantara

DELTA

Pi-Ramses

Memphis

EGYPT

SINAI

Mt.
Sinai

Red Sea

Nile

Koptos

Thebes

Quseir

500 km

1

Ramses was alone, awaiting a sign from the Invisible.

Alone, facing the vast scorched stretches of desert. Alone, facing the destiny still just beyond his grasp.

At twenty-three, Prince Ramses was tall and athletic, with well-defined, powerful muscles and a magnificent head of red-gold hair. A broad, high forehead, thick brows arching over small, bright eyes, a long, slightly hooked nose, rounded, delicately lobed ears, full lips and a strong chin added up to a commanding, attractive countenance.

He had already been through so much – younger son of Pharaoh Seti, royal scribe, army officer, finally named co-regent by his father and initiated into the mysteries of Abydos.

Seti had been a great ruler, an irreplaceable sovereign whose reign had brought peace and prosperity. But now Seti was dead after fifteen remarkable years on the throne, fifteen all-too-brief years which had flown like an ibis in the summer twilight.

Ramses had at first not even been aware that his distant, demanding, awe-inspiring father was gradually grooming him for kingship. Seti had put him through several demanding tests, beginning with a face-to-face encounter with a wild bull, the symbol of pharaonic power. At fourteen, Ramses had had the courage to confront the beast, but not the strength to overcome it. He would have been gored to death if Seti hadn't roped the charging bull, leaving Ramses indelibly impressed with the understanding of a pharaoh's first duty: protecting the weak.

The king alone held the key to true power. Through the magic of experience, he communicated it to Ramses, stage by stage, without revealing his master plan. Over the years, father and son had grown closer, united in faith and purpose. Reserved, unbending, Seti was a man of few words, but he had granted Ramses the unique privilege of long conversations, in the course of which he did all he could to pass on to Ramses a thorough grounding in the skills of the kingship of Upper and Lower Egypt.

Those golden hours, those blessed moments, had now vanished into the silence of death.

Pharaoh's words had poured like a blessed elixir into Ramses' heart, where they were stored as precious treasure, infusing his thoughts and actions. But Seti had departed, gone to commune with his fellow gods, and Ramses was alone, bereft of his father's guiding presence.

He felt defenceless, unable to bear the weight thrust upon his young shoulders. To govern Egypt . . . at thirteen it had been his dream, a childish longing for a prize that could never be his. Convinced that his elder brother, Shaanar, was his father's chosen successor, he had finally surrendered the foolish notion.

But Pharaoh Seti and Tuya, the Great Royal Wife, had decided otherwise. After observing the conduct of their two sons, their choice had fallen on Ramses. Why hadn't they found someone stronger and abler, someone as great as Seti? Ramses felt prepared to meet any challenger face to face, but not to steer the ship of state through the uncertain waters of the future. He had proven himself in combat, campaigning with Seti in Nubia; his boundless energy would see him through a war in defence of his country, if the need arose; but he had

2

no idea how to command an army of bureaucrats, dignitaries and priests, all of whom could outmanoeuvre him.

The founder of their dynasty, the first Ramses, had been an elderly vizier, who had become pharaoh only reluctantly. When Seti inherited the throne, he was mature and experienced. Ramses had been content to live in his father's shadow, following his directives and responding to the least of his demands. It had been wonderful to have a trusted guide. To work under Seti's orders, to serve Egypt by obeying the pharaoh, to have him available with the answer to every question – a paradise now lost.

Now fate had unfairly dictated that Ramses, a spirited, even rash, young man, should take Seti's place. It might be better if he fled, laughing, so far into the desert that no one would ever find him.

Of course, he could count on his supporters: his mother, Tuya, an exacting and faithful ally; Nefertari, his beautiful, calm young wife; and his four boyhood friends. Moses, the Hebrew, now supervised royal construction projects; Ahsha was in the diplomatic corps; Setau was a snake-charmer; Ahmeni had devoted his life to Ramses as his private secretary and sandal-bearer.

However, he could count far more enemies. Shaanar had still not given up on claiming the throne for himself. It was anyone's guess what plots he was currently hatching. If Shaanar appeared before him this very instant, Ramses would offer no resistance. His brother might as well wear the double crown if he coveted it so desperately.

But did Ramses have the right to betray his father and abdicate the responsibility with which he had been entrusted? It would be so simple to conclude that Seti had been mistaken, that in the end he might have changed his mind. Ramses would not lie to himself. His fate depended on the answer he received from the Invisible.

It was here, in the desert, the heart of this 'red land'

3

charged with a dangerous energy, that the answer would come to him.

Sitting cross-legged in the classic scribe's pose, Ramses waited. The vast and solitary desert was the place for a pharaoh. The rocks and sand harboured a fire that would either strengthen his soul or break him. Let the fire pass judgment!

The sun approached its zenith, the wind died down. A gazelle leaped from dune to dune. Danger was near.

It came out of nowhere: an enormous lion, twice as big as a normal specimen. Its blazing mane gave it the air of a triumphant warrior; its sleek dark-brown body rippled with muscles.

At the sight of Ramses, it loosed a fearful roar that echoed far into the distance. Teeth flashing, claws bared, the big cat studied its prey.

Seti's son had no way to escape him.

The lion came closer, then stopped a few yards from Ramses, who noted its golden eyes. For a few seconds, they stared challengingly at each other.

Flicking its tail at a fly, the lion loped forward, suddenly tense.

Ramses rose to his feet, still staring hard.

'Invincible, it's you. Come, boy. I saved your life. What do you intend to do to me?'

Forgetting the danger, Ramses remembered plucking the baby lion from the brush as his army left Nubia. His remarkable constitution had allowed him to survive a snakebite. Cured by Setau's remedies, the cub grew to colossal proportions as Ramses' pet.

For the first time, Invincible had escaped from the pen where he was kept in his master's absence. Reverting to the wild, he was ready to pounce on the man who had raised him.

'It's up to you, boy. Fight at my side for life, or kill me now.'

The lion reared on his hind legs and set his paws on Ramses' shoulders, nearly knocking him over. The prince held steady. Invincible's claws retracted. He sniffed Ramses' face. There was friendship, trust and respect between them.

'You've sealed my fate, boy.'

There was no longer any choice for the young man Seti had named 'Son of the Light'.

He would fight like a lion.

2

In Memphis, the palace was deep in mourning. Men stopped shaving, women wore their hair down. The mummification process took seventy days, and during that time the country was in limbo. The king was dead. The throne remained vacant until his successor was officially proclaimed, which could happen only after Seti was entombed and his mummy united with the heavenly light.

The frontier posts were on alert, troops ready to check any attempted invasion, at the order of the Regent and the Great Royal Wife, Tuya. The principal threat was from the Hittites, to the north in Asia Minor. While there appeared to be no imminent danger, a surprise attack was always possible. For centuries, the rich agricultural provinces of Egypt's Delta had been tempting prey for the 'sand-runners', the nomadic Bedu of the Sinai desert, as well as Asian princes who occasionally managed to form coalitions and storm the north-eastern border.

Seti's departure for the Land of the West was cause for alarm. Whenever a pharaoh passed away, the forces of chaos threatened to engulf Egypt, destroying a civilization that had lasted through eighteen dynasties. Would young Ramses be able to keep the Two Lands safe from danger? Some of the notables were less than sure he could and wished he would step aside in favour of Shaanar, his less rash and craftier brother.

The Great Royal Wife, Tuya, had not changed her habits since Seti's death. She was forty-two years old, slender and regal, with a fine, straight nose, piercing almond eyes, and a nearly square jaw – and her moral authority was unquestionable. She had always been Seti's full partner; when he was forced to leave the country on state business, it was she who ruled Egypt, and ruled it firmly.

At daybreak, Tuya liked to stroll briefly in her garden, among the tamarisk and sycamore trees, organizing her working day as she walked. Her time was divided between secular and religious duties.

With Seti gone, all her activity seemed devoid of meaning. Tuya's sole desire was to join her husband in a world without conflict, far from the vanity of men; yet she was resigned to serving out her time on earth. Great happiness had been hers. She must repay her country by serving until she drew her last breath.

Nefertari's elegant silhouette emerged from the morning mist. 'More beautiful than the palace beauties', as the common folk said, Ramses' wife had shiny black hair and sublime blue-green eyes. An accomplished musician who played at the goddess Hathor's temple in Memphis, a gifted weaver, educated in literature (including her husband's favourite, the sage Ptah-hotep), Nefertari was not of noble birth; but Ramses had fallen madly in love with her, with her beauty, intelligence and unusual maturity for her age. Nefertari never sought to charm, yet she was charm itself. Tuya had recruited the girl to oversee her household, a position Nefertari continued to fill even after her marriage to the Regent. The two women were very close, almost reading each other's thoughts.

'The dew is thick this morning, Majesty. A blessing on our fair land.'

'Why are you up so early, Nefertari?'

'You're the one who needs rest, don't you think?'

'I can't sleep any more.'

'What can we do to ease your pain, Majesty?'

A sad smile fluttered on Tuya's lips. 'Seti is irreplaceable. The rest of my life will be bearable only if Ramses prospers in his reign. The thought of it is all that keeps me going.'

'I'm worried, Majesty.'

'Tell me what you fear.'

'That Seti's wishes will not be respected.'

'Who would dare go against them?'

Nefertari remained silent.

'You're thinking of Shaanar aren't you? I know he's vain and ambitious, but he would never be so foolish as to defy his father's will.' The soft gold of dawn began to light the queen's garden. 'Do you think I'm naive, Nefertari? You don't seem to share my opinion.'

'Majesty . . .'

'Has something happened to . . . ?'

'No, it's only a feeling.'

'Daughter, you're intuitive and quick as lightning. I know you never speak ill of others. But at this point nothing can stop Ramses from being crowned, short of killing him.'

'That's exactly what I fear, Majesty.'

Tuya stroked the branch of a tamarisk. 'Would Shaanar resort to murder as his stepping stone to power?'

'I hate the idea as much as you do, but I can't get it out of my mind. You may think I'm a fool and tell me it's all in my imagination. Even so, I had to say something.'

'What security measures has Ramses taken?'

'His lion and watchdog are always on duty, along with Serramanna, the head of his personal bodyguard. Since he came back from the desert, I've managed to convince him of the need for constant protection.'

'We're only ten days into the mourning period. In two months, Seti's body will be placed in his tomb, preserved for eternity. Then Ramses will be crowned and you will become Queen of Egypt.'

Ramses bowed to his mother, then pressed her tenderly to him. Seemingly so fragile, she was a lesson in dignity and nobility.

'Why has God put us to such a cruel test?' he asked.

'Seti's spirit lives on in you, my son. His time is over, yours is beginning. He will never die if you continue his work.'

'His shadow dwarfs me.'

'You, the Son of the Light? You must dispel the darkness around us, overcome the chaos that looms around us.'

The young man pulled away from his mother. 'My lion was loose in the desert. He approached me as a friend.'

'That's the sign you were hoping for, isn't it?'

'Definitely, but may I ask you a favour?'

Tuya inclined her head in acquiescence.

'Whenever my father went abroad, it was you who ruled.'

'Yes, according to tradition.'

'You have experience. You have everyone's respect and admiration. What keeps you from succeeding him now?'

'You know that was not Seti's wish. He embodied the law we must all try to follow. *You* are the one he chose, my son, and you must succeed him. I'll help all I can and advise when you ask.'

Ramses did not press her. His mother was the only person who could alter his destiny and lift this burden from him, but she would never swerve from the course her late husband had set. Despite his misgivings, Ramses would have to make his own way.

Serramanna, Ramses' Sardinian bodyguard, stuck close to the king-to-be, never leaving his wing of the royal palace. Naming the former pirate to this prestigious position had been a controversial move. Some were convinced that sooner or later the mustachioed giant would turn on Seti's son.

For the time being, no one entered the palace without his permission. The Great Royal Wife had urged him to send unauthorised visitors packing and to feel free to use his sword if danger threatened.

Hearing distant shouts, Serramanna hurried towards the entry.

'What's going on here?'

'This one was trying to force his way in,' replied a guard, gesturing towards a tall, broad-shouldered man with flowing hair.

'Who are you?' challenged Serramanna.

'Moses the Hebrew, royal construction supervisor and friend of the prince.'

'What do you want?'

'Ramses never refuses to see me.'

'Today I'm the one who'll decide.'

'Is he in seclusion?'

'Security measures. State the reason for your visit.'

'None of your business.'

'Then you'd better leave and stay away from here, or I'll have you thrown in jail.'

It took no fewer than four guards to restrain Moses.

'Tell Ramses I'm here, or he'll have your hide!'

'Your threats don't scare me.'

'Listen, you idiot! My friend is expecting me. Go and ask Ramses.'

Years as a pirate captain and scores of fierce battles had honed Serramanna's ability to read situations. Despite this Hebrew's muscle and swagger, he seemed to be genuine.

Ramses and Moses embraced.

'Is this a palace or a fortress?' Moses asked.

'My mother, my wife, Ahmeni and Serramanna all fear the worst.'

'What is that supposed to mean?'

'An attempt on my life.'

The Regent's audience chamber looked out on the gardens. In the doorway, his huge pet lion dozed, with Wideawake, the golden-yellow dog, curled between his front paws.

'With them to guard you, you ought to feel safe enough.'

'Nefertari is convinced that Shaanar still thinks he should be king.'

'A coup before your father's laid to rest? Hardly his style. He likes to work away in the background and bank on making his move at the right time.'

'He's running out of time.'

'You're right. But he won't risk a confrontation.'

'God forbid! It would only bring harm to Egypt. What do you hear at Karnak?'

'Opinion is running against you.'

Moses had been running Seti's vast construction site at Karnak, where the royal architects had been instructed to add a huge Hall of Pillars to the temple. The pharaoh's death had brought the work to a halt.

'Whose opinion?'

'The priesthood of Amon, some nobles, the Vizier of the South . . . Your sister Dolora and her husband Sary have stirred them up. They didn't take kindly to being exiled from Memphis.'

'Sary tried to have me and Ahmeni killed. He and my sister could have faced a much stiffer punishment than being sent to Thebes.'

'The southern sun did nothing to dry up their poison. You should have banished them from Egypt once and for all.'

'Dolora is my sister. Sary practically raised me.'

'Should a king have different standards for his relatives?'

Ramses was cut to the quick. 'I'm not king yet, Moses.'

'I still think you should have let justice take its course.'

'If the two of them pull any more tricks, I'll show no mercy.'

'I wish I believed you. You don't realize how ruthless your enemies can be.'

'Right now I'm grieving for my father.'

'And forgetting your duty to your country. If Seti is looking down from heaven, do you think he approves of your feebleness?'

If Moses hadn't been his best friend, Ramses would have hit him.

'You want me to be hard and impersonal?'

'You've suffered a great loss, but keep your eyes open. Shaanar approached me, even knowing how close to you I am. He tried to turn me against you. Does that give you some sense of the danger you're in?'

Ramses was speechless.

'You're facing a tough opponent,' Moses continued. 'Wake up, my friend.'

3

Memphis, situated where the Nile Valley began branching out into the Delta, was the country's economic capital. Now it slumbered. In the harbour, called 'Safe Journey', merchant ships stayed in their moorings. For the seventy-day mourning period, trade was suspended, and the nobles stopped entertaining.

Seti's death had sent the town into a state of shock. His reign had brought increased prosperity, but the most prominent businessmen feared that the trend would be reversed under an irresolute pharaoh who made Egypt vulnerable and weak. And who could be strong as Seti? Shaanar, his elder son, would run the country capably, but the ailing Seti had favoured the young and fiery Ramses, who seemed more like a wastrel than a head of state. The most clear-sighted of leaders could make mistakes, the businessmen reasoned, and Memphis quietly agreed with Thebes that Seti might have chosen the wrong son to succeed him.

Shaanar restlessly paced Meba's receiving-room. A fit-looking man of sixty with a broad, calm face, Meba was Seti's long-time minister for foreign affairs. He had secretly worked against Ramses, supporting Shaanar, whose political and economic views more closely resembled his own. Opening the Mediterranean and Asian markets, strengthening commercial ties, was the way to a healthy economic future,

13

even if it meant forgetting a few traditional principles. After all, he felt, the arms trade was preferable to armed conflict.

'Will he come?' asked Shaanar.

'He's on our side, rest assured.'

'That could change at any moment. You can't trust a bully.'

Seti's elder son was short, stocky and overweight, with a round face and plump cheeks. His thick, sensual lips betrayed his love of good food, while his dark, beady eyes were perpetually nervous. He avoided the sun and all forms of exertion. A cultivated voice failed to mask his uneven temper.

Shaanar was a pacifist for financial reasons. Egypt's economic isolationism was folly, in his opinion. 'Treason' was a term for moralizers without a nose for profit. Ramses, brought up in the old ways, didn't deserve to be king – and was unfit to be. Shaanar had no compunction about fomenting the plot that would bring him to power: Egypt would thank him for it.

But he still needed his most important ally.

'A drink,' Shaanar demanded. Meba served his illustrious guest a cup of cool beer. 'We never should have trusted him,' said the prince.

'I'm sure he'll come. Don't forget how eager he is to get home.'

At last, the minister's door-keeper announced the long-awaited caller.

Blond, sharp-eyed Menelaus, son of Atreus and King of Sparta, was lucky in war. He wore a double cuirasse and a wide belt with golden buckles that had served him well in the victory over Troy. With his fleet in tatters, he had sought refuge in Egypt. Now his wife, Helen, refused to leave the land of the pharaohs, fearing bitter treatment from her husband once they reached home. Since Queen Tuya had taken Helen under her wing, Menelaus was unable to coerce his wife. Fortunately, Shaanar had stepped in to enlist

14

his cooperation in overthrowing Ramses, promising to hand over Helen in return. The moment Shaanar became pharaoh, Menelaus would be able to leave for Greece with Helen.

For several months, his troops had settled in, the officers joining the Egyptian army, the soldiers and sailors finding ways to make a living, all seeming content with their good fortune. In reality, they anxiously awaited their commander's order to spring into action, like a new and improved Trojan Horse.

The Greek eyed Meba suspiciously. 'Tell him to leave,' he ordered Shaanar. 'You and I talk, no one else.'

'The minister is one of us.'

'Don't make me repeat myself.'

Shaanar waved the older man out of the room.

'Where do we stand?' asked Menelaus.

'It's time to act.'

'Are you sure? This infernal mummy-making takes so long I'm beginning to wonder about you people.'

'We need to act before my father's mummy is laid in his tomb.'

'My men are ready.'

'I don't want any unnecessary violence or . . .' Shaanar hesitated.

'Out with it, man! You Egyptians are afraid of a good fight. We Greeks kept after the Trojans for years until we destroyed them. If you want Ramses dead, say so. My sword will do the rest.'

'Ramses is my brother, and sometimes deceit is more effective than brute force.'

'They go hand in hand. And who are you to be lecturing me, a hero of the Trojan wars, on strategy?'

'You need to win Helen back.'

'Helen!' he spat. 'The woman makes me sick, but I can't go home without her.'

'Then let's try my plan.'

'What is your plan?'

Shaanar smiled. Luck was with him this time. With the Greek's help, it would work. 'Only two things stand in our way: the lion and Serramanna. We'll poison the first and cut down the second. Then we capture Ramses and you carry him off to Greece.'

'Why not just kill him?'

'I don't want blood on my hands when I take the throne. The official story will be that Ramses renounced his claim and decided to see the world. Unfortunately, a tragic accident will occur during his travels.'

'What about Helen?'

'Once I'm crowned, my mother will have to obey my orders and stop protecting her. If Tuya resists, she'll be placed under house arrest in a temple.'

Menelaus nodded. 'Not bad, for an Egyptian. Do you have the poison to hand?'

'Of course.'

'Our man in Ramses' guard is one of my best officers. He'll have no trouble slitting Serramanna's throat while he sleeps. When do we act?'

'It won't be long. I have business in Thebes. As soon as I'm back, we'll strike.'

Helen relished every moment of a happiness she had thought lost for ever. In a light, nectar-scented dress, with a veil on her head to protect her from the sun, she reflected that her life in Tuya's household was a wonderful dream. She had managed to escape from that vicious, cowardly tyrant Menelaus, whose greatest pleasure was to humiliate her; even his men called her 'evil bitch'.

Tuya and her daughter-in-law, Nefertari, had given Helen friendship and employment. It was a pleasure to live in a country where women were not forced to live as prisoners in their homes, even if that home was a palace.

Was Helen truly to blame for the deaths of thousands of

Greeks and Trojans? She had never wanted the long years of frenzied killing, yet somehow she had been tried and convicted without ever having had the chance to defend herself. Here in Memphis no one condemned her. She wove, she listened to music and played it, she swam in the palace pools, strolled in the endlessly delightful gardens. The clash of weapons grew distant, yielding to birdsong.

Several times a day, white-armed Helen prayed to the gods that her dream might continue. Her only wish was to leave the past, her country, her husband, behind her.

On a sandy path lined by persea trees, she spotted a dead crane. Walking closer, she saw that the bird's handsome body had been torn open. Helen knelt and examined the entrails; her gift for prophecy had been acknowledged by both the Greeks and the Trojans.

It was a long while before she struggled to her feet.

What she read in the crane's entrails appalled her.

4

Thebes, the southern capital, was home to the cult of Amon, the god credited with helping to drive out the Hyskos, a cruel, barbarian Asiatic people who had occupied the country several centuries earlier. Since Egypt's liberation, every pharaoh for generations had paid tribute to Amon and further embellished his temple at Karnak until it became the greatest and richest of temples, a sort of state within the state. The High Priest of Amon was now more a powerful administrator than a man of prayer.

Upon his arrival in Thebes, Shaanar immediately requested an audience with the High Priest. The two men talked in the shade of an arbour dripping with wisteria and honeysuckle. A cooling breeze blew from the sacred lake nearby.

'You came without an entourage?' the High Priest asked in wonder.

'Very few people are aware I'm here.'

'I see. I'll be discreet then.'

'Are you still opposed to Ramses?'

'More firmly than ever. He's too young and hot-headed to be pharaoh. His reign would be disastrous. Seti made a mistake designating him.'

'Will you take me into your confidence?'

'What rank would you grant the Temple of Amon, if you wore the crown?'

18

'The first, naturally.'

'Your father favoured other priesthoods like those of Heliopolis and Memphis. Karnak must no longer be second best; that's all I ask.'

'That's Ramses' intention, not mine.'

'What do you have in mind, Shaanar?'

'We must act, and act quickly.'

'In other words, before Seti's funeral rites.'

'Yes. It's our last chance.'

What Shaanar did not know was that the High Priest of Amon was seriously ill. His doctor had told him he had only months, perhaps weeks, to live. A speedy resolution would be a final blessing from the gods. Before he died, he would see Ramses deposed and Karnak saved.

'I cannot condone violence,' the High Priest decreed. 'Amon gave us peace, which must be preserved.'

'I agree completely. Unfit as he may be to rule, Ramses is my brother, and I hold him dear. I have never for one second intended him any harm.'

'What are your plans for him?'

'He's an energetic man, in love with adventure and wide-open spaces. An extended trip abroad will be a welcome prospect once he's freed from his crushing responsibilities. When he returns, his first-hand observations will be extremely valuable.'

'I would also like to see your mother remain as your close adviser.'

'That goes without saying.'

'Be faithful to Amon, my son, and your future will be assured.'

Shaanar bowed deferentially. This old priest's gullibility was a wonderful stroke of luck.

Dolora, Ramses' elder sister, rubbed soothing unguents into her oily skin. Plain, lanky, always tired, she hated Thebes, hated the South. A princess belonged in Memphis, in the thick of court gossip.

Thebes was boring. High society had welcomed her with open arms, of course, and showered her with invitations; she was, after all, a member of the royal family. But fashionable life lagged behind that of Memphis and, besides, her husband was slowly sinking into a deep depression. Affable, paunchy Sary had been Ramses' tutor, then head of the Kap, the royal school where Egypt's top students were sent. His talents were wasted here, and it was all her brother's fault.

Yes, Sary had come up with a feeble plot to have Ramses killed. And yes, she, Dolora, had thrown in her lot with Shaanar. Yes, they had both made mistakes. Even so, shouldn't Ramses grant them his pardon, considering Seti had died?

Revenge was the only possible response to his cruelty. Ramses' luck would turn eventually, and when it did, she and Sary would be ready. Meanwhile, she attended to her skin while her husband read or dozed.

Shaanar's unannounced arrival shook them out of their torpor.

'My dear brother!' exclaimed Dolora, kissing him. 'Bearing glad tidings, I hope!'

'Possibly.'

'Don't keep us in suspense!' Sary demanded.

'I'm going to be king.'

'Our day is coming soon, then?'

'Come back to Memphis with me. I'll find a place for you until we can dispose of Ramses.'

Dolora blanched. 'Dispose of him, you say?'

'Don't worry, little sister. I'm only sending him on a grand tour.'

'Will you have a job for me?' asked Sary. 'Something important?'

'You've made it just a bit awkward,' replied Shaanar. 'But

I can use a man of your intelligence. Be loyal to me and the rewards will be great.'

'You have my word, Shaanar.'

Iset the Fair was biding her time. Before she gave birth to their son, Ramses had sent her to Thebes; now she was raising her beloved Kha in the royal palace. A striking young woman with green eyes, a small, straight nose and finely drawn lips, she was energetic, vivacious, Ramses' first lover and now his lesser wife.

Lesser wife – hard to accept the title and the status it implied. Yet Iset found it impossible to be envious of Nefertari, so lovely, gentle and serious, with the bearing of a queen, though quite devoid of worldly ambition.

It would have been easier if she were consumed with hate, if she could lash out at the two of them, but she still loved the man who had given her so much happiness and pleasure, the man to whom she had given his firstborn son.

Iset cared nothing for power and prestige. She loved Ramses for himself, his intensity and verve. But the pain of living apart from him was sometimes unbearable. Why didn't he realize how much it hurt her?

Soon Ramses would be king and come to see her only rarely. Each time, she knew, she would give in to her love for him. If only she could meet someone else – but other men paled in comparison to Ramses.

When her steward announced Shaanar, Iset was amazed. What was Seti's elder son doing in Thebes before the funeral?

She received him in a room with narrow slits of windows high in the walls, letting in fresh air but little direct sunlight.

'You look magnificent, Iset.'

'What do you want?'

'I know you don't care for me,' he said, 'but I also know you're intelligent enough to look out for your own best interests. I think you have the makings of a Great Royal Wife.'

'Ramses doesn't share your opinion.'

'What if it weren't up to him?'

'What do you mean?'

'My brother isn't a complete fool. He finally sees that he's not fit to govern Egypt.'

'Meaning . . . ?'

'Meaning that for the good of our country I'll take over and you can be Lady of the Two Lands.'

'Ramses would never step down. You're lying.'

'It's the truth, dear lady. He's planning to leave the country with Menelaus and has asked me to be Seti's successor, out of respect for the memory of our father. When he's done travelling, he'll be treated with all the respect due to a member of the royal family.'

'Has he said anything about me?'

'I'm afraid he's forgotten you and his little son. All he can think of is seeing the world.'

'Is he taking Nefertari?'

'No, no . . . too many fish in the sea,' laughed Shaanar. 'When it comes to pleasure, he's insatiable.'

Iset seemed distraught. Shaanar would have liked to take her hand, but it was too soon. He mustn't frighten her away. First he needed to offer comfort, then slowly begin to woo her.

'Kha will have the finest education,' he promised. 'You won't have to worry. After Seti is laid to rest, we'll go back to Memphis together.'

'Ramses . . . Will Ramses be gone by then?'

'Of course.'

'He's not attending the funeral rites?'

'It's a shame, but there's nothing to be done about it. Menelaus refuses to wait any longer. Forget Ramses, Iset. Concentrate on becoming queen.'

5

Iset spent a sleepless night.

Shaanar was lying. Ramses would never leave Egypt to numb his grief in foreign travels. If he missed Seti's funeral, it would be against his will.

Ramses had treated her badly, true, but she would never betray him by throwing herself into Shaanar's arms. Iset had no desire to be queen, no matter what Shaanar thought. The moon-faced, smooth-talking, ambitious, conceited fool! She hated him.

She knew what she had to do: warn Ramses of the plot being hatched against him and of his elder brother's plans for him.

On fresh papyrus, she composed a long letter relating her conversation with Shaanar. Then she summoned the local head of the royal courier service.

'This needs to reach Memphis as soon as possible.'

'I'll see to it personally,' he assured her.

River traffic at Thebes had slowed considerably, as in Memphis, while the country was in mourning. Guards dozed at the river landing where boats for the North customarily docked. Iset's messenger hailed a sailor.

'Weigh anchor – we're leaving for Memphis.'

'Sorry, can't leave port.'

'Why?'

'The High Priest of Amon at Karnak has the boat reserved.'

'Without going through my office?'

'Just got the order.'

'Well, weigh anchor anyway. I've got an urgent message for the royal palace at Memphis.'

A man appeared on the bridge of the boat in question.

'Orders are orders, my good man and you must obey them.'

'Keep your nose out of this, whoever you are.'

'I'm Shaanar, Seti's elder son.'

The official bowed. 'Forgive my insolence, Your Highness.'

'All right, if you give me the message Iset the Fair wants delivered.'

'But—'

'It goes to the royal palace in Memphis, correct?'

'Yes, to your brother Ramses.'

'That's where I'm heading tonight. Or don't I meet your standards as a courier?'

The official handed the letter to Shaanar.

As soon as the boat pulled away from Thebes, Shaanar tore Iset's letter to shreds and scattered them in the wind.

The night was warm and fragrant. It didn't seem possible that Seti had left his people and that the very soul of Egypt mourned the death of a king as great as those of the Old Kingdom. Usually the evenings were cheerful and lively. In village squares and city streets, people danced, sang and told stories – often fables of animals taking the place of humans and acting more wisely than humans. But, during the time of mourning and mummification, laughter and games had disappeared.

Wideawake, Ramses's yellow dog, slept with his head against Invincible, the huge lion that patrolled the Regent's private garden. After the gardeners finished the evening watering, the two pets liked to stretch out on the cool grass.

Among the gardeners was a Greek, one of Menelaus' men. Before leaving for the night, he had tucked poisoned chunks of meat into one of the lily beds, where the greedy beasts would surely find them. Even if the lion took hours to die, no treatment could save him.

Wideawake was the first to pick up the unfamiliar scent. Yawning, he stretched, sniffed the air, and trotted over to the lilies. His snout quickly led him to the meat; he nosed and pawed it thoroughly, then backtracked. This was too good a find not to share with his friend.

The three soldiers perched on the garden wall smiled as the lion sleepily trailed the yellow dog back to the flower bed. Just a little longer and the coast would be clear. They could slip into Ramses's bedchamber, take him by surprise while he slept, and carry him off to Menelaus's waiting ship.

The lion and dog lay with their heads in the foliage. Before long they seemed to go limp. Ten minutes later one of the Greeks jumped down from the wall. Given how deadly the poison was and how much had been put in the meat, the big cat must already be paralysed.

The scout motioned to his companions, who followed him down the path towards the Regent's suite. They were about to go inside when a growl made them wheel round.

Invincible and Wideawake stood behind them, staring at them. Among the trampled lilies lay the tainted meat, which the lion had shredded after confirming his friend's suspicions.

The three Greek soldiers huddled together, daggers raised.

Claws extended and fangs bared, Invincible sprang at them.

The Greek officer who had infiltrated Ramses's royal body-guard crept through the silent palace towards the Regent's room. He was assigned to patrol the hallways and warn of any intruders, so the other soldiers on duty, who knew him well, let him pass and thought nothing of it.

He headed towards the granite threshold where Serramanna slept. The Sard always boasted that anyone coming after Ramses would have to slit his throat first. Once he was dead, the Regent would have lost his principal protector, and all his bodyguards would be won over to Shaanar, the new ruler of Egypt.

The Greek stopped and listened. Not a sound, except for the steady breathing of deep sleep. Even a giant had to sleep sometimes. But he might have a cat's reflexes and suddenly wake, sensing danger. The Greek must move swiftly and surely, allowing the Sard no time to react.

Cautiously, he listened a while longer. There could be no doubt: Serramanna was at his mercy. Holding his breath, he unsheathed his dagger, then struck furiously at the sleeping figure's throat.

'Nice try, for a sneaking coward,' a deep voice snarled from behind him. He whirled round.

'You've just killed a dummy,' said Serramanna. 'The breathing was real, though. I had a hunch that something was up tonight.'

Menelaus' man gripped the handle of his dagger.

'Drop it.'

'I'm still going to slit your throat.'

'Try it.' The Sard loomed over him. The Greek's dagger connected with air. For his size, Serramanna was surprisingly quick on his feet.

'You don't even know how to fight,' he jeered.

The Greek tried a feint, stepping aside, then rushed forward, blade pointing at his opponent's stomach.

The Sard's right hand chopped at his wrist, breaking it, as his left hand slammed into the Greek's temple. Tongue dangling, eyes glazed, he collapsed and was dead before he even hit the floor.

26

'One coward fewer to deal with,' muttered Serramanna.

Ramses considered the two-pronged attack. In the garden, three Greeks had died under the lion's claws; in the corridor lay another dead Greek, a member of his personal bodyguard.

'They were after you,' Serramanna said flatly.

'Did the one you killed say anything?'

'I didn't have time to ask questions. No great loss – he wasn't much of a soldier.'

'Weren't they Menelaus' men?'

'Just let me at that bully! I'll send him off to meet all the heroes he's always lamenting.'

'For the moment, just double the watch.'

'Defence is a bad strategy, Prince. Only attacking leads to victory.'

'First we need to know who the enemy is.'

'Menelaus and his Greeks. They're liars and cheats. Send them all packing before they try again!'

Ramses laid a hand on Serramanna's right shoulder.

'With you on my side, I don't have to worry.'

Ramses spent the rest of the night in the garden with his pets. Invincible was fast asleep; Wideawake dozed fitfully. The prince contemplated human folly. The struggle for power had begun even before Seti's mummy could be laid in his tomb.

Moses was right. Lenience towards his enemies had only made them more likely to keep up their attacks, convinced he would not retaliate.

With the dawn, the prince's spirits rose. No one could take Seti's place, but it was time for Ramses to start acting like a pharaoh.

6

In Seti's Egypt, temples were responsible for redistributing excess donations, as well as the food produced on their extensive domains. As long as there had been pharaohs, the law of Ma'at, the fragile goddess of truth and justice, maintained that each child of this blessed land of plenty should be free from want. What god could bless a feast day if even the humblest soul went hungry?

As head of state, the pharaoh was both the rudder that steered a steady course and the captain who held his crew together. He must inspire the cooperation essential to any lasting society.

A key government department maintained strict control over the redistribution of goods. However, the temples were allowed to commission a few independent merchants to travel the length of the country, trading freely.

One such trader was Raia, a Syrian who had lived in Egypt for over ten years. With his cargo ship and herd of donkeys, he was constantly on the move, selling wine, preserved meat, and vases imported from Asia. He was of average height and build, sporting a small pointed beard and dressed in a striped tunic. Polite, discreet and honest, he attracted a faithful clientele with quality merchandise at reasonable prices. His work permit was renewed year after year in recognition of his service to his adopted country. Like many other immigrants, the Syrian had become practically indistinguishable from the natives.

No one knew that Raia was a spy in the pay of the Hittites.

They had ordered him to gather all the information he could and send it to them as quickly as possible. The warlike Anatolians would then decide when to attack Pharaoh's foreign dominions, seize their land, then invade Egypt itself. Raia had cultivated contacts in the military, the customs department, the police. Titbits from their dinner conversation ended up in Hattusa, the Hittite capital, by way of coded messages inserted into the alabaster vases Raia exported to southern Syria, Egypt's official ally. Customs had searched his shipments more than once, finding only what appeared to be routine business letters and invoices. The importer, who belonged to the spy ring, made a profit selling the vases and a bonus for delivering the messages to an agent in Hittite-controlled northern Syria, who relayed them directly to Hattusa.

It was a simple way for the Near East's greatest military power to receive monthly briefings on Egyptian politics from a primary source.

Seti's death and the subsequent mourning period would be the perfect opportunity to attack Egypt, but Raia had argued forcefully against it, telling the Hittite generals it would be madness. If they thought the Egyptian army had been demobilized, they were sadly mistaken. Fearing a possible invasion before the ascension of Seti's successor, the Egyptians had reinforced their border patrols.

Furthermore, the king's loose-tongued daughter had made it plain that Shaanar, elder brother of the future king, was not resigned to being relegated to the second rank. In other words, he was planning to seize power before the coronation.

Raia had made a thorough study of the disgruntled

prince. Ambitious, clever, devious – and ruthless when his self-interest was at stake – he was altogether different from his father and brother. That he should become pharaoh was devoutly to be wished, for he seemed to have fallen into the Hittite's trap, believing their claims to want closer diplomatic and trade relations, which would bring an end to the old hostilities. Even Seti had failed to take the key fortress of Kadesh when he had the chance, suing for peace instead. The King of the Hittites had announced that he was abandoning his expansionist plans. He hoped the new pharaoh would believe him and let down the country's defences.

Raia next began to identify Shaanar's co-conspirators and determine how he planned to proceed. His unerring instinct led him to the Greeks who had recently settled in Memphis. Menelaus was no more than a cruel mercenary whose most cherished memories were of the slaughter at Troy. Rumour had it that the bloodthirsty Greek was restless, eager to sail home to Sparta as a conquering hero with his wife, Helen, in tow. Shaanar had paid the Greek contingent handsomely to eliminate Ramses and help him reclaim his rightful place as Seti's successor.

Raia had become convinced that Ramses would mean trouble for the Hittites. Unafraid to fight, he had inherited his father's determination. He was young, hot-blooded, unpredictable. Shaanar, on the other hand, was a known quantity, reasonable, open-minded: clearly the better choice.

Unfortunately, a palace servant in Raia's employ had just brought the information that several Greek mercenaries had been killed while attempting to enter Ramses' bedchamber. The attempted coup had apparently failed.

The next few hours would be telling. If Shaanar managed to avoid being implicated, he still had a future. If not, he'd have to be crossed off the list.

Menelaus stamped on the shield that had warded off so many

blows on the battlefield. He broke one of the spears that had dispatched many a Trojan, then grabbed a vase and threw it against the wall of his antechamber.

Still fuming, he turned to face Shaanar.

'A complete failure! How can it be? My men never fail. It took us ten years to beat the Trojans, but we did it.'

'I sympathize, but the fact is that Ramses' lion got your three soldiers and Serramanna killed the fourth.'

'They were betrayed.'

'No, simply not up to the job you gave them. Ramses suspects you now. He'll probably order you out of the country.

'Without Helen.'

'Yes. You have failed, Menelaus.'

'Your plan was stupid.'

'You seemed to think it would work.'

'Get out!'

'You'd better be prepared to leave soon.'

'I know what I have to do.'

Ahmeni was Ramses's sandal-bearer and private secretary, but first and foremost his lifelong friend. He had sworn allegiance to the Regent and linked his own destiny to his – whatever it might be. Short, slight, with thinning hair, his frail physique did not prevent him from being a tireless worker and peerless scribe, forever studying official documents and briefing Ramses – as he was doing now – on their contents. Devoid of personal ambition, Ahmeni was nevertheless a strict taskmaster, holding his administrative staff of twenty to the highest standards, prizing accuracy and discipline above all else.

Although he had little use for a brute like Serramanna, Ahmeni admitted that the bodyguard had dealt effectively with the Greek assassin. Ramses' reaction to the attack was surprising. The future pharaoh had simply asked his secretary for a thorough description of the main branches of government, how they worked, how they related to one another.

When Serramanna came in to announce Shaanar, Ahmeni was irritated. He did not want to be interrupted as he pored over documents concerning the reform of outdated laws regulating public ferries.

'Don't let him in,' Ahmeni urged Ramses.

'Shaanar is my brother.'

'He's a self-centred schemer.'

'I think I should hear what he has to say.'

Ramses had his brother shown into the garden, where Invincible lazed in the shade of a sycamore tree and Wideawake gnawed on a bone.

'Your security is much tighter than Seti's!' exclaimed Shaanar. 'It's almost impossible to get near you.'

'Haven't you heard that some Greeks broke in here last night? They were after me.'

'I heard. I've come to tell you who was behind it.'

'How do you know that?'

'Menelaus tried to bribe me.'

'What did he offer?'

'To put me on the throne.'

'And you turned him down?'

'I do love power, Ramses, but I know my limitations. No one but you can be the next pharaoh. Our father's wishes were clear; they must be respected.'

'Why would Menelaus risk his neck?'

'He's dying to go home to Sparta as a conquering hero, but to do that he needs to take Helen with him. He's convinced that you're holding her against her will. In exchange for making me king, he wanted me to banish you to the desert, hand over Helen, and clear him for departure.'

'Helen is free to do whatever she chooses.'

'To a Greek that's inconceivable – she must be being controlled by a man.'

'Is he really that stupid?'

'Menelaus is stubborn and dangerous. He's acting like a Greek hero.'

'What would you advise?'

'He's violated our hospitality. It's time that he left for good.'

7

The poet Homer lived in a fine new residence not far from the palace. Ramses had also provided a cook, maid and gardener to look after him. The cellar was stocked with Delta wine which Homer spiced with anise and coriander. There was also a supply of the fragrant olive oil he liked to rub on his skin. The old poet was so comfortable that he rarely left his garden, seeking inspiration in the shade of his beloved lemon tree.

He would smoke crushed sage leaves in a pipe fashioned from a giant snail shell and a hollow reed. Hector, his black and white cat, purred in his lap as he dictated verse after verse of his *Iliad* to Ahmeni or one of the scribe's assistants.

Ramses' visit was an added pleasure. The cook brought a Cretan wine jug with a very thin spout, pouring just a trickle of cool spiced wine. The garden pavilion – four acacia columns with a palm-frond roof – gave some relief from the summer heat.

'This nice hot weather helps my aching bones,' said Homer, stroking the flowing white beard that was such a contrast to his lined and craggy face. 'Do you have storms like we do in Greece?'

'Tremendous ones,' answered Ramses. 'When our god Set unleashes his fury, dark clouds fill the sky, lightning flashes, thunder rumbles, and bolts crash to the ground. The rain floods dry riverbeds, sweeping rocks through the wadis. People are terrified, and some think it's the end of the world.'

'Wasn't your father named after Set?'

'For a long time I couldn't understand why a pharaoh would place himself under the protection of the god who murdered Osiris, his own brother. Then I realized that Seti wanted to harness the powers of darkness and use them to do good.'

'What a strange country Egypt is! And it seems you've been having your own stormy weather.'

'I didn't know you could see from your garden to mine.'

'My eyesight is failing, but my hearing is excellent.'

'So you heard that your countrymen tried to kill me.'

'The other day I wrote these lines: "I greatly fear that you will be caught tight in the enemy's net, that you will all become their prey and spoils of war. They will sack your cities. Think on it night and day, fight on, if you wish to hold your heads high."'

'Are you a seer?'

'I can guess why the future pharaoh should take time from his official duties to seek the opinion of an obscure old poet – not that I don't appreciate your visits.'

Ramses smiled. He liked the way Homer spoke his mind.

'All right. Do you think the soldiers who came after me were acting alone or on orders from Menelaus?'

'Beware of Greeks, my friend! Hatching plots is their favourite pastime. Menelaus wants Helen, and you're standing in his way: violence is the only answer.'

'But I'm still here.'

'Menelaus is as single-minded as he is unprincipled. He'll keep trying, attack you in your own back yard, without a thought for the consequences.'

'What do you recommend?'

'Pack him off to Greece with Helen.'

'She won't go.'

'Through no fault of her own, that woman sows death and destruction in her wake. If you think you can alter the course of her destiny, you're sadly mistaken.'

'She's free to choose where she lives.'

'Don't say I didn't warn you. By the way, I could use some new papyrus and more of that wonderful olive oil.'

Some might have said the white-bearded poet should be less brusque with his royal patron. Ramses, however, valued the old man's frankness. There were yes-men to spare in the royal court.

The moment Ramses walked through the gate to his wing of the palace, Ahmeni came running, in a most uncharacteristic state of agitation.

'What's happening?'

'Menelaus,' Ahmeni panted.

'What now?'

'He's taken hostages down at the harbour – dock workers, women and children. Says he'll kill them unless you deliver Helen to him today.'

'Where is he?'

'On his ship, with the hostages. His whole fleet is ready to sail. Not one of his mercenaries is left in town.'

'And where were our naval police when all this happened?'

'Don't be too hard on them. Menelaus took the guards on duty by surprise.'

'Has anyone told my mother?'

'She's waiting for you, with Nefertari and Helen.'

Seti's widow, Ramses' wife, and Menelaus' reluctant spouse were all looking anxious. Tuya sat on a low gilded chair, Nefertari on a folding stool. Helen stood, her back against a light-green column with a lotus capital.

The Great Royal Wife's audience chamber was cool and

restful, with subtle, pleasing scents in the air. On Pharaoh's throne, a bouquet of flowers marked the temporary absence of a monarch.

Ramses bowed to his mother, kissed his wife gently, and greeted Helen.

'How much do you know?' asked Tuya.

'Only that it's serious. How many hostages?'

'Around fifty.'

'Even one life is more than I'm willing to sacrifice.'

Ramses turned to Helen. 'If we attack, will Menelaus really kill the hostages?'

'He'll slit their throats with his own dagger.'

'How could he live with innocent blood on his hands?'

'He wants me back. If he can't have me, he'll kill before he gets killed.'

'It's barbaric.'

'Menelaus is a warrior. To him, everyone is either friend or foe.'

'And his own men – doesn't he realize none of them will survive if the hostages are executed?'

'They'll die as heroes, with their honour intact.'

'Heroes? Murderers of defenceless bystanders?'

'Menelaus knows only one law: kill or be killed.'

'There must be a special hell reserved for Greek heroes.'

'Frightening as that may be, the need to fight is more intense than the simple desire to survive.'

Nefertari drew closer to Ramses. 'What will you do?'

'I'll board Menelaus' ship alone and unarmed and try to reason with him.'

'You must be joking,' Helen said with a bitter laugh.

'The least I can do is try.'

'He'll take you hostage too!' Nefertari interjected.

'You have no right to put yourself in such danger,' Tuya told him. 'Won't you just be falling into his trap?'

'He'll take you away to Greece,' Nefertari prophesied, 'and

someone else will be pharaoh – someone who'll use Helen as a pawn in trade negotiations.'

Ramses shot a questioning look at his mother. She seemed to agree with Nefertari.

'If persuasion won't work with Menelaus, we'll have to resort to violence.'

Helen approached the Regent.

'No,' he said, 'we won't let you sacrifice yourself. Protecting a guest is a sacred duty.'

'Ramses is right,' the Great Royal Wife agreed. 'Giving in to your husband's blackmail would be in violation of the law of Ma'at. It could only bring unhappiness to Egypt.'

'But I'm the one who's responsible for all this and it's—'

'Don't, Helen. Since you've chosen to live among us, we're bound to help you stay free.'

'I'll think of something,' Seti's son concluded.

Trembling and sweating, Meba, the late pharaoh's minister for foreign affairs, stood on the pier shouting back and forth with Menelaus and fearing that a Greek archer's arrow would pierce him at any moment. However, he did win one concession from the King of Sparta: Ramses would be allowed one night to host a farewell banquet in Helen's honour.

Menelaus stipulated that the hostages would be given no food whatsoever until Helen boarded the ship. He would release them once he had sailed clear and was sure no Egyptian warships were trailing his fleet.

Unharmed, Meba walked briskly away from the flagship, not minding the Greek soldiers' taunts. Ramses' praise for his able negotiating was some consolation.

The prince now had one night to find a way of freeing the hostages.

8

Average in height, strong as an ox, dark-haired, swarthy Setau the snake-charmer was making love to his lissome Nubian wife, Lotus, whose slender curves kept him constantly on the brink of arousal. Their large home on the edge of the desert, far from the centre of Memphis, also served as their laboratory and workshop. Several rooms were filled with flasks and vials of various sizes and the strange contraptions they used to process the venom and prepare the medicines the doctors needed.

Lotus was an amazingly agile and willing participant in her husband's seemingly endless variations on a theme. Since he had brought her to Egypt after marrying her, she had never ceased to amaze him with her deep, subtle knowledge of reptiles. Their shared passion for snakes led to important discoveries and the creation of new remedies, after a great deal of experimentation.

As Setau caressed his wife's breasts, tender as flower buds, their pet cobra which lay coiled in the doorway, suddenly lifted its head.

'We have a visitor,' said Setau.

Lotus glanced at the splendid reptile. Its swaying told her whether their visitor was a friend or a stranger. Tonight it did not seem alarmed.

Setau slid off the cosy bed and grabbed a club. Though he

trusted the cobra's judgment, at this time of night it was best to be careful.

A galloping horse pulled up in front of the house. The rider jumped off.

'Ramses! What are you doing here in the middle of the night?'

'Hope I'm not disturbing you.'

'As a matter of fact, Lotus and I were just—'

'Sorry, but I need your help.'

The two had attended the Royal Academy together, but Setau had shunned the traditional administrative career to devote himself to the study of snakes, unlocking the secrets of life and death. When they were still in their teens, he had dared Ramses to face the master of the desert, a lethal species of cobra. Setau was immunized against the cobra's bite, but the prince was not. Their friendship survived the challenge, and Setau belonged to the limited circle of Ramses' closest confidants.

'Is the kingdom in danger?'

'Menelaus has taken hostages and threatens to kill them unless we hand Helen back to him.'

'A fine mess. But why not let her go? The woman did cause the destruction of an entire city.'

'Violating the laws of hospitality would make us no better than barbarians.'

'Let the barbarians sort it out between them.'

'Helen is a queen. She wants to stay in Egypt. It's my duty to keep her out of Menelaus' clutches.'

'You really sound like a pharaoh. It must be your destiny. But then it's a job only a madman or a fool would want.'

'I need to storm Menelaus' ship without harming the hostages.'

'You've always liked beating impossible odds.'

'The commanding officers of the regiments stationed in

Memphis haven't come up with one worthwhile idea. Every plan they suggest would end in a massacre.'

'Does that surprise you?'

'No. That's why I thought of you.'

'You think I'm going to storm Greek warships?'

'Not you – your snakes.'

'Let's hear it.'

'Before dawn, we'll send swimmers to climb up the sides of the ship, carrying bags with snakes in them. When they reach the bridge, they'll release the snakes and throw them at the soldiers guarding the hostages. A few of the guards will be bitten, and in the confusion our men can free the hostages.'

'Original, but awfully risky. What makes you think the cobras will be selective about their victims?'

'I'm fully aware of the enormous risk we'll be taking.'

'We?'

'You and I will be leading the raid, of course.'

'You expect me to risk my life for some Greek woman I've never met?'

'No, for Egyptian hostages.'

'What will happen to my wife and my snakes if I die in the process?'

'They'll be taken care of.'

'No, it's too dangerous. And how many snakes would you expect me to sacrifice to fighting these bloodthirsty foreigners?'

'You'll be paid triple their value, and I'll designate your laboratory as an official research centre.'

Setau looked back towards Lotus, so appealing in the warm summer darkness.

'Enough talk. We'd better start bagging the snakes.'

Menelaus paced the bridge of his flagship. The lookouts had noted no unusual activity on the riverbanks. Just as he supposed, the Egyptians were too afraid of bloodshed to make a move, the cowards. Taking hostages was hardly honourable, but it had worked. There was no other way to pry Helen loose from Tuya and Nefertari.

The hostages had stopped their crying and moaning. Hands tied behind their backs, they huddled on the poop deck, guarded by ten soldiers who were relieved every two hours.

One of Menelaus' officers came up to the bridge.

'Do you think they'll attack?' he asked.

'It would be counterproductive. We'd have to slaughter the hostages.'

'In that case, we'd have no buffer.'

'We'd kill a lot of Egyptians before we were back at sea. But don't worry, they won't endanger their countrymen's lives. I'll get Helen back at dawn and we'll sail home.'

'I'll miss this place.'

'Have you lost your mind?'

'Didn't you think life was good in Memphis? Peace at last.'

'We were born to fight, not for idleness.'

'How safe will you be when you do get home? By now there must be plenty of pretenders to your throne.'

'I can still handle a sword. When they see Helen under my thumb, they'll realize who's in charge.'

Ramses had selected thirty of his best soldiers, all strong swimmers. Setau showed them how to avoid being bitten when they released their snakes. The volunteers' faces were tense. The Regent made a rousing speech. His strength of conviction, along with Setau's obvious competence, convinced the raiding party they would win the day.

Ramses hated keeping secrets from his wife and mother, but neither of them would have wanted him to take part in the raid, thinking it put him in too much danger. He assumed full responsibility for the surprise attack. If he was truly meant to be pharaoh, fate would see him through.

Setau talked to the snakes inside their sacks and chanted spells to calm them. Lotus had taught him the sounds which, though meaningless to humans, had a magical effect on snakes.

Once the secret weapon was ready, the raiders moved quietly down to the far end of the harbour, out of the Greek lookouts' sight.

Setau touched Ramses' wrist.

'Wait. Am I seeing things, or is Menelaus casting off ?'

Setau was right.

'Stay here,' Ramses said, dropping his sack, which contained a sand viper, and running towards the Greek flagship. In the silvery moonlight, he saw the King of Sparta standing on the prow, holding Helen in front of him.

'Menelaus!' Ramses shouted.

The Greek, who was wearing his double cuirasse and belt with golden clasps, recognized the prince's voice immediately.

'Ramses! You came to see me off. It will be a second honeymoon for me and Helen. She'll be glad she decided to come. Believe me, in Sparta she'll be the happiest woman alive!' Menelaus snorted with laughter.

'Free the hostages!'

'Never fear, you'll get them back alive.'

Ramses trailed behind the Greek fleet in a small boat with two sails. When the sun rose, Menelaus's soldiers raised a racket, beating on their shields with swords and spears.

Under orders from the Regent and the Great Royal Wife, the Egyptian Navy made no move, giving the Greeks free passage to the Mediterranean. Menelaus could start his northward crossing.

For a second, Ramses thought he had been fooled, and that the King of Sparta was about to slit his prisoners' throats. But then a boat was lowered and the hostages climbed down a rope ladder to board it. The able-bodied men among them took the oars and rowed away from their floating prison as fast as they could.

On the prow of her husband's ship, white-armed Helen, wearing a purple cloak, a white veil, and a golden necklace, gazed at the coast of Egypt, the country where she had known a few months of happiness hoping that she was free of Menelaus.

Once the hostages were beyond the Greek archers' range, Helen twisted the amethyst in the ring on her right hand and drank the contents of the minuscule vial it concealed: poison stolen from a Memphis laboratory. She had sworn never again to become her husband's slave; she refused to end her days beaten and humiliated in the palace gynoecium, the women's apartments. Returning with nothing but her corpse, the black-hearted conqueror of Troy would be a laughing stock.

She gloried in the touch of the summer sun, wishing her fair skin would turn a warm Egyptian copper, that she could be like her new-found friends, free to love, satisfied body and soul.

Helen quietly slumped, her head rolling on to her shoulder, her eyes wide open and fixed on the bright blue sky.

9

By the time the young diplomat Ahsha returned from a brief information-gathering mission in southern Syria, Memphis had already been in mourning for forty days. The next day, Tuya, Ramses, Nefertari and key government figures were set to depart for Thebes, where Seti's mummy would be laid to rest and the new king and queen would be crowned.

The only son of a wealthy family, well-bred, elegant, with a long, fine-featured face, a pencil moustache, lively, intelligent eyes and a spellbinding, sometimes haughty, manner of speaking, Ahsha had also been a fellow student of Ramses. Somewhat distant and dispassionate, he was both friend and critic. Ahsha knew several languages and from an early age had loved to travel and study other cultures. A diplomatic career was a natural choice for him. Thanks to some notable successes, which had surprised diplomats of greater experience, his professional advancement was assured. At twenty-three, he was considered one of the leading specialists on Asia. He was brilliant in the field and a gifted analyst as well, qualities rarely combined in one man. Some of his colleagues even suspected he was clairvoyant. Be that as it may, Egypt's security hinged on correctly assessing the intentions of Egypt's main enemy, the Hittite Empire.

When he reported to Meba, Ahsha found the minister on the defensive, offering little comment and recommending only that he try to see Ramses as soon as possible, since the pharaoh-to-be was asking to meet all high-level diplomats.

Ahsha was admitted by Ahmeni, the Regent's private secretary. The two old schoolfriends greeted each other warmly.

'Still thin as a reed,' Ahsha noted.

'And you're wearing the latest fashion, as usual.'

'One of my many vices. It's a long time since we were students . . . It's good to see that your talents are appreciated, Ahmeni.'

'I pledged my loyalty to Ramses and I've kept my oath.'

'Wise choice. It won't be long before Ramses is crowned, if the gods are willing.'

'They are. Did you hear he's already survived one assassination attempt? Our Greek visitor, Menelaus, sent his henchmen after Ramses.'

'Menelaus is a minor king and a scoundrel.'

'To put it mildly. He took hostages and threatened to kill them unless we handed Helen over.'

'What did Ramses do?'

'He refused to violate the laws of hospitality and planned a counterattack.'

'Risky.'

'What else could he have done?'

'Negotiate, then negotiate some more. Though I admit it would be almost impossible to get through to a ruffian like Menelaus. His plan worked, then?'

'No, Helen gave herself up without his knowledge. She felt responsible for the hostages. As soon as they were free and Menelaus' ship headed out to sea, she took her life.'

'A grand gesture, but rather final.'

'Ironic as ever, I see.'

'I find that making fun of everything, including oneself, helps keep things in perspective.'

'Helen's death doesn't seem to affect you.'

'Getting rid of Menelaus and his crew is to Egypt's benefit.

If we're looking for allies in Greece, we'll have to do better than that.'

'Homer stayed behind, though.'

'Ramses' charming old poet,' Ahsha said with a smile. 'Still writing his account of the Trojan War?'

'I've had the honour of taking it down for him. His verse is tragic, but not lacking in nobility.'

'Literature will be your downfall, Ahmeni! Do you know what plans Ramses has for you once he's pharaoh?'

'No. I like what I'm doing now.'

'You deserve better.'

'What about you? What are you hoping for?'

'My first concern is to meet Ramses.'

'Urgent business?'

'Do you mind if I save it for him?'

Ahmeni blushed. 'Sorry. You'll find him in the stables. No matter what he's doing, he'll want to see you.'

Ramses seemed strikingly different. The prince was regal and sure of himself, driving his chariot with consummate skill, leading his horses through incredibly complex manoeuvres that left the old stable-hands gaping.

The tall adolescent had become a powerfully built athlete with the incontestable authority of a monarch. However, Ahsha noted a rashness and over-excitement that might lead to errors in judgment. But what use would it be recommending moderation to someone burning with so much energy?

As soon as he caught sight of Ahsha, the prince drove towards him. The horses pulled up short only a length or two from the young diplomat, splattering his spotless tunic.

'Sorry, Ahsha! These young warhorses can be a bit hard to handle.'

Ramses jumped down, called two grooms to look after the horses, and took Ahsha by the shoulders.

'More trouble brewing in Asia?'

'I'm afraid so, Majesty.'

'Wait, I'm not pharaoh yet!'

'A good diplomat always looks towards the future. As it happens, your future is fairly easy to predict.'

'You're the only one who thinks so.'

'Does that bother you?'

'Asia, my friend – I asked you about Asia.'

'Outwardly, all is calm. Our protectorates are ready to welcome you as pharaoh. The Hittites are making no move to expand their territory.'

'Outwardly, you say.'

'That's what the official reports will tell you.'

'But you don't see it that way.'

'There's always a calm before the storm – but how long before?'

'Come, have a drink with me.'

Ramses checked on his horses, then sat down with Ahsha under a sloping roof with a view of the desert. A servant instantly appeared with cool beer and scented towels.

'Do you believe that the Hittites really want peace?'

Ahsha considered this, enjoying the delicious brew. 'The Hittites are fighters and conquerors. To them, the word "peace" is a sort of poetic image with no concrete meaning attached.'

'So they're lying.'

'They hope that a young, peace-loving leader will place less emphasis on defence, gradually weakening the country.'

'Like Akhenaton.'

'A prime example.'

'Are they still manufacturing arms?'

'In fact, they've stepped up production.'

'Do you think war is inevitable?'

'A diplomat's job is to make sure it isn't.'

'How would you go about stopping them?'

'I can't answer that question. My current duties don't

afford me a broad enough view to suggest effective counter-measures.'

'You'd like to take on other duties?'

'It's not up to me.'

Ramses looked out at the desert.

'When I was a boy, Ahsha, I dreamed of becoming pharaoh like my father, because I thought power was the best game of all. Then Seti had me face the wild bull – the traditional test of will, you know. He opened my eyes to the perils of ultimate power. Then I found another dream world: living in my father's shadow, relying on his strength. Now his death has brought reality crashing in on me. I prayed to the Invisible to be relieved of the burden of power I no longer sought, and I looked for a sign from the gods. Menelaus sent his men to kill me; my lion, my dog, and my bodyguard saved me as I communed with my father's soul. Since then I have decided not to try to fight against my destiny. What Seti has ordained will come to pass.'

'Do you remember that night just before graduation, when we discussed true power with Setau, Moses, and Ahmeni?'

'Of course. Ahmeni found it in serving his country, Moses in building monuments, Setau in studying snakes, and you in the diplomatic secretariat.'

'You're still the only one who will have true power.'

'No, Ahsha, it will pass through me, come to life in my heart, my sword arm, but leave me if I misuse it.'

'Living only for Egypt – it's a terrible price to pay.'

'I'm no longer free to choose my destiny.'

'Your words are almost frightening, Ramses.'

'Do you think I'm never afraid? No matter what stands in my way, I shall rule and continue my father's work. I need to leave Egypt stronger and more beautiful than ever. Will you help me, Ahsha?'

'Yes, Majesty.'

10

Shaanar was dejected.

The Greeks had failed him miserably; Menelaus, obsessed with getting Helen back, had lost sight of their goal of eliminating Ramses. The only consolation, which was not inconsiderable, was being able to convince his brother he was not involved in the coup. Now that Menelaus and his men were gone, no one would dare point a finger at Shaanar.

But Ramses would ascend to the throne and rule Egypt single-handedly – and he, Seti's elder son, would be forced to bow and scrape to his brother. No, he refused to accept this reversal of fortune.

That was why he had arranged a meeting with his one remaining ally, a friend of Ramses, a man above suspicion, who might help him fight his brother from within and undermine his authority.

At dusk, business was still brisk at the pottery stands. Strollers and serious shoppers passed the displays, eyeing vases of all different sizes and prices. At the end of an alley-way, a water-bearer hawked his thirst-quenching product.

That was where Ahsha waited, almost unrecognizable in an ordinary kilt and common wig. Shaanar, too, was carefully disguised. The two men bought a water-skin and shared a bunch of grapes like simple peasants, sitting side by side against a wall.

'Have you been to see Ramses again?' asked Shaanar.

'I no longer work for the Foreign Affairs secretariat. I report directly to our future pharaoh.'

'What does that mean?'

'A promotion.'

'To what?'

'I'm not sure yet. Ramses is forming his government. Since he's a loyal friend, Moses, Ahmeni and I should be given high-level positions.'

'Who else?'

'His only other close friend is Setau, but he's so devoted to his beloved snakes that he refuses to take on public duties.'

'Did Ramses seem determined to rule?' asked Shaanar.

'He realizes that it's a crushing responsibility and admits he's not fully prepared, but he won't give up now. Don't expect him to change his mind.'

'Did he mention the High Priest of Amon?'

'No.'

'Good. Then he underestimates the man's influence and potential to do him harm.'

'I heard the old fellow was rather intimidated by royalty,' said Ahsha.

'He was afraid of Seti – but Ramses is young, with little experience of power struggles. Now, as far as getting help from Ahmeni is concerned, it's hopeless. That damned little scribe is as devoted to Ramses as a dog to its master. On the other hand, I think I may be able to inveigle Moses into our camp.'

'Have you tried?'

'He wouldn't have anything to do with me, but it was only my first try. That Hebrew's a tortured soul, seeking some personal truth that may end up clashing with Ramses' views. If we offer him what he needs, he'll switch sides.'

'That makes sense.'

'Do you have any influence with Moses, Ahsha?'

'I don't think so, but give me long enough and I'll find his weak spot.'

'And Ahmeni?'

'He seems incorruptible,' Ahsha commented, 'but one never knows. In time, he may develop weaknesses. If he does, we'll be there to exploit them.'

'I don't intend to wait until Ramses has his network firmly in place.'

'Nor do I, Shaanar, nor do I. But we must be patient. Your experience with Menelaus should teach you that a successful strategy leaves no room for guesswork.'

'How long do I have to wait?'

'Let Ramses get settled on the throne. Power and his own rashness will turn his head. What's more, I'll be one of his advisers on Asia, the one he'll listen to most closely.'

'What's your plan, Ahsha?'

'You want the throne, don't you?'

'It's my birthright. I know how to lead.'

'Therefore, Ramses must be overthrown or killed.'

'I see no other way.'

'Two avenues are open to us: a coup or a foreign war. For the first, we would need to enlist a number of influential people. The onus would fall largely on you. The second would depend on determining the Hittites' true intentions and preparing a conflict that would ruin Ramses, but not Egypt. If the country is devastated, a Hittite king will take over the Two Lands.'

Shaanar's displeasure was obvious. 'It sounds too risky.'

'Ramses is no mean adversary. You won't find it easy to take power.'

'If the Hittites win, they'll invade Egypt.'

'That's not certain.'

'Do you have a miracle up your sleeve?'

'Not a miracle, but a trap that we'll set for Ramses, without our country being involved. Either he'll be killed or else he'll be blamed for the defeat, in which case, he'll no longer be a credible ruler. Then you can step in to save the day.'

'It sounds too easy.'

'I've built my reputation on accurate predictions. When I know exactly what my role in the government will be, I'll set things in motion. Unless you'd rather stop before we begin.'

'Never! I want Ramses out of my way, dead or alive.'

'If our plan works, I hope you won't prove ungrateful.'

'Don't worry. My right-hand man will be richly rewarded.'

'Can I really be sure?'

Shaanar was taken aback. 'Don't you trust me?'

'Not in the least.'

'But . . .'

'Don't pretend you're surprised. If I were that naive, you'd have got rid of me long ago. When a man is ambitious like you, no one ought to believe his promises. The sole basis for his behaviour is personal interest.'

'Are you a cynic, Ahsha?'

'I'm a realist. When you become pharaoh, you'll form a government based on your needs at the time. There may be no room for those who, like me, have paved your way to the throne.'

Shaanar smiled. 'Your intelligence is exceptional, Ahsha.'

'In my travels, I've encountered a great many cultures and all sorts of different people, but wherever I've been it comes down to the survival of the fittest.'

'Not in Seti's Egypt.'

'Seti is dead now, and Ramses can't wait to flex his military muscle. We must find him the right war.'

'In exchange for your research, I suppose you want immediate compensation.'

'Your own intelligence is pretty good, Shaanar.'

'Tell me exactly what you expect.'

'My family is well off, of course, but who's ever rich

enough? Since I'm constantly on the move, having several residences would be both a help and a pleasure. I'd like villas in Upper and Lower Egypt. Three houses in the Delta, two in Memphis, two in Middle Egypt, two near Thebes and one in Aswan ought to meet my needs when I'm here at home.'

'That would cost me a small fortune.'

'A trifle, Shaanar, a mere trifle when you consider what I'll be doing for you.'

'I suppose you want precious metals and gemstones as well.'

'It goes without saying.'

'I wouldn't have thought you so venal, Ahsha.'

'I like luxury – great luxury. A collector of fine vases like you must understand what I mean.'

'Yes, but so many houses . . .'

'Beautifully decorated houses, serving as a background for fine furniture! They'll be my earthly paradise, pleasure palaces where I'll be the absolute master while you climb the steps to the throne of Egypt.'

'When do we get under way?'

'Immediately.'

'You haven't been appointed yet.'

'When I am, I'm certain to have considerable responsibilities. Encourage me to serve you well, Shaanar.'

'Where do we start?'

'With a villa in the north-eastern Delta, near the border. A sizeable estate, a small lake, a vineyard and attentive servants. Even if I spend only a few days a year there, I want to be treated like a prince.'

'Anything else?'

'Well, women. When I'm on a mission, the pickings can be rather slim. I have to make up for that here in Egypt. Yes, a good supply of women. As long as they're attractive and willing, I'm not particular about where they come from.'

'I agree to your conditions.'

'I won't disappoint you, Shaanar. Just one more thing: we'll continue to meet in the strictest secrecy and you will mention it to no one. If Ramses were to learn of our dealings, my career would be finished.'

'Your best interest is my best interest, Ahsha.'

'There's no better guarantee of friendship. Farewell, Shaanar.'

As he watched the young diplomat merge into the crowd, Ramses' elder brother mused that luck was still with him. Ahsha made a first-rate partner. The day he had to be done away with would be a sad one.

11

Tuya, the late pharaoh's Great Royal Wife, sailed at the head of the fleet leaving Memphis for Thebes and the Valley of the Kings, where Seti's mummy would be entombed. Nefertari never left Tuya's side, sensing the pain beneath her usual serenity. Simply spending time with the great king's widow taught Nefertari how a queen should behave when faced with the cruellest of losses. The young woman's quiet presence was a tremendous comfort. Neither of them felt a need to express her sorrow, but their unspoken communion was deep and intense.

All through the voyage, Ramses worked.

Ahmeni, though highly susceptible to the heat, had prepared an impressive stack of dossiers on foreign policy, the safety of the kingdom, public health, public works (including dykes and canals), food management and a host of other more or less complex subjects.

Ramses was fully aware of the magnitude of his responsibilities. An army of civil servants would be helping him, but he needed detailed knowledge of how each department worked, in order to keep the government under his control. Otherwise Egypt was likely to pitch and sink like a rudderless boat. Time was against the pharaoh-to-be; the moment he assumed power, he would be expected to make informed decisions and function as the Lord of the Two Lands. The prospect of serious mistakes plagued him.

His mood lifted at the thought of his mother, a precious ally who would help him to avoid many errors and teach him how to deal with the tricks the notables would use to preserve their status. So many officials had already called on him to plead for their departments!

After long hours of work with the incomparably thorough and meticulous Ahmeni, Ramses liked to stand in the prow of the boat, contemplating the Nile, source of Egypt's prosperity, and enjoying the brisk wind – the breath of the Divine. In these stolen moments Ramses had the feeling that all Egypt belonged to him, from the mouth of the Nile to the desert reaches of Nubia. Would he be able to satisfy her needs?

At dinner his guests of honour were Moses, Setau, Ahsha, and Ahmeni. It was like the old days when they studied together at the Kap, the country's elite school. Even then they'd thirsted for power as well as knowledge. The pleasant reunion did not disperse the melancholy caused by Seti's death. Each of them sensed that difficult days might lie in store for Egypt.

'This time,' Moses told Ramses, 'your dream is about to come true.'

'It's not a dream any more, but a frightening obligation.'

'What?' objected Ahsha. 'You're not afraid of anything!'

'It's the last job you'd ever get *me* to take,' muttered Setau.

'I hesitated for a long time. But what would you have thought if I'd betrayed my father's wishes.'

'That you'd come to your senses. Your father's funeral may not be the only one we end up attending on this trip.'

'Have you got wind of another plot?' asked Ahmeni worriedly.

'A plot? There'll be ten of them, or twenty, or a hundred!' said Setau. 'That's why I'm here – with a few of my trusted assistants.'

'Setau a bodyguard,' said Ahsha ironically. 'Who'd have thought it.'

'At least I have something concrete to contribute.'

'Criticizing diplomacy, are we?'

'It complicates everything, when life is basically simple: good on one side, evil on the other, and nothing in between.'

'Your simplistic outlook is the problem,' retorted Ahsha.

'It suits me,' Ahmeni chimed in. 'People are either for Ramses or against him.'

'And what if the balance tips the wrong way?' asked Moses.

'My position will never change.'

'Soon Ramses will no longer be our friend but Pharaoh of Egypt. He'll see us differently.'

Moses' words were disturbing. Everyone waited to hear how Ramses would answer.

'Moses is right. Since this burden has fallen to me, I accept it. And since you're my friends, I'll call on you for help.'

'What will you have us do?' asked the Hebrew.

'The four of you have already gone far. I'll ask you to join me on a new journey, seeking the greater good of Egypt.'

'You know where I stand,' declared Setau. 'The minute you're safe on the throne, I shall go back to my snakes.'

'I still plan to try to persuade you to work with me.'

'A waste of time. When this security mission is over, I leave. Moses can be your masterbuilder, Ahsha can be head of Foreign Affairs, and more power to them!'

'Are you forming my government for me?'

Setau shrugged.

'Why don't we try the wine?' suggested Ahsha.

'I propose a toast,' said Ahmeni. 'To Ramses' health, and a long, full life in which to enjoy it, by the grace of the gods.'

Shaanar had sailed not with the Regent, but on his own ship, a splendid vessel with a crew of forty. As Head of Protocol, he had invited a party of notables, most of whom were no friends of Ramses. Seti's elder son carefully refrained from joining in their criticism, merely compiling a mental list of future supporters. The courtiers thought Ramses' youth and inexperience were insurmountable handicaps.

He smugly noted that his own excellent reputation remained intact, while his brother would continue to suffer from the comparison to Seti. The breach already open, the trick would be to widen it, taking every opportunity to weaken the young pharaoh's power.

Shaanar's guests sampled jojoba fruit and cool beer. His easy manner and moderate opinions made him a favourite with the courtiers, who enjoyed basking in the public gaze with a great man, whose brother would have to award him a prominent role.

For more than an hour, a man of average stature, with a neat pointed beard and a brightly striped tunic, had been waiting for an audience. He looked humble, almost submissive, yet calm and collected.

When he had a free moment, Shaanar motioned the man forward. He approached, bowing deferentially.

'Who are you?'

'My name is Raia. I come from Syria, but I've been a travelling merchant in Egypt for a number of years now.'

'Dealing in what?'

'Preserved meats and the finest Asian vases.'

Shaanar lifted an eyebrow. 'Vases?'

'Yes, Prince, I'm the exclusive distributor for some very fine manufacturers.'

'Do you know that I'm a collector?'

'So I was told just recently. I came here in hope of arranging a private showing for you.'

'Are your prices high?'

'That depends.'

Shaanar was curious. 'On what?'

From a sturdy cloth sack, Raia extracted a small, thin-lipped vase of solid silver, with a palmetto design. 'What do you think of this, Prince?'

Shaanar's eyes widened. Beads of sweat broke out on his forehead, his hands grew damp. 'A masterpiece . . . an unbelievable masterpiece. How much?'

'Is it permitted to offer a gift to the future Pharaoh of Egypt.'

Could he be hearing things? 'My brother Ramses is the future pharaoh, not me. You're mistaken, merchant. So name your price.'

'I never make mistakes, Prince. In my profession, there's no room for mistakes.'

Shaanar tore his eyes away from the stunning vase. 'What are you trying to tell me?'

'That many people don't want Ramses for king.'

'He'll be crowned in a matter of days.'

'Perhaps, but will that end the dissatisfaction?'

'Who are you, really, Raia?'

'A man who believes in your future and wants to see you on the throne of Egypt.'

'What do you know of my intentions?'

'That you clearly wish to expand foreign trade, make Egypt less arrogantly insular, and improve economic relations with the most powerful kingdom in Asia.'

'You mean . . . the Hittites?'

'We understand each other.'

'Ah. You're spying for them. And your employers like what they see in me?'

Raia nodded.

'What are you proposing?' asked Shaanar, as excited as if he were being offered another rare vase.

'Ramses is rash and war-loving. Like his father, he wants to maintain Egypt's grandeur and supremacy. You, Prince, are a reasonable man, better able to come to terms with foreign powers.'

'If I betray Egypt, Raia, I'm risking my life.'

Shaanar recalled how Tutankhamon's widow had been condemned to death for her dealings with the Hittites, even though she was attempting to protect the throne.

'A certain amount of risk is to be expected on the way to the top.'

Shaanar closed his eyes. The Hittites . . . Naturally, he'd considered using them against Ramses, but that had been no more than idle speculation. Now, suddenly, the idea sprang to life in the form of this ordinary, harmless-looking merchant.

'I love my country . . .'

'No one would doubt it. But you love power more. And only an alliance with the Hittites will guarantee it to you.'

'I need to think this over.'

'I'm afraid I can't indulge you.'

'You want my answer now?'

'My own safety is at stake, now that you know who I am.'

'And if I refuse?'

Raia did not answer, but his expression became fixed and unreadable.

Shaanar had little trouble convincing himself that it was meant to be. He would handle his powerful new partner with the utmost care, exploiting the Hittites without endangering Egypt. Ahsha, of course, would have to be kept in the dark, though he could still be of use.

'I accept, Raia.'

The merchant smiled faintly.

'You live up to your reputation, Prince. I'll be in touch with you every now and again. Now that I'm supplying vases for your collection, no one will be surprised if I visit you. Take this one, please, to seal our bargain.'

Shaanar closed his hands around the silver curves. The future was already looking brighter.

12

Ramses had memorized every parched and rocky inch of the Valley of the Kings, the 'Great Place' he had first visited with his father. Seti had shown him the tomb of his own father, the first Ramses, their dynasty's founder, an elderly vizier selected by a council of wise men to succeed the childless Horemheb. He had reigned for only two years, entrusting to his son the mission of reasserting Egypt's power, a power now invested in Ramses II.

The stifling summer heat felled some of the servants carrying furnishings for Seti's tomb, but it seemed to have no effect on Ramses. Grim-faced, he marched at the head of the procession transporting his father's mummy to its final resting-place.

Ramses felt a rush of hatred for the place that was claiming his father, leaving him so alone. Then the magic of the Valley took hold of him again, a magic that radiated life, not death.

The stony silence rang with the voices of the old ones. They spoke of light, transfiguration, resurrection. They demanded worship and respect for the celestial world that gave birth to all forms of life.

Ramses was the first to set foot inside Seti's vast tomb, the longest and deepest in the Valley. Once he was pharaoh, he planned to decree that no other tomb might surpass it. In the eyes of posterity, Seti would remain without equal.

Twelve priests carried in the mummy. Clad in a panther skin, Ramses was to conduct the rites for Seti's journey into the beyond and rebirth in the land of the gods. Ritual texts on the walls of the tomb would guide his father on the journey and serve his soul through all eternity.

Seti's mummy was a masterpiece of the embalmers' art. He looked perfectly at peace with himself and his life on earth, as if at any minute his eyes might open, his lips might speak . . . The priests placed the lid on the sarcophagus, to be enclosed in a House of Gold where Isis would work her alchemy, making the mortal immortal.

'Seti was a just ruler,' murmured Ramses. 'He upheld the Rule of Ma'at and was beloved of the light. He walks living into the West.'

All over Egypt barbers toiled, shaving off beards now that the official mourning was over. Women pinned up their hair, society ladies summoned their hairdressers.

On the eve of the coronation, Ramses and Nefertari gathered their thoughts in the Temple of Gurnah, where prayers for Seti would henceforth be said every day, maintaining his *ka* – his spiritual essence – and affirming the transfigured pharaoh's presence among the living. Then the couple proceeded to the temple of Karnak to see the High Priest, who welcomed them with cold formality. After a frugal dinner, the Regent and his wife withdrew to the royal quarters within the god Amon's earthly residence. Each of them meditated before a separate throne, symbolizing the primordial mound that emerged from the ocean of chaos at the beginning of time. It figured in the hieroglyph for Ma'at, the timeless Rule, 'That Which Is Right Will Give The Best Direction', the Rule that they must embody and impart to their subjects.

Ramses had the feeling his father was close at hand, seeing

him through these last tense hours before his life changed for ever. As king, his life would no longer be his own. His only care would be for his people's welfare and his nation's prosperity.

Once again, the prospect overwhelmed him.

He wished he could flee this palace, take refuge in his lost youth, in Iset the Fair, and the carefree pleasure they once knew. But now he was Seti's designated successor and Nefertari's husband. He would have to master his fear and ride out this one last night before his coronation.

The shadows parted and dawn came forth, announcing the sun's rebirth. Once more it had won the nightly struggle with the monster from the depths. Two masked priests, one in the guise of a falcon, the other an ibis, stood on either side of Ramses. They symbolized the gods Horus, protector of royalty, and Thoth, master of hieroglyphs and sacred learning. Pouring the contents of two tall vases over the prince's naked body, they cleansed him of his humanity. Then they remade him in the image of the gods, applying from head to toe the nine different unguents that would open his energy centres and give him a perception of reality different from other men's.

The ritual garments also helped construct his new and unique identity. The two priests dressed the prince in a kilt of white and gold, the same as the first pharaohs wore. On the sash, they hung a bull's tail, the emblem of royal potency. Ramses recalled the terrifying encounter with a wild bull his father had arranged as a test of his youthful courage. Now he would embody the bull's power, which he must learn to exercise wisely.

Then the ritualists fastened a large jewelled collar, with seven rows of coloured beads, round his neck, placed copper bracelets on his wrists and upper arms, and shod him in white sandals. They presented him with the white club he would use to strike down his enemies and make the darkness into light. Around his forehead they tied the golden band called *sia*, meaning 'intuitive seeing'.

'Do you accept the ordeal of power?' asked the Horus priest.

'I do.'

Horus and Thoth took Ramses by the hands and led him into another room. On a throne were the crowns of the Two Lands. Protecting them was a priest wearing the mask of the god Set.

Thoth stepped aside as the brothers Horus and Set embraced. Despite their eternal rivalry, they were obliged to be reunited in one being: Pharaoh.

Horus lifted the Red Crown of Lower Egypt, basket-shaped and surmounted by a spiral, and placed it on Ramses' head. On top of it, Set placed the White Crown of Upper Egypt whose oval form tapered up into the shape of a lotus bulb.

'The Two Powers are united in you,' declared Thoth. 'You govern and unify the black land and the red land, you are the rushes of the South and the beehive of the North, you make both lands green.'

'You alone will be able to lay a hand on these two crowns,' revealed Set. 'Within them is thunder to strike down any usurper.'

Horus gave the pharaoh two sceptres. The first was called 'Mastery of Power' and was used to bless offerings. The other, 'Magic', was a shepherd's crook serving to keep his people together.

'The time has come to appear in glory,' Thoth decreed.

Preceded by the three god-priests, Pharaoh left the temple's hidden rooms, heading for the huge inner courtyard where the privileged few allowed within the temple gates had gathered.

On a platform, beneath a dais, was a gilded wooden throne, rather modest and squarely built: Seti's throne, the one he had used for official ceremonies.

Sensing her son's hesitation, Tuya took three steps in his direction and bowed low.

'May Your Majesty rise like a new sun and take his place on the throne of the living.'

Ramses was deeply moved by this welcome from the pharaoh's widow, the mother he would venerate until the end of his days.

'This is the testament of the gods that Seti left you. As it legitimized his reign, so will it yours, so will it your successor's.' Tuya handed Ramses a leather case containing a papyrus written in Thoth's own hand, at the dawn of civilization, declaring Pharaoh the heir to Egypt.

'Here are your five royal names,' continued Tuya in her clear, steady voice. 'Strong Bull, Beloved of Ma'at. Protector of Egypt, Who Binds Foreign Countries. Rich in Armies, He of Stupendous Victories. Chosen of the God of Light, Powerful in His Rule. Ra-Begot-Him: Son of the Light.'

Total silence greeted these words. Even Shaanar felt the poison of ambition drain from him as he surrendered to the magic of the moment.

'A royal couple rules the Two Lands,' continued Tuya. 'Step forward, Nefertari, and take your place beside the king as his Great Royal Wife and Queen of Egypt.'

Despite the solemnity of the occasion, Ramses was so entranced by his bride's fresh beauty that he wished he could take her in his arms. In a long linen gown, with a golden collar, amethyst earrings and jasper bracelets, she gazed at the king and repeated the time-honoured formula:

'I recognize Horus and Set united in one being. I sing your name, Pharaoh: you are yesterday, today, and tomorrow. I live through your word and will keep you from evil and danger.'

'I recognize you as Queen of the North and South and of all lands, lady of utmost sweetness who pleases the gods, who is mother and wife of the god, who has my love.'

Ramses set a crown on Nefertari's head. Its two tall plumes declared her Great Royal Wife and associate ruler.

Like a blot on the sun, a falcon spread its great wings, circling above the new king and queen, then dived for them so suddenly that no royal archer had time to react.

A cry of horror and disbelief rose from the onlookers as the raptor landed on the new king's back, digging its claws into his shoulders. Ramses stood absolutely still; Nefertari stared.

Time stood still as the awe-struck courtiers registered the miracle. The falcon was Horus, protector of the monarchy. This man was truly chosen to govern Egypt!

The falcon flew back towards the sun, strong and serene.

A single cheer proclaimed Ramses' accession to the throne, on this twenty-seventh day of the third month of summer.*

* Early June, 1279 BC, according to one of the most commonly used estimates.

13

As soon as the ceremony was over, Ramses was swept up in a whirlwind of activity.

The head steward of the pharaoh's household had him inspect his palace at Thebes, both public rooms and private quarters. As head of state, he toured the pillared grand reception room whose floor and walls were adorned with mosaics and paintings of lotus, papyrus, fish and birds; the smaller private audience chambers; the scribes' offices; the balcony for official appearances, a winged solar disc above its window; the dining room with a table in the middle laden night and day with baskets of fruit and flower arrangements; the bedchamber with coloured pillows piled high on the bed; the tiled bathing room.

Ramses was introduced to the members of his household: the priests in charge of secret rituals, the scribes of the House of Life, the physicians, the chamberlain who superintended the private quarters, the heads of the royal messenger service, the royal treasury, the granary, livestock, and so on, all eager to meet their brand-new pharaoh and assure him of their undying devotion.

'And this is—'

Ramses got to his feet. 'That's enough.'

'Majesty, please!' the head steward spluttered. 'So many important people . . .'

'More important than I am?'

'Forgive me, I didn't mean—'

'Take me to the kitchens.'

'That's no place for you!'

'Who would know better than I where I belong?'

'Forgive me, I—'

'Let's not waste any more time on excuses. I'd rather hear why the vizier and the High Priest of Amon weren't here to pay their respects to me.'

'I have no idea, Majesty. That's completely beyond the scope of my authority.'

'To the kitchens, then.'

Butchers, bakers, pastry chefs, brewers, vegetable peelers, makers of preserved foods – Remet, the palace cook, commanded a small army of specialized workers, jealously guarding their prerogatives and as pernickety about their hours of work as about their days off. Jolly, round-cheeked, slow-moving Remet never worried about his triple chin and bulging belly. He'd do something about his weight when he retired. For now, he concentrated on ruling his domain with an iron fist, preparing delicious and flawless meals, keeping the peace among his staff of prima donnas. A stickler for cleanliness and fresh ingredients, Remet personally tasted each dish that left his kitchens. Whether or not Pharaoh and the members of his court were in Thebes, the cook never settled for less than perfection.

When the head steward appeared with a young man in tow, impressively built and dressed in an immaculate white kilt, Remet groaned inwardly. The head steward must be planning to saddle him with yet another useless worker in exchange for some favour from the boy's family.

'Greetings, Remet! I want to introduce you—'

'I can guess who he is.'

'Then bow, as is fitting.'

'That's rich!' guffawed Remet, hands on ample hips. 'Why should I bow to this young buck? First let's find out if he can even wash dishes.'

Scarlet with embarrassment, the steward turned to the king. 'I *beg* your forgiveness . . .'

'I can wash dishes,' Ramses said. 'Do you know how to cook?'

'Who do you think you are, questioning my expertise like that?'

'Ramses, Pharaoh of Egypt.'

Remet froze, convinced his career was over. Then he crisply removed his leather apron, folded it, and laid it on a low table. An insult to the king, confirmed as such by the vizier's court, carried a heavy penalty.

'What's on the menu for lunch?' asked Ramses.

'Quail,' Remet managed. 'Roast quail, nile perch with herb sauce, fig purée, honey cakes.'

'Tempting, but will it taste as good as it sounds?'

'I stake my reputation on it Majesty!' Remet protested.

'Your reputation means nothing to me. Let me try some food.'

'I'll have the staff prepare the dining room,' the steward said unctuously.

'Don't bother. I'll eat right here.'

Ramses lunched heartily under the steward's anxious gaze.

'Excellent,' he pronounced. 'What is your name, cook?'

'Remet, Majesty.'

'Remet. *Man.* It fits. All right, Remet, you're my new head steward, cup-bearer, and director of royal kitchens throughout the land. Follow me. I have a few questions for you.'

Stunned, the former chief steward stammered, 'Majesty? Pardon me, but where will I—'

'I have no use for inefficiency and meanness. There's always a shortage of dishwashers, though.'

The king and Remet strolled together in the shade of a covered portico.

'You'll report to my private secretary, Ahmeni. He looks frail and doesn't much care what he eats, but he's a tireless worker. Above all, he honours me with his friendship.'

'That's a huge responsibility for a mere cook,' said Remet in astonishment.

'My father taught me to judge men according to my instincts. If I'm wrong, that's just too bad. To govern, I shall need loyal followers. Do you think I'll find them at court?'

'To tell the truth—'

'Do, Remet. That's all I ask.'

'Then I can say that Your Majesty's court is the biggest collection of hypocrites and self-seekers in the entire kingdom. In fact, they seem to think they own the place. Your father kept them in line, but as soon as he was gone they started showing their true colours, like desert flowers after a rainstorm.'

'They hate me, don't they?'

'That's an understatement.'

'What do they hope will happen?'

'That you'll trip yourself up before long.'

'If you're with me, Remet, I demand your total loyalty.'

'Do you think I'm up to it?'

'A good cook isn't thin. A talented cook has everyone trying to steal his recipes. Rumours fly through his kitchen and he has to sort through them with the same care he takes in selecting ingredients. What are the main factions against me?'

'Almost the whole court is against you. The general opinion is that *anyone* would be ineffectual in comparison to a pharaoh of Seti's stature. They see you as a transitional figure until a serious contender appears.'

'Will you risk leaving your own little kingdom here in Thebes to run my households?'

Remet smiled broadly. 'Safety has both good and bad sides. As long as I can still cook good food, I'm willing to try. But I do have one reservation.'

'Tell me.'

'With all due respect, Majesty, you don't stand a chance.'

'Why this pessimism?'

'You're young and inexperienced. You don't intend to play a bit part in an administration run by the High Priest of Amon and dozens of experienced officials who know all the tricks of government. The balance of power is too unequal.'

'A pharaoh doesn't wield much power, according to you.'

'Of course he does. That's why everyone wants to take a shot at him. What chance does one man have against an army?'

'Pharaoh is supposed to be endowed with the might of the bull.'

'Not even a wild bull can move mountains, Majesty.'

'Am I to understand that you're advising me to abdicate, on the day of my coronation?'

'If you let the powers that be take charge, who will even notice, and who would blame you?'

'You, Remet?'

'I'm only the best cook in the country. What I think isn't important.'

'You're chief steward now, aren't you?'

'Would you listen, Majesty, if I offered some advice?'

'It all depends on what it is.'

'Never let yourself be served food or drink that's less than the best. It's the beginning of the end. Now, if you don't mind, I think I should get to work. Starting here in Thebes, there's a great deal to be done.'

Ramses had made no mistake. Remet was the man for the job.

Relieved, he headed for the palace garden.

14

Nefertari tried her hardest not to cry.

What she most feared had finally come to pass. She had dreamed of a quiet, cloistered life; now she felt as if she'd been swept away by a monstrous wave. Immediately after the coronation, she had been separated from Ramses to begin fulfilling her duties as Great Royal Wife, visiting the temples, schools, and weavers' guilds she officially sponsored.

Tuya introduced Nefertari to the managers of the queen's various estates, directors of harems where young women were educated, scribes in charge of administering her affairs, tax-collectors, priests and priestesses who would perform in her name the rites of 'the Wife of God', which were intended to preserve the creative force on earth.

For several days, Nefertari kept up a gruelling pace, meeting hundreds of people, finding the right thing to say to each of them, smiling constantly, never showing the slightest sign of fatigue.

Each morning a hairdresser, make-up artist, manicurist and pedicurist worked to make her even lovelier than the day before. The good of Egypt depended as much on her charm as on her husband's power. No queen could be more beautiful than Nefertari in her elegant, red-belted linen gown.

She lay exhausted on a narrow bed, unable to face the

evening's banquet or the thought of being presented with more jars of perfumed unguents.

Tuya's slight figure moved towards her through the gathering dusk.

'Are you ill, Nefertari?'

'I haven't the strength to go on.'

Seti's widow sat on the edge of the bed and took the young queen's right hand in her own hands.

'I know what you're going through. It was the same for me. Two things will help: a special tonic and the magnetizing force Ramses inherited from his father.'

'I wasn't meant to be queen.'

'Do you love Ramses?'

'More than myself.'

'Then you'll stand by him. He wed a queen, and a queen will fight at his side.'

'What if he chose the wrong woman?'

'He didn't. Don't you think there were times when I felt as tired and discouraged as you are now? The demands placed on a Great Royal Wife are beyond any woman. So it has been since the creation of Egypt, and it cannot be otherwise.'

'Didn't you want to give up?'

'A dozen times, a hundred times a day, at first. I begged Seti to take someone else as his chief consort and let me become his lesser wife. His answer was always the same: he took me in his arms and comforted me, yet did nothing to ease my burden of work.'

'If I can't perform my duties, aren't I unworthy of Ramses' faith in me?'

'Good, Nefertari. You take nothing for granted. Now listen. I'm not going to say this twice.'

The young queen's eyes filled with uncertainty. Tuya's clear gaze locked on hers.

'You're condemned to reign, Nefertari. Don't fight your

destiny. Let yourself glide with it, like a swimmer in the river.'

In less than three days, Ahmeni and Remet had begun a far-reaching reform of the government of Thebes, following Ramses' directives. He had met a wide range of officials, from the mayor to the head ferryman. Owing to its distance from Memphis and the fact that Seti had taken up near-permanent residence in the North, the Southern capital had grown increasingly independent. The High Priest of Amon, with the force of his temple's immense wealth behind him, was beginning to consider himself a kind of monarch, whose decrees took precedence over the king's. Ramses' meetings with local officials made him aware of how dangerous the situation was. Unless he acted quickly, Upper and Lower Egypt might split into two different, even opposing, countries, and the division would lead to disaster.

From the beginning, Ahmeni and Remet worked well together. Physical and mental opposites, they complemented each other *because* of their differences. They shared a deep respect for Ramses as well as the conviction that he was heading in the right direction. Turning a deaf ear to hidebound courtiers, they forged ahead with their sweeping reforms, making a number of unexpected appointments with the king's approval.

Two weeks after the coronation, Thebes was in turmoil. Some officials had predicted that the new pharaoh would prove incompetent. Others saw him as an adolescent, in love with hunting and sporting exploits. Yet Ramses had spent his days in the palace, holding meetings and issuing decrees with a vigour and authority worthy of Seti.

Ramses waited for the inevitable reaction, but it never came. Thebes seemed stunned into inertia.

Summoned by the king, the Vizier of the South was

deferential, noting His Majesty's directives with assurances that they would be carried out at once.

Ramses did not share in Ahmeni's boyish excitement or Remet's amused satisfaction. His enemies might have been taken by surprise, but they were far from defeated. They would regroup and come back at him stronger than ever. The king would have preferred an open fight to their insidious plotting in the shadows, but that was a childish wish, he knew.

Just before sunset he always walked the paths of the palace garden, as twenty-odd workers began watering the trees and flower beds in the cool of the evening. On his left trotted Wideawake, the yellow dog, wearing a collar of blue flowers; on his right loped Invincible, the gigantic lion. And at the entrance to the garden was Serramanna, the Sardinian captain of the Royal Bodyguard, sitting beneath an arbour, alert and ready to act at the smallest sign of danger.

Ramses felt an intense affection for the sycamores, pomegranates, perseas, figs, and other trees that made the garden a paradise and a comfort to his soul. He wished all of Egypt could be like this haven where a wealth of essences lived in harmony.

One evening, Ramses was planting a tiny sycamore, mounding soil around the seedling and watering it carefully.

'Your Majesty should wait half an hour, then give it another jug of water, almost drop by drop.'

He looked up to see a gardener of indeterminate age. The back of his neck showed a healing ulcer where the weight of his yoke rested. Two heavy earthenware water jugs hung from it – one at either end.

'Wise advice,' Ramses told him. 'What's your name, gardener?'

'Nedjem.'

'"The mild one." Tell me, Nedjem, are you married?'

'Married to this garden, you might say. The trees, plants, and flowers are my family, my ancestors and descendants. The sycamore you just planted will outlive you, even if you spend a hundred and ten years on earth like the wise men.'

'You can be sure of that,' said Ramses with a smile.

'It can't be easy to be a king and be wise. The human race are too perverse and devious.'

'You're a member of it. Don't you share those faults?'

'I dare not say, Majesty.'

'Have you trained any of the younger men?'

'That's up to the superintendent, not me.'

'Is he a better gardener than you?'

'How would I know? He never comes here.'

'Do you think the tree population is adequate in Egypt?'

'It's the only population that can never be too large.'

'I agree.'

'A tree is a gift,' the gardener said emphatically. 'During its lifetime, it offers us shade, flowers, and fruit; after its death comes wood. Thanks to trees, we eat, we build, we feel blessed when the soft north wind fans us through the branches. I dream of a country of trees where the only other inhabitants are birds and the souls of the dead.'

'I intend to have trees planted in every province,' revealed Ramses. 'Every village square will have a patch of shade where the generations can meet and the young can listen to the wisdom of their elders.'

'May the gods smile upon your work, Majesty. No government programme could be more useful.'

'Will you help me make it a reality?'

'How could I?'

'The Agriculture secretariat is full of hard-working, competent scribes. But to steer them in the right direction, I need a man who loves nature and knows its secrets.'

'I'm only a gardener, Majesty, a—'

'You have the makings of an excellent minister for

agriculture. Come to the palace tomorrow and ask to see Ahmeni. He'll know what I want you to do and help you get started.'

Ramses went on his way, leaving Nedjem amazed and stunned. At the edge of the huge garden, between two fig trees, the king thought he saw a slim, white figure. Had a goddess just appeared in this magical spot?

He hurried towards the apparition, which hadn't moved.

In the soft glow of sunset he made out shining dark hair and a long white gown. How could a woman be so beautiful, at once aloof and enticing?

'Nefertari . . .'

She ran into his arms. 'I managed to slip away,' she confessed. 'Your mother agreed to stand in for me at the lute concert tonight. Have you forgotten me yet?'

'Your mouth is a lotus bud and your lips cast magic spells, but all I want to do right now is kiss you.'

Their kiss renewed them. As they clung together, their devotion to each other was reborn.

'I'm a wild bird you've trapped in the net of your hair,' said Ramses. 'You're a garden of a thousand different flowers, whose perfumes intoxicate me.'

Nefertari let down her hair, Ramses slipped the straps of her linen dress off her shoulders. In the warmth of a peaceful, sweet-smelling summer night, they came together.

15

The first ray of sunlight woke Ramses. He stroked his sleeping wife's delicious back and kissed her on the neck. Without opening her eyes, she twined round him, fitting her body to his powerful frame.

'I'm so happy.'

'Happiness is what you are, Nefertari.'

'Let's never stay apart so long again.'

'Neither of us has any choice in the matter.'

'Won't our lives ever be our own?' Ramses held her tight. 'You aren't answering,' she said.

'Because you know the answer, Nefertari. You're the Great Royal Wife, and I'm Pharaoh. We can't escape the fact, even in our dreams.'

Ramses rose and walked to the window, looking out over the Theban countryside, lush green in the summer sun.

'I love you, Nefertari, but I'm wed to my country as well. I have to keep this land fertile and prosperous. When Egypt calls, I must not ignore it.'

'Is there so much left to do?'

'I thought I'd be ruling a peaceful country, and I forgot that it's inhabited by men. A few weeks is all it would take to overturn the rule of Ma'at and undo the work of Seti and all our ancestors. Harmony is the most fragile of treasures. If I relax my vigilance, Egypt will soon be conquered by evil and darkness.'

Nefertari crossed to meet him, pressing her naked body to his. The merest touch of her scented skin told him their understanding was complete.

Someone knocked urgently at the bedchamber door. Before they answered, it flew open, and a wild-eyed Ahmeni entered. As soon as he noticed the queen, he looked away.

'It's serious, Ramses, very serious.'

'Isn't it a bit early to come bursting in like this?'

'Come with me. There isn't a moment to lose.'

'No time to wash and have some breakfast?'

'Not this morning.'

Ramses could not ignore Ahmeni's warning, especially when the young scribe, usually so imperturbable, had lost his self-possession.

The king drove his own two-horse chariot. The one behind him carried Serramanna and an archer. The ride made Ahmeni queasy, but he was glad Ramses drove so fast. They came to a halt in front of one of the gates to the temple of Karnak, jumped down and studied the stele covered with hieroglyph inscriptions any literate passer-by would be able to read.

'Look,' said Ahmeni. 'There, the third line down.'

The drawing of three animal pelts, signifying 'Birth' and designating Ramses as the 'Son' of the Light, was incorrect. The error robbed the inscription of its protective magic and damaged the Pharaoh's secret identity.

'I checked,' a shattered Ahmeni informed them, 'and the same mistake is on statue pedestals, and steles like this one, which can be seen by all and sundry. It's deliberate malice, Ramses!'

'Who could have done such a thing?'

'The High Priest of Amon and his sculptors. They carved

80

all the inscriptions proclaiming your coronation. If you hadn't seen for yourself, you'd never have believed me.'

Although the general meaning of the proclamations was unchanged, the altered royal name was definitely a serious matter.

'Call in the sculptors,' ordered Ramses, 'and have the inscriptions put right.'

'Aren't you going to prosecute the culprits?'

'They were only following orders.'

'The High Priest of Amon is ill; that's why he hasn't come to pay his respects to you.'

'Have you any proof that he's behind this? He's an important religious leader.'

'His guilt is obvious!'

'Don't trust in the obvious, Ahmeni.'

'Is he to go unpunished? No matter how rich and powerful he is, he's still your servant.'

'Compile a list of his possessions for me, will you?'

Remet had no complaints about his new duties. After appointing strict, diligent men to oversee sanitation, to ensure the palace's cleanliness, he turned his attention to the royal menagerie, consisting of three wild cats, two gazelles, a hyena and two grey cranes.

One animal remained beyond his control, however. Wide-awake, the pharaoh's yellow-gold dog, was in the annoying habit of snacking on fish from the royal pond. Since the king's pet lion was his partner in crime, there was no way of stopping him.

Early in the morning, Remet had helped Ahmeni haul in a heavy crate of papyrus. He wondered where the puny young scribe, who barely ate and slept only three or four hours a night, found so much energy. He spent the greater part of his days at his desk poring over papers, never showing the slightest sign of fatigue.

Ahmeni conferred with Ramses while Remet made his

daily inspection of the kitchen. Pharaoh's health, and therefore the health of the entire nation, depended on the quality of his food, he maintained.

Ahmeni unrolled several papyrus scrolls on low tables.

'Here's the information on Karnak,' he said with a hint of pride.

'Was it hard to gather?'

'Yes and no. The temple administrators weren't particularly happy to see me or answer my questions, but they didn't dare stop me checking their figures.'

'And is Karnak as rich as we thought?'

'Richer. Eighty thousand employees, forty-six building sites on its outlying properties, four hundred and fifty gardens, orchards and vineyards, four hundred and twenty thousand head of livestock, ninety boats, and sixty-five settlements of various sizes directly dependent on the largest religious establishment in Egypt. The High Priest commands a veritable army of scribes and farm workers. Add to all this the property belonging to the god Amon, which the clergy controls, and the total is six million head of cattle and as many goats, twelve million donkeys, eight million mules, and several million fowl.'

'Amon is the god of victory and the protector of the empire,' said Ramses.

'No one's denying that, but his priests are only men. Managing such enormous wealth exposes them to overwhelming temptations. I didn't have time to investigate any further, but the situation worries me.'

'Anything specific?'

'The Theban authorities are anxious for Your Majesty to go north again. You're disrupting their peace and upsetting their routine. All they want is to fatten Karnak's coffers and keep it growing like a state within a state, until the day the High Priest of Amon proclaims himself King of the South and secedes from the union.'

'That would mean the death of Egypt, Ahmeni.'

'And misery for the people.'

'I'd need solid proof that there's been corruption. If I'm to move against the High Priest of Amon, I can't afford any mistakes.'

'Leave it to me, Ramses.'

Serramanna was uneasy. Ever since Menelaus' bungled coup, he was aware that Ramses' life was in danger. The Greeks might have left the country, but the threat remained.

He kept a close eye on what he considered the trouble spots in Thebes: the military base, palace police headquarters, the barracks for the guard detachment. If a revolt was in the making, it would come from one of those places. The Sard trusted his pirate's instincts, remaining wary of enlisted men and officers alike. In a number of instances, he had survived only by striking the first blow against an enemy who'd pretended to be a friend.

Despite his huge size, Serramanna moved like a cat. He liked to eavesdrop and observe from the shadows. No matter how hot it was, he wore a metal breastplate. In his belt he carried a dagger and a short, sharp-tipped sword. A frizzy moustache and side-whiskers made his massive face even more frightening; he used this to his advantage.

Career army officers, most of whom came from a wealthy background, hated Serramanna and wondered why Ramses had put such a lout in charge of his personal bodyguard. The Sard blithely ignored them. He didn't care about popularity. It wouldn't help him be the best fighter serving a good leader.

And Ramses was a good leader, captain of an enormous ship on a treacherous and adventure-filled course.

In short, his job was everything a Sardinian pirate could have wished for, and he was determined to keep it. He enjoyed his villa, fine food, Egyptian beauties with breasts round as love-apples, but these were not enough to satisfy

83

him. Nothing could replace the thrill of proving himself in combat.

The palace guard was changed on the first, eleventh, and twenty-first of each month. The men received their food and wine rations and were paid in grain. Each time the troops were relieved, Serramanna looked the new men over carefully before he assigned them. Any lapse in discipline, any slackening, resulted in a flogging and immediate dismissal.

The Sard walked slowly down the single row of soldiers. He stopped in front of a fair-haired boy who seemed slightly nervous.

'Where do you come from?'

'A village in the Delta, sir.'

'Your favourite weapon?'

'The sword.'

'Have a drink, soldier. You look thirsty.'

Serramanna handed the fair-haired boy a flask of anise-flavoured wine. He took two quick swallows.

'I'll post you in the hallway to the royal office. Your job is keeping everyone out of there during the last watch of the night.'

'Yes, sir.'

Serramanna had the men present arms, checked their uniforms, exchanged a few words with other soldiers, then sent them on their way.

The palace architects had set windows high in the walls so that cool air could circulate through the corridors on hot summer nights.

Everything was quiet. Outside, the frogs sang their mating songs.

Serramanna crept soundlessly down the tiled hallway leading to Ramses's office.

As he had suspected, the boy from the Delta was not at his post. Instead, he was fiddling with the latch on the office door. The Sard reached out one broad hand and lifted him by the scruff of the neck.

'A Greek, eh? Only a Greek could drink anise wine without flinching. Which faction do you belong to, my lad? One of Menelaus' leftovers, or part of some new plot? Answer me!'

The fair-haired boy twitched briefly, but made no sound.

Feeling the Greek go limp, Serramanna put him down on the floor, where he sprawled like a rag doll. Without meaning to, he had broken the boy's neck.

16

Written reports were not Serramanna's province. He simply stated the facts to Ahmeni, who put them down on papyrus and alerted Ramses. No one knew anything about the young Greek, who had been recruited on the strength of his skill with a sword. His brutal death made it impossible to trace the real instigator, but the king, more grateful than ever for Serramanna's vigilance, refrained from reprimanding his bodyguard.

This time, the object of the break-in was not the pharaoh but his office, meaning affairs of state. Someone wanted confidential documents and information about the new king's future policies.

Menelaus' attack had been motivated by revenge; this incident was far murkier. Who had hired the young Greek to slink through the shadows and compromise Ramses at the beginning of his reign? Of course, there was Shaanar, the embittered brother, strangely inactive and quiet since the coronation. Could he be working behind the scenes, much more effectively than in the past?

Remet bowed to the king. 'Majesty, your visitor has arrived.'

'Show him to the garden pavilion.'

Ramses wore only a simple white kilt and a single piece of jewellery, a gold bracelet on his right wrist. He collected his thoughts for a few moments, aware that the fate of Egypt would hinge on the interview he was about to conduct.

The king had had an elegant wooden pavilion put up in the garden, in the shade of a willow tree. A low table was spread with silvery green grapes and fresh figs. Cups of light, refreshing beer would be ideal in the summer heat.

The High Priest of Amon sat in an armchair with plump cushions and a matching footstool. He was resplendent in his wig, linen robe, bib necklace of pearls and lapis lazuli, and his silver bracelets.

As soon as he saw his sovereign, the High Priest rose and bowed to him.

'I trust this place is to your liking,' Ramses said.

'Majesty, I thank you for considering an old man's health.'

'You're not feeling well?'

'I'm no longer a young man. It's very hard to accept.'

'I was beginning to think we'd never meet.'

'Heavens, no, Majesty. For one thing, I was confined to my bed for a time. For another, I hoped to bring the Viziers of the North and the South along with me, and the Viceroy of Nubia.'

'What a delegation! Did they reject your proposal?'

'At first, no; later they did.'

'What made them change their minds?'

'They're high-ranking officials – they did not wish to displease Your Majesty. Still, their presence would have given my words added weight.'

'If your cause is just, you have nothing to fear.'

'Do you think it is?'

'Let me decide that, with Ma'at to guide me.'

'I'm worried, Majesty.'

'What can I do to ease your mind?'

'You asked for an accounting of Karnak's riches.'

'And I got it.'

'What do you conclude?'

'That you're a remarkable administrator.'

'Should I take that as criticism?'

'Certainly not. Our ancestors taught, did they not, that spiritual and material welfare go hand in hand. Pharaoh endows Karnak, and you make it prosper.'

'I still sense criticism in your tone, Majesty.'

'Puzzlement, nothing more. Why don't we discuss your concerns instead?'

'It's rumoured that Karnak's wealth and glory offend Your Majesty, and you wish to redistribute some of its privileges.'

'Where have you heard this?'

'Here and there.'

'And you believe these rumours?'

'When they are persistent, one cannot ignore them.'

'What do you yourself think?'

'That Your Majesty would be well advised to leave things as they are. That the wisest course would be to follow in your esteemed father's footsteps.'

'Unfortunately, his reign was cut short before he had time to enact a great many necessary reforms.'

'Karnak needs no reforms.'

'That's not what I think.'

'Then my worries were justified.'

'Perhaps mine are, too.'

'Majesty, I don't understand.'

'Is the High Priest of Amon still Pharaoh's faithful servant?'

The prelate averted his eyes. To regain his composure, he ate a fig and drank some beer. The king was as direct in his questioning as he was unpretentious in dress, and the priest had not been prepared for either. However, the young pharaoh was careful not to push him, allowing him time to gather his wits.

'How can you doubt my loyalty, Majesty?' he said at length.

88

'Because of Ahmeni's investigation.'

The High Priest reddened. 'That snivelling little scribe, that sneak, that rat, that—'

'Ahmeni is my friend, and his only ambition is to serve Egypt. I will not tolerate any insult to him, no matter who utters it.'

'Forgive me, Majesty,' stammered the priest. 'But his methods . . .'

'Did he use undue force?'

'No, but he was more relentless than a jackal devouring its kill!'

'He's conscientious and thorough.'

'For what are you criticizing me?'

Ramses looked the High Priest square in the face. 'Don't you know?'

Again, the prelate looked away.

'Egypt and everything in it belongs to the pharaoh, does it not?' asked Ramses.

'According to the testament of the gods.'

'But the pharaoh may grant land to men who have proved themselves worthy.'

'According to custom.'

'Is the High Priest of Amon authorized to act in Pharaoh's stead?'

'The High Priest is his delegate and his representative at Karnak.'

'Haven't you taken being his delegate too far?'

'I don't see—'

'You've deeded land to secular individuals, putting them in your debt. Military officers, for instance, whose loyalty to me might then be compromised. Perhaps you need an army to defend your private domain?'

'Mere circumstance, Majesty! You can't be thinking—'

'There are three major centres of worship in Egypt. Heliopolis is the holy city of Ra, the God of Light. Memphis worships Ptah, who created the Word, and inspires the work of craftsmen. Thebes is the home of Amon, the hidden god, whose true form no one knows. My father strove to maintain these three cities in harmony. Your policies, however, have thrown them out of balance, giving Thebes a disproportionate importance.'

'Majesty! Would you see Amon slighted?'

'Never. Amon's worldly representative is the one I question. As of today, I suspend you from your administrative responsibilities so that you may concentrate on religious devotions.'

The prelate struggled to his feet. 'You know very well I can't do that.'

'Why not?'

'Because my duties are both spiritual and administrative, exactly like yours.'

'Karnak belongs to Pharaoh.'

'No one would deny that, but who will manage its affairs.'

'I'll appoint an administrator.'

'That would destroy our whole priestly order. Majesty, I beg you to reconsider. Turning the priesthood of Amon against you would be most unwise.'

'Is that a threat?'

'The advice of an experienced man to a young monarch.'

'Do you think I'll follow it?'

'Ruling is a difficult art which requires a number of alliances, including that with the priests of Amon. Of course, as your faithful servant I shall follow your orders, whatever they may be.'

Though visibly weary, the High Priest had regained his confidence.

'Don't fight a pointless battle, Majesty. You could lose much by doing so. When the excitement of coming to power has passed, come to your senses again and don't turn everything upside-down. The gods abhor excess – remember Akhenaton's appalling conduct towards Thebes.'

'Your net is tightly woven,' Ramses told him, 'but a falcon's beak can tear holes in it.'

'Such a waste of energy! You belong in Memphis, not here. Egypt needs your strength to push back the barbarians who long to invade us. Let me take care of Thebes, and I'll support you.'

'I'll think it over.'

The High Priest smiled. 'You have intelligence to match your spirit: you'll be a great pharaoh, Ramses.'

17

Each and every Theban notable had only one thing in mind: pleading his cause with the new king in order to retain existing privileges. Ramses was an unknown quantity, aligned with no particular faction. Who knew what unpleasant surprises he might have in store for even the best-connected courtiers? But to meet with the pharaoh one had to get past Ahmeni, who refused to let anyone waste his own time, much less Ramses'. Then there was the little matter of Serramanna's insistence on searching each visitor for hidden weapons.

Ramses cancelled the rest of the morning's appointments, including one with the dykes inspector Ahmeni had recommended. Well, let Ahmeni take care of him. The king needed the advice of the Great Royal Wife.

After a refreshing dip, they sat on the edge of the pool, their naked bodies basking in the sun that filtered through the sycamores. The palace gardens were more beautiful than ever since Nedjem had been made minister for agriculture.

'I finally met the High Priest of Amon this morning,' Ramses confessed.

'Is his hostility implacable?'

'Absolutely. Either I fall in with his wishes or I enforce my own.'

'What does he want you to do?'

'Leave Karnak as the most powerful temple in Egypt. He'll rule the South and let me keep the North.'

'Out of the question.'

Ramses looked at Nefertari in amazement. 'I was certain you'd preach moderation!'

'If moderation leads to the country's ruin, it's no longer a virtue. This priest is trying to impose his rule on Pharaoh, to protect his own interests with no concern for the general welfare. If you give in, the throne will be shaken and everything Seti built will be destroyed.'

Nefertari spoke calmly, in her soft, soothing voice, yet her views were clear and firm.

'Can you imagine the consequences of conflict between the king and the High Priest of Amon?' Ramses asked her.

'If you show weakness at the beginning of your reign, ambitious and unworthy men will rise up against you. The High Priest will head the rebellion and assert his own authority at the expense of Pharaoh's.'

'I'm not afraid to take him on, but—'

'You're afraid it's for selfish reasons. That you have to prove your strength from the beginning.'

Ramses gazed at her reflection in the blue water of the pool. 'Are you a mind-reader?'

'I'm your wife.'

'Tell me what you think, Nefertari.'

'A pharaoh is larger than life. You are all that is generous, eager and strong. You're acting on those qualities – acting as a ruler.'

'But am I choosing the right way?'

'The High Priest wants to divide and conquer. There is no evil greater than civil war. As pharaoh, you must not cede him a single cubit of ground.'

Ramses laid his head on Nefertari's breast. She gently stroked his hair as all around them swallows dived, rustling the silken air.

The sound of a scuffle at the gates to the garden broke the

spell. A woman was arguing with the guards, her voice growing ever louder.

Ramses threw on his kilt and headed towards the group.

'What's going on here?'

The guards stepped aside and there stood Iset the Fair, blooming and vivacious as ever.

'Majesty!' she exclaimed. 'Let me speak to you, I beg of you.'

'Who's stopping you?'

'Your police, your army, your secretary, your—'

'Come with me, Iset.'

A small boy stepped out from behind her.

'Here's our son, Ramses.'

'Kha!' Ramses picked him up and lifted him over his head. The frightened child burst into tears.

'He's very shy,' said Iset.

The king sat the boy astride his shoulders. Soon Kha forgot his fear and began to laugh.

'Four years old . . . He's getting to be a big boy! What does his tutor say?'

'That he's too serious. Kha doesn't play much; he'd rather be reading. He already knows a lot of hieroglyphs; he can even write a few.'

'He'll catch up with me before long! Come and sit by the pool. I'm going to teach Kha to swim.'

'Is she . . . is Nefertari with you?'

'Of course.'

'Why have I had so much trouble getting in to see you? You shouldn't treat me like a stranger. You'd be dead if it weren't for me.'

'What do you mean?'

'I sent that letter to warn you about the coup.'

'What are you talking about?'

Iset hung her head. 'All right, I admit there was a time when I resented being left in Thebes. I was so alone. But I never stopped loving you, and I refused to join forces with the members of your own family working against you.'

'I never got your letter.'

Iset turned white. 'Then you thought I was against you, too?'

'Was I wrong?'

'Yes, you were! By the name of Pharaoh, I swear I never betrayed you!'

'Why should I believe you?'

Iset took Ramses's arm. 'How could I lie to you?'

Now they approached Nefertari, and her beauty took Iset's breath away. It was not so much her outward perfection as her true radiance that disarmed and conquered everyone around her. Nefertari was truly a Great Royal Wife. No one could touch her.

Iset was untroubled by jealousy. Nefertari shone like the summer sky; her nobility inspired only respect.

'Iset! I'm so happy to see you.' As lesser wife, Iset bowed to her. 'Please don't. Come, Iset, have a swim. It's so hot today.'

Iset had not expected such a welcome. Without a word, she acquiesced, removing her clothes. Naked as Nefertari, she dived into the blue water.

As they swam, Ramses watched the two women he loved. How could his feelings for them be so different, yet so intense and sincere? Nefertari was the great love of his life, an exceptional person, a queen. Neither adversity nor the ravages of time could weaken the passion that illuminated their lives. Iset the Fair was his carefree youth – desire, sensuality, passion. Still, she had lied and plotted against him; he had no choice but to punish her.

'Is it true I'm your son?' piped Kha.

'Yes, it is.'

'The hieroglyph for "son" has a duck in it.' The little boy carefully drew a duck in the sand with his finger.

'Do you know the one for "pharaoh"?'

Kha drew a house, then a column.

'The house means protection, the column means greatness. *Per-ah*, great house – that's the real meaning of the word. Do you know why they call me Pharaoh?'

'Because you're taller than everybody and you live in a great big house.'

'That's right, my son, but the house is all Egypt, and each person must find a home in it.'

'Will you teach me some more hieroglyphs?'

'Wouldn't you like to play another game?'

Kha pouted.

'All right then,' Ramses told him, and the boy brightened. The king traced a circle with a dot in its centre.

'The sun,' he explained. 'The sun is called Ra. His name is made of a mouth and an arm, because he's both word and deed. Now you draw it.'

The child drew a series of suns, each one closer to a perfect circle. Fresh from their swim, Iset and Nefertari inspected Kha's hieroglyphs and were astonished.

'He's very advanced for his age,' said the queen.

'It almost frightens me sometimes,' said Iset. 'His tutor doesn't know what to do with him.'

'Then he needs another tutor,' said Ramses. 'My son should develop his talents, no matter what other children his age do. His ability is a gift from the gods. We mustn't hold him back. Wait here.'

The king left the garden and went into the palace.

Kha began to cry; his finger was sore. 'May I pick him up?' Nefertari asked Iset.

'Yes. Yes, of course.'

The boy quietened almost at once. Nefertari's eyes were full of tenderness. Iset felt bold enough to ask the question tormenting her.

'Despite the loss of your daughter, are you planning to have more children?'

'In fact, I've just begun to suspect I'm pregnant again.'

'Ah . . . may the gods of childbirth smile upon you.'

'Thank you, Iset. Your kind words will help me when my time comes.'

Iset hid her dismay. She did not dispute that Nefertari was Ramses' queen and hardly envied her the crushing responsibilities that came with the position of Great Royal Wife. What she did want was more children with Ramses, many more, and the honour attached to being their mother. For the time being, she remained the mother of his firstborn son, but, if Nefertari gave birth to a boy, he would probably be given precedence over Kha.

Ramses returned with a miniature scribe's palette, complete with two tiny cakes of ink, one red, the other black, and three miniature brushes. When he handed it to his son, Kha's face lit up and he clutched the precious things to his heart.

'Thank you, Daddy!'

Once Iset and Kha had gone, Ramses again spoke his mind to Nefertari.

'I'm convinced she had something to do with the coup.'

'Did you question her?'

'She admits she was upset with me, but she claims she tried to warn me that an attack was being planned. If she did, I never got her message.'

'Why don't you believe her?'

'I think she is lying, and that she hasn't forgiven me for making you my consort.'

'You're wrong.'

'Her offence should be punished.'

'What offence? A pharaoh can't hand out punishments based on fleeting impressions. Iset has given you a fine son. She wishes you no harm. Forgive the offence, if she ever committed one, and forget the punishment.'

18

Setau's outfit stood out from those of the palace courtiers and scribes. His thick antelope-skin garment, cut like a winter tunic, had been treated with antivenom preparations. In an emergency, Setau could whip off his tunic, soak it in water, and produce a satisfactory snakebite remedy.

'This isn't the desert,' Ramses told him. 'You hardly need that portable pharmacy in Memphis.'

'It's more dangerous here than in deepest Nubia. Snakes and scorpions everywhere, though you might not recognize them at first glance. Are you ready?'

'I fasted, just as you told me to.'

'The treatments have gone well so far. You've built up an immunity to most kinds of snakebite, even certain cobras. Do you really want this added protection?'

'I gave you my consent.'

'It's not without risk.'

'Let's get on with it.'

'Did you ask Nefertari about it?'

'Did you ask Lotus?'

'She says I'm slightly mad, but we see eye to eye.'

Unshaven, square-jawed, refusing to wear a wig, Setau would have sent an ordinary patient running.

'If I've got the dose wrong,' he warned his friend, 'you could end up an imbecile.'

'No use trying to scare me off.'

'Drink this, then.'

Ramses drank the potion.

'What do you think?'

'Tastes good.'

'That's because of the carob juice. The other ingredients are less appetizing: extracts of several different stinging plants and diluted cobra blood. Now you're protected against any bite there is. You'll only need to take this mixture every six months to keep up that defence.'

'Setau, when will you come to work for me?'

'Never. And when will you stop being so naive? I could have poisoned you, just now.'

'You're not a murderer.'

'As if you'd know!'

'I learned a few things from Menelaus. What's more, you've been screened by Serramanna, my lion and my dog.'

'What a threesome. But are you forgetting that Thebes can't wait to see you leave and most of the notables hope to see you fail?'

'Nature has endowed me with a good memory.'

'Men are a far more dangerous species than snakes, Ramses.'

'Yes, but men are what a pharaoh has to work with, if his goal is to build a just and harmonious world.'

'Humph! You must be living in a dream world. Beware, my friend. You're surrounded by schemers and villains. Still, you have one advantage: you feel the same mysterious force I do when I work with cobras. It brought you Nefertari, the most wonderful partner any king could have. I think you'll make it.'

'It will be harder without your help.'

'Flattery didn't use to be one of your faults. I'm heading north now, with a load of venom. Take care, Ramses.'

Despite his brother's early show of strength, Shaanar was not discouraged. Who could tell what would happen when the young pharaoh locked horns with the High Priest of Amon? It would probably end in a stalemate, undermining Ramses' authority. His word was far from carrying the weight of Seti's.

Shaanar was beginning to get the measure of his brother.

A frontal attack was certain to fail, since Ramses would defend himself so forcefully that he would turn the situation to his advantage. It would be better to lay a series of traps, using trickery, lies and betrayal. As long as Ramses could not identify his enemies, he would waste his energy flailing at shadows. Once he was exhausted, it would be easy to finish him off.

While the new king was busy forming his government and bringing Thebes to heel, his brother had been quiet and discreet as if these events were nothing to do with him. Soon he would have to make himself heard, or else be suspected of plotting in the background.

After much thought, Shaanar had concluded that his best course was to play an apparently crude game, blatantly exploiting Ramses, who would react in his usual hot-headed way, without realizing that it was exactly the reaction his brother wanted. If his little experiment worked, Shaanar would know that Ramses could be manipulated.

In that case, the future would be bright.

For the tenth time, Ramses was lecturing Wideawake about his fishing expeditions. It wasn't nice to steal from the palace ponds. It *was* nice to share his catch with Invincible, but didn't they both get enough to eat as it was? The yellow-gold dog listened attentively, yet his expression told the king he was wasting his breath. With the lion as his accomplice, Wideawake knew he could get away with murder.

The towering figure of Serramanna appeared in the doorway of Ramses' office.

'Your brother wants to see you, but he refuses to be searched.'

'Let him in.'

Serramanna stepped aside. Shaanar shot him an icy look in passing.

'Would Your Majesty be so good as to grant me a private interview?'

The yellow dog tagged after Serramanna, who always had a treat for him.

'It's a long time since we talked, Shaanar.'

'You have so much to do. I didn't want to be a nuisance.'

Ramses circled his brother, inspecting him.

'Why are you looking at me like that?' Shaanar said anxiously.

'You're thinner, dear brother.'

'I've been trying to cut back these last few weeks.'

Despite his dieting, Shaanar was still plump. His small dark eyes shone in a moon face with the pudgy cheeks and the full lips of a true food-lover.

'Why have you kept your beard?'

'I'll never stop mourning Seti,' he said. 'How could I ever forget our father?'

'I sympathize,' Ramses said feelingly.

'I'm sure you do, but your duties leave you little time to dwell on it. It's not the same for me.'

'What brings you here today?'

'You've been expecting me, haven't you?'

The king made no comment.

'I'm your elder brother and my reputation is excellent. I've put our differences behind me; I can live with the fact that I was passed over for the throne. But I can't resign myself to being a rich, idle courtier, of no real use to my country.'

'I understand how you feel.'

'My work as Head of Protocol is no longer enough for me, especially since Remet, the new head steward, has been handling most of it.'

'What do you want, Shaanar?'

'I've thought long and hard before approaching you. I had to swallow my pride.'

'There should be no question of such a thing between brothers.'

'Will you meet my demands?'

'Not when I have no idea what they are.'

'Will you hear me out?'

'Please go ahead.'

Shaanar began to pace. 'Could I ask to become vizier? Impossible. You'd be accused of favouritism. Head of the police? The bureaucracy is too complicated. Head royal scribe? Too demanding – not enough rest and leisure time. What about overseeing your construction projects? No, I have no experience. Agriculture? You've already filled the position. Finance? You kept the incumbent. You plan to reform the temples, but I have no taste for the religious life.'

'What does that leave?'

'The one job I'm suited for: minister for foreign affairs. You're aware of my interest in trade relations. Instead of concentrating on negotiations for my personal gain, I want to work towards strengthening diplomatic ties with our neighbours, as well as within our dependent territories.' Shaanar finally came to a halt, asking, 'Does my proposal shock you?'

'It's a tremendous responsibility.'

'Would you authorise me to do everything possible to prevent war with the Hittites? No one wants bloodshed. If Pharaoh appoints his elder brother minister for foreign affairs, it will show just how important peace is to him.'

Ramses pondered. 'I'll grant your request, Shanaar, but you'll need help.'

'I know. Who do you have in mind?'

'My friend Ahsha, a professional diplomat.'

'A supervisor?'

'A partner, I hope.'

'As Your Majesty wishes.'

'Meet him as soon as possible, then let me have details of your plans.'

On his way out of the palace, Shaanar could barely contain a whoop of joy.

Ramses had reacted just as he'd hoped.

19

Dolora prostrated herself and kissed her brother's feet.

'Forgive me, I beg of you,' she sobbed. 'Forgive my husband and me!'

'Get up, Dolora. Don't make a spectacle of yourself.'

Dolora let Ramses help her to her feet, but was still afraid to look at him. Tall and listless, she seemed about to swoon.

'Forgive us, Ramses. We didn't know what we were doing!'

'You wanted me dead. Twice your husband tried to have me killed. Sary, who practically raised me!'

'It was wrong of him, very wrong, and I was just as bad. But we were used as catspaws.'

'By whom, dear sister?'

'The High Priest at Karnak. He convinced us you'd be a bad king, that you'd lead the country into a civil war.'

'You didn't have much faith in me at all.'

'My husband knew you as an impetuous boy, always itching for a fight. Now he sees the error of his ways – if you only knew how truly sorry he is!'

'And did our dear brother also try to convince you?'

'No,' lied Dolora. 'He's the one we should have listened to. Once he was reconciled to our father's decision to name you as his successor, Shaanar became one of your staunchest supporters. His only thought now is of serving Egypt in a position worthy of his talents.'

'Why didn't Sary come with you?'

Dolora hung her head. 'He fears the wrath of Pharaoh.'

'You're very lucky, sister. Our mother and Nefertari have pleaded fervently that you shouldn't be punished harshly. They want to keep peace in the family, out of respect for Seti's memory.'

'Are you pardoning me?'

'I'm appointing you honorary superior of the harem at Thebes. A grand title, but not too tiring for you. Just make sure you behave yourself, Dolora.'

'And . . . my husband?'

'He's going to head the brickyard at Karnak. He'll be doing something useful, and can learn how to build instead of destroy.'

'But Sary has always been a scribe, an academic. He can't do manual labour!'

'Remember the teachings of the sages, Dolora. The hand and the mind must work together, or men turn to evil. Now hurry and take up your new posts, both of you. There's work to be done.'

Leaving the palace, Dolora breathed a sigh of relief. Just as Shaanar had predicted, she and Sary had escaped the worst. Having just come to power, still under the influence of his mother and his wife, Ramses was inclined to be merciful.

Being forced to work was a real punishment to her, but less harsh than house arrest in some desert outpost or exile in the wilds of Nubia. As for Sary, his pride would suffer, but, considering he could have been sentenced to death for treason, becoming a brickmaker was better than the alternative.

Their disgrace would be short-lived. Dolora's lies had enhanced Shaanar's credibility as a supportive and respectful brother to the king. Ramses, preoccupied with his new responsibilities, would believe that his old enemies, including his brother and sister, had finally fallen in line.

Moses was overjoyed to be back in Karnak at the works where bricks were being made for the great Hall of Pillars. Once the period of mourning for Seti was over, Ramses had decided to continue work on his father's great project. The young Hebrew had a powerful build, broad shoulders, flowing hair, a full beard on his craggy face. He also had the respect and affection of his crew of stone-cutters and hieroglyph-carvers.

Moses had refused the post of masterbuilder that Ramses had offered him, feeling unequal to such responsibility. He could coordinate the work of experts and motivate workers, yes, but draw architectural plans like the brotherhood at Deir el-Medina, no. By gaining practical experience, listening to those more knowledgeable than himself and becoming familiar with the qualities of different building materials, the young Hebrew would become a skilled builder.

The rough working conditions and hard physical labour helped calm his soul. Every night, tossing in bed as sleep refused to come, Moses tried to understand why his mind was so troubled. He was living in a prosperous country, had a promising career, and was one of Pharaoh's closest friends. He could have any woman he wanted, earned a good living . . . No matter how many blessings he counted, it was no use. Why did he always feel incomplete? Why this unwarranted internal torment?

In the morning, he found relief in the bustle of the work site, the clang of mallet and chisel, the sight of huge blocks of stone sliding along a moistened track on wooden sledges, the constant alertness to danger, the slow satisfaction of raising a column.

Work was usually halted in the hot summer months, but Seti's death and Ramses's coronation had changed that.

Moses had come up with a plan after consulting with the leaders of the various work gangs from Deir el-Medina, as well as the Karnak masterbuilder, who explained his drawings in detail. Each day two sessions would be scheduled, the first from dawn to mid-morning, the second from late afternoon to nightfall, to keep the men out of the heat of day and allow them to rest. Furthermore, awnings would be rigged to provide some shade.

Moses had just passed the guardpost at the entry to the hall of pillars when the head stone-cutter approached him.

'No one can work under these conditions,' the man said flatly.

'Come on, the heat isn't that bad yet.'

'It's not the heat. I'm talking about the brickmakers building the scaffolding for us. It's their new head man.'

'Do I know him?'

'His name is Sary. Married to the pharaoh's sister, Dolora. That's why he thinks he can do as he pleases!'

'What's the problem?'

'It's too rough for him out here, so he only wants his gang to work every other day, but without the afternoon break or any extra water. Does he think he can treat his men like slaves? This is Egypt, not somewhere in Greece or Hittite territory. I stand by the brickmakers!'

'I don't blame you! Where can I find this Sary?'

'Sitting in the shade,' the man said, gesturing towards the foremen's tent.

Sary seemed a different man. The affable, portly tutor he had known was now almost gaunt, sharp-featured, jumpy. He alternately fiddled with a copper band on his left wrist, almost falling off now, and rubbed ointment into the big toe of his right foot, which was gnarled with arthritis. The only sign of his former station in life was an elegant white linen robe, the customary dress of successful scribes.

Reclining against a pile of cushions, Sary was sipping

cool beer. He glanced up absently when Moses entered the tent.

'Why, hello, Sary! Do you remember me?'

'How could I forget Moses, Ramses' brilliant fellow student? So you too are condemned to sweat it out in this brickyard. I thought he'd do better by his old friends.'

'I have no complaints.'

'You ought to try for something better.'

'What could be better than helping to build a monument like this? It's like a wonderful dream.'

'A dream? The heat, the dust, the sweat and toil, the awful noise, and even worse, rubbing elbows with illiterate labourers. A nightmare more like! You're wasting your talents, Moses.'

'Seti entrusted me with a mission. I plan to accomplish it.'

'A noble attitude. But when you get fed up, you'll change your tune.'

'And what is your mission at Karnak?'

A scowl darkened Sary's face.

'Running the brickyard – now there's a plum assignment.'

'The brickmakers are solid, respectable men. I'd take them over a bunch of self-indulgent scribes any day!'

'That's an odd thing to say, Moses. Are you rebelling agains the social order?'

'Against your contempt for other people.'

'Are you lecturing me, by any chance?'

'Look, Sary, I set the schedule here. It's the same in the brickyard as anywhere else, and I want you to follow it.'

'I have made my decision.'

'It doesn't tally with mine. You'll have to give way, Sary.'

'I shan't.'

'As you like. I'll pass on your refusal to the master builder, who'll take it up with the vizier, and he'll go to Ramses.'

'Is that a threat?'

'The usual procedure in a case of insubordination at a royal construction site.'

'You like humiliating me, don't you?'

'All I want is to be part of building this temple, and to see that nothing hinders it.'

'Don't make me laugh,' sneered Sary.

'We're colleagues,' Moses told him. 'Cooperation is the best answer.'

'Ramses will drop you, just like me.'

'Listen, Sary. Get your brickmakers to work on the scaffolding, give them the midday break they're entitled to, and make sure they have all the water they want.'

20

The wine was exceptional, the beef tasty, the bean purée pleasantly spicy. Say what you will about Shaanar, thought Meba, he certainly knows how to entertain.

'Is everything to your liking?' asked Ramses' elder brother.

'Simply wonderful! My dear fellow, your cooks are the finest in Egypt.'

Despite his long years in charge of the Foreign secretariat, Meba was not merely being diplomatic. Shaanar treated his guests to the very best.

'Don't the king's politics strike you as inconsistent?' asked Meba.

'He's not an easy man to understand.'

This veiled criticism satisfied Meba. His broad, kindly face had begun to show rare signs of strain. How could he be sure that Shaanar had not gone over to Ramses' side in order to live in peace and safeguard his own privileges? Still, the words he had just spoken seemed to prove the opposite.

'I can hardly approve of this new rash of ill-timed appointments, turning excellent state officials out of their offices and relegating them to lesser positions.'

'I quite agree, Meba.'

'Naming a gardener to the Agriculture secretariat – what a farce! It makes me wonder what on earth Ramses plans to do with *my* secretariat.'

'That's exactly what I wanted to discuss with you today.'

Meba squared his shoulders and adjusted the costly wig he wore year-round, even in the hottest weather.

'Are you trying to tell me something?'

'Let me give you all the details so that you can fully appreciate the situation. Yesterday, Ramses sent for me, out of the blue. I had to drop everything and go to the palace, where I was made to wait for over an hour.'

'Weren't you . . . concerned?'

'I admit I was. His Sardinian even searched me, despite my protest.'

'You, the king's brother! Has it come to that?'

'I'm afraid so, Meba.'

'Did you complain to the king?'

'He wouldn't let me. Apparently his security takes precedence over family feeling.'

'Seti would never have stood for it!'

'Unfortunately, Seti is no longer with us.'

'Men come and go, institutions remain. A prince of your stature must one day rise to the highest office.'

'It's in the hands of the gods, Meba.'

'Weren't you going to tell me about my secretariat?'

'I'm coming to that. Now there I was, trembling with shame and indignation after the bodyguard searched me, when in walked Ramses, telling me he was making me minister for foreign affairs!'

Meba blanched. 'You, in my job? It's beyond comprehension!'

'You'll understand better when you hear that he plans to monitor my every move. He wouldn't be able to control you, Meba, but I'll make a perfect figurehead. Our allies will be honoured that Ramses cares enough about foreign policy to appoint his own brother to the Foreign Affairs secretariat. They won't realize I'm tied hand and foot.'

Meba was crestfallen. 'So much for me . . .'

111

'And for me, despite appearances.'

'This king is a monster.'

'As other men of rank will soon discover. That's why we mustn't allow ourselves to be too discouraged.'

'What are you suggesting?'

'What would you rather do, retire or help me keep fighting?'

'I can make trouble for Ramses.'

'Pretend to step aside gracefully and wait for my instructions.'

Meba smiled. 'Ramses may have made a mistake in underestimating you. Heading that secretariat will give you plenty of opportunities, even with his supporters around you.'

'You're still sharp, old friend. Now why don't you explain how you've kept the secretariat running so smoothly all these years?'

Meba was more than willing. Shaanar did not mention that he had an invaluable ally, affording him control of the situation. Ahsha's treachery must remain his most closely guarded secret.

Holding Lita by the hand, the sorcerer Ofir walked slowly down the main street of the city of the Horizon of Aton, the abandoned capital where the heretic pharaoh Akhenaton had reigned with his wife Nefertiti. The buildings were intact but, through the open doors and windows, sand blew in from the desert.

The Horizon of Aton, situated many leagues to the north of Thebes, had been deserted for more than fifty years. After Akhenaton's death, the court had abandoned his grandiose Middle Egyptian capital and returned to Thebes, centre of the worship of Amon some three hundred miles to the south. Akhenaton's cult of the One God Aton, the golden orb, was repudiated in favour of worship of the old gods.

In Ofir's opinion, Akhenaton had not gone far enough. Sun-worship was a travesty: God was beyond any representation, any symbol. God dwelt in the heavens, man on earth. Egyptians believed that their gods walked the earth; they rejected the notion of a single god. Therefore Egypt must be destroyed.

Ofir was descended from one of Akhenaton's advisers, a Libyan who had spent countless hours with the king, transcribing his mystic poems. He had later circulated them throughout the Near East, even among the tribes of Sinai, particularly the Hebrews.

General Horemheb – the true founder of the dynasty to which Seti and Ramses belonged – had ordered the execution of Ofir's great-grandfather, branding him a dangerous agitator and practitioner of black magic who had led Akhenaton astray and distracted him from kingly duties.

That was indeed what the Libyan intended: to avenge the humiliation his people had suffered, to undermine Egypt, to take advantage of Akhenaton's failing health, persuading him to abandon any semblance of a defence policy. And he had very nearly succeeded.

Today, Ofir had taken up his great-grandfather's torch. He had inherited his forebear's magical lore and talent for sorcery, as well as the hatred for Egypt that fuelled his destructive fury. Bringing Egypt to its knees meant defeating the pharaoh – defeating Ramses.

Lita stared blankly, yet Ofir continued to describe each public building, each private residence, the shops and craft establishments, the menagerie where Akhenaton had housed his collection of rare animals. They had already spent hours wandering through the empty palace where the king and Nefertiti had played with their six daughters, one of whom was Lita's grandmother.

On this new visit, Ofir noted that Lita was more attentive, as if her interest in the outside world was finally awakening. She lingered in Akhenaton and Nefertiti's bed-chamber, slumped over an empty cradle and wept.

When her tears were spent, Ofir took her by the hand and led her to a sculptor's workshop. In crates lay plaster heads of women, models for more permanent works in stone.

The sorcerer began pulling them out, one after the other.

Suddenly, Lita reached out for a statue, stroking its sub-limely beautiful face. 'Nefertiti,' she murmured.

Then her hand darted towards another, smaller head, with remarkably delicate features.

'Meritaton, "Beloved of Aton", my grandmother. And her sister . . . and her other sisters . . . my lost family! I've finally found my family.'

Lita clutched the plaster heads to her chest. One tumbled out of her grip and shattered on the floor.

Ofir braced himself for an outburst, but Lita stood mute and rigid. Then she dashed the rest of the heads against a wall and ground the pieces beneath her feet.

'The past is past. Let me kill it dead,' she said with her vacant stare.

'No,' objected the sorcerer, 'the past never dies. Your grand-mother and mother were persecuted because they believed in Aton. But I found you, Lita. I rescued you from exile and certain death.'

'It's true, I remember now. My grandmother and mother are buried out there in the hills, and I should have joined them long ago. But you've been like a father to me.'

'The time for revenge is at hand, Lita. What you suffered as a child was caused by Seti. Seti is dead, but he left his son to oppress us. Ramses must be humbled. You must punish him.'

'I want to walk through my city,' said Lita.

This time she was eager to touch the gates of temples, the doors of houses, as if taking possession of the empty town. At sunset, she climbed on to the terrace of Nefertiti's palace and contemplated her ghostly domain.

'My soul is empty, Ofir. Your thoughts will fill it.'

'I want you to be queen, Lita, so that you can impose worship of the One God.'

'Words, Ofir. Only words. Hatred is what drives you. I can feel it. You're evil inside.'

'Are you refusing to help me?'

'My soul is empty. You've filled it with your desire to do harm. You've patiently moulded me into an avenger. Now I'm ready to fight for your revenge and mine, to cut like a sword.'

Ofir knelt and gave thanks to God. His prayers would be answered.

21

There was entertainment in the Theban tavern: a troupe of dancers, enticing Egyptian girls from the Delta and lissome, ebony-skinned Nubians. Moses looked on in fascination from his table at the back of the room, sipping a cup of palm wine. After a hard day's work, marked by two near-accidents, he felt the need to be alone in a noisy crowd, to be surrounded by people yet remain aloof.

Not far away sat an unusual couple.

The young woman was blonde, full-figured, attractive. The man, much older, had a disturbing countenance: gaunt, with jutting cheekbones, a prominent nose, very thin lips, a strong chin, he looked like a bird of prey. In the din, Moses could not overhear their conversation. He heard only meaningless snatches of the man's droning bass.

The Nubians were pulling patrons in to join in the fun. A tipsy middle-aged man laid a hand on the blonde's right shoulder, asking her to dance. Startled, she pushed him away. When the man persisted, her hawk-faced companion extended his right arm and the drunk was instantly blasted back a good five paces, as if he'd been punched. Muttering an apology, he slunk away.

The gesture had been swift and unobtrusive, but Moses knew he'd seen correctly. This remarkable-looking character seemed to be gifted with extraordinary powers.

When the pair left the tavern, Moses followed them. They walked towards the southern edge of Thebes, disappearing among the workmen's hovels, cramped lanes of single-storey dwellings. For a moment he thought he'd lost them. Then he heard the man's firm footsteps.

This late at night, the streets were deserted. A dog barked. Bats swooped. The farther Moses went, the more curious he grew. He glimpsed the couple threading their way through hovels that would soon be pulled down to make way for new construction. No one lived here.

The woman opened a door with a loud creak, rending the still of the night. The man was nowhere in sight.

Moses hesitated.

Should he go in and question her, ask who they were, what they were doing here? He realized how ludicrous he would seem, with no connection to the police and no business mixing in other people's private lives. What evil genius had inspired him to shadow them? Furious with himself, he wheeled – to find the hawk-faced man directly in his path.

'Were you following us, Moses?'

'How do you know my name?'

'I only had to inquire at the tavern. You're a well-known figure, friend of the pharaoh's and all.'

'And who might you be?'

'First tell me why you were following us.'

'An impulse, nothing more.'

'That's a feeble explanation.'

'Perhaps, but it's the truth.'

'I don't believe you.'

'Let me pass.'

The man held out his hand.

In front of Moses, the dusty street quaked. A horned viper slithered out, its tongue darting furiously.

'A magic trick!' protested Moses.

'Don't go near it. It's real enough; I merely roused it.' The Hebrew turned round. Another snake was behind him.

'If you value your life, go into the house.'

The creaking door opened.

In the narrow street, there was no escaping the reptiles. Where was Setau when he needed him? Moses entered a room with a low ceiling and a floor of beaten earth. The man followed and shut the door behind him.

'Don't try to run. The vipers will get you. When I decide it's time, I'll send them back to sleep.'

'What do you want?'

'To talk.'

'I could flatten you with one punch.'

The man smiled. 'I wouldn't try it if I were you. Remember what happened in the tavern.'

The young blonde woman was huddled in a corner of the room, a cloth covering her face.

'Is she sick?' Moses asked.

'She can't bear the darkness. Once the sun comes up, she'll feel better.'

'Are you ever going to tell me what you expect of me?'

'My name is Ofir. I was born in Libya, and I practise magic.'

'At which temple?'

'None.'

'You're outside the law, then.'

'My young companion and I live in hiding, always on the move.'

'What other offence have you committed?'

'Not sharing the faith of Seti and Ramses.'

Moses was bewildered. 'I don't understand . . .'

'This fragile and wounded young woman is named Lita. She's the granddaughter of Meritaton, one of the great Akhenaton's six daughters. He's been dead these fifty years, his royal city abandoned, his name expunged from the annals

– all because he tried to make Egypt worship Aton as the One True God.'

'None of his followers was persecuted!'

'No, only forgotten, which is far worse. Queen Ankhese-namon, Tutankhamon's widow and heir to the throne of Egypt, was unjustly sentenced to death. Then Horemheb and his impious successors gained control of the Two Lands. If there were any justice, Lita would be Queen of Egypt.'

'You want to overthrow Ramses?'

Ofir smiled again. 'I'm only an ageing sorcerer, Lita is weak and despairing; the powerful Pharaoh of Egypt has nothing to fear from us. But there is one force that can topple him and impose its own law.'

'What force is that?'

'The true God, Moses, the one true God whose wrath will soon be felt by all those who fail to bow down before him!'

Ofir's deep, rumbling voice shook the walls of the hovel. Moses was filled with an uneasy mixture of dread and fascination.

'You're a Hebrew, Moses.'

'I was born in Egypt.'

'You and I are alike: both exiles. We're looking for a purer land, untainted by crowds of gods. You're a Hebrew, Moses. Your people suffer. They wish to revive the faith of their fathers, to revive Akhenaton's grand design.'

'The Hebrews are happy in Egypt. They are well-paid and well-fed.'

'Their material needs are being met, perhaps, but that's no longer enough for them.'

'If you're so sure, why don't you become their prophet?'

'I'm only a Libyan, with neither your credentials nor your influence.'

'You're nothing but a madman, Ofir! Turning the Hebrew community against Ramses would end in their utter ruin. They have no desire to rebel and leave the country. As for

119

me, I'm the friend of a pharaoh whose reign promises great things.'

'A fire burns within you, Moses, as it burned in the heart of Akhenaton. He still has followers. We're beginning to find one another.'

'So you and Lita aren't alone?'

'We have to be very careful, but our movement is growing day by day. Akhenaton's way is the religion of the future.'

'I doubt that Ramses would agree.'

'You're his friend, Moses. You can make him see the light.'

'Have *I* seen it?'

'The Hebrews will impose their belief in the One God throughout the world, and you will become their leader.'

'Your prophecy is absurd!'

'It will come true.'

'I have no intention whatsoever of opposing the king.'

'Let him stay out of our way, and no harm will come to him.'

'Stop your raving and go back to Libya, Ofir.'

'The new land I spoke of doesn't exist yet. You'll be its founder.'

'I have other plans.'

'You believe in the One God, don't you?'

Moses was uneasy. 'I don't have to answer that.'

'Don't run away from your destiny.'

'I've had enough of you, Ofir.'

Moses headed for the door. Ofir made no move to stop him.

'The snakes are back underground,' the sorcerer declared.

'Goodbye, Ofir.'

'I'll see you again soon, Moses.'

120

22

Shortly before dawn, Bakhen left his priest's cell, washed his shaven body, and put on a white kilt. Carrying a water-jug, he walked to the sacred lake, where swallows circling overhead announced the new day. The broad lake, accessible by stone steps at its four corners, contained the water of Nun, the watery chaos from which all life emerged. Bakhen drew off a bit of the precious liquid, which would be used in the many purification rites performed within the sanctuary.

'Bakhen? We meet again.'

The priest turned to the man who had greeted him, dressed as a simple 'pure priest'.

'Ramses . . .'

'When I joined the army and you were my combat instructor, we fought. More or less to a draw, as I recall.'

Bakhen bowed. 'My past is dead, Majesty. Today I belong to Karnak.'

The former supervisor of the royal stables and renowned cavalryman still had his rugged, square-jawed face, harsh voice, and forbidding manner; otherwise, he was very much the priest.

'Does Karnak belong to the crown?' asked Ramses.

'Is someone claiming that it doesn't?'

'I'm sorry to disturb you, Bakhen, but I need to know whether you're a friend or a foe.'

121

'Why would I oppose Pharaoh?'

'The High Priest of Amon is fighting me, or didn't you know?'

'Quarrels in high places—'

'Don't evade the issue, Bakhen. There isn't room for two masters in this country.'

The ex-supervisor was taken aback. 'I've just finished my novitiate and I—'

'If you're my friend, Bakhen, you must join me in this fight.'

'What can I do?'

'Like every other temple in the land, Karnak should be an example of rectitude. If that were not the case, what would your reaction be?'

'I'd tan the culprits' hides, as sure as I trained my horses!'

'That's how you can help me, Bakhen. Bring me proof that no one here is breaking the law of Ma'at.'

Ramses left him, taking the path round the sacred lake as calmly as the other 'pure priests' who had come to fill their vessels with holy water.

Bakhen was unable to reach an immediate decision. Karnak had become his home, his world. Still, he thought, doing Pharaoh's bidding was the highest calling of all.

In Thebes, the Syrian merchant Raia had acquired three fine market stalls in the centre of town. Cooks from noble families bought his excellent preserved meats, while their mistresses fought over his latest Asian vases, which were exquisite and beautifully made.

Since the end of official mourning, business had picked up again. Courteous, enjoying an excellent reputation, Raia had a faithful and growing clientele. He paid his employees well and praised them lavishly, so they always spoke highly of him.

After seeing his barber out, the merchant stroked his newly

trimmed beard and set to work on his accounts. His staff were instructed not to disturb him for any reason.

Raia mopped his brow. The summer heat was hard on him. Even worse was the setback he had just suffered. The young Greek he had hired had failed to break into Ramses' office and report on which matters were receiving the new king's attention. A predictable enough outcome, however: Raia's main objective had, after all, been to test Ramses and Serramanna's security measures. Unfortunately, they appeared highly effective. Obtaining accurate information would not be easy, although bribery was always a useful weapon.

The merchant pressed an ear to his office door. He heard nothing in the antechamber; no one was spying on him. Just to be sure, he hopped on a stool and peered through a tiny hole in the dividing wall.

Reassured, he entered the storeroom full of small alabaster vases from southern Syria, an ally of Egypt. His ladies were especially fond of these, so Raia displayed only one at a time to whet their appetite. He searched for the one with a tiny red dot beneath the lip. Inside was an oblong fragment of wood with the vase's dimensions and price marked on it.

The code was easy to decipher, and the message from his Hittite employers was clear: oppose Ramses and back Shaanar.

'A beautiful piece,' cooed Shaanar, lovingly stroking the vase that Raia was showing him, in full view of wealthy clients who would never dare outbid the king's elder brother.

'The masterpiece of an old craftsman who'll take his secrets to the grave with him,' said Raia.

'I can offer you six milch-cows, an ebony bed, eight chairs, twenty pairs of sandals and a bronze mirror.'

The merchant bowed. 'A most generous offer, Your Highness. Would you do me the honour of affixing your seal to my accounts scroll?'

123

Raia steered the prince towards his office at the back of the shop, where they could talk without being overheard.

'I have excellent news,' he said once the door was shut. 'Our foreign friends are most receptive to your plan and would like to back you.'

'What are their conditions?'

'No conditions, no restrictions.'

'It sounds too good to be true.'

'We'll discuss the details later. For the moment, we have an agreement in principle. Consider this an important victory. Congratulations, my lord: I feel as if I'm talking to Egypt's next pharaoh, no matter how long the road we may have to travel.'

For Shaanar, it was a heady sensation. This secret alliance with the Hittites was as effective and dangerous as a deadly poison. He must determine how it could be used to destroy Ramses without harming himself or weakening Egypt too much. It was like walking a tightrope across a precipice. He knew he could do it.

'What is your reply?' asked Raia.

'Send my thanks and tell them I'm hard at work – as the newly appointed minister for foreign affairs.'

'You've been given that position?' said Raia, clearly astonished.

'Under close supervision.'

'My friends and I will count on you to make the most of the situation.'

'What your friends should do is make raids into the weaker Egyptian protectorates, buy up princes and tribes Egypt thinks it controls, and spread as many false rumours as possible.'

'For instance?'

'Oh, suggesting that they plan to expand their borders, annex Syria, invade the ports of Canaan. Say morale is low among Egyptian troops in the territories . . . We must bait Ramses until he loses his head.'

'Allow me to express my admiration.'

'I'm full of ideas, Raia. Your friends won't regret their decision to work with me.'

'Perhaps it's forward of me to hope that my own recommendations may have played some part?'

'On top of the payment you record for the vase, there will be a sack of Nubian gold.'

Shaanar returned to the front of the shop. A man of his rank would never linger in a merchant's office, no matter how well-known his penchant for exotic vases.

Should he tell Ahsha about this secret alliance with Egypt's major enemy? No, that would be a mistake. Shaanar judged it better to keep his networks of supporters strictly apart. That way, he could manipulate them more effectively and compensate for any possible weaknesses.

In the pleasant shade of a sycamore, Queen Tuya was chronicling her late husband's reign, commemorating the essential dates in a blessed era of peace and prosperity for Egypt. Seti's every thought, every deed, was fresh in her mind. She had been attuned to his hopes and fears. She treasured the memory of the intimate moments when their souls had communed.

In this frail woman, Seti lived on.

Watching Ramses come towards her, Tuya saw the stamp of his father's authority. The new pharaoh was all of a piece, without the inconsistencies that plagued most men. Like an obelisk, he seemed able to withstand the strongest tempest. His youth and strength added to the impression of invulnerability.

Ramses kissed his mother's hands and sat down on her right.

'You write all day long.'

'All night, too. Would you forgive me if I left anything out? You look worried, my son.'

Tuya could always read his mood in a minute.

'The High Priest of Amon is challenging my authority.'

'Seti saw it coming. Sooner or later, the clash was inevitable.'

'What would my father have done?'

'You know perfectly well. There's only one possible course of action.'

'Nefertari said as much.'

'She's Queen of Egypt, and, like every queen, is the guardian of the Rule of Ma'at.'

'You don't urge moderation?'

'When it's a matter of preserving the country's unity, there's no room for compromise.'

'Dismissing a High Priest of Amon will have serious repercussions.'

'Who rules Egypt, my son, you or him?'

23

The donkeys followed their grizzled leader through the gates of the temple enclosure. The old one's hooves knew every step from the weaving workshops to the temple warehouses. He held the others to a steady, dignified pace.

It was a full shipment. Bakhen had been sent to help another priest with the receiving. Each length of linen, to be used for vestments, was supposed to be tagged with a number and entered in the accounts with a note on its origin and quality.

'Good stuff,' said Bakhen's colleague, a foxy-looking little man. 'Been here at Karnak long?'

'A few months.'

'You like the life here?'

'It's what I expected.'

'What do you do on the outside?'

'Nothing. I'm a fully fledged priest now.'

'I serve two months at a time here in the warehouses, then go back to town and work as a ferry inspector. It's not too hard. Here, though, we never stop!'

'Then why do you do it?'

'That's my business. Listen, I'll pick out the first-quality material. You record the rest.'

When each donkey was unloaded, warehouse workers carefully laid the linen on a cloth-covered sledge. Bakhen inspected it and made entries on a wooden writing-board, including the date of delivery. It seemed to him that his fellow receiver was not as busy as he claimed. The greater part of his time was spent glancing furtively in all directions.

'I'm thirsty,' he said. 'Care for a drink?'

'Gladly.'

The foxy little lay priest left the storeroom. He'd set his writing-board on the back of the lead donkey, where Bakhen could see it. There were only scribbled approximations of hieroglyphs, nothing to do with shipments of first-quality linen.

When the lay priest returned, carrying a skin of cool water, Bakhen was already back at work.

'Here, have some. Making us work in this heat is inhuman, anyhow.'

'I don't hear the donkeys complaining.'

'Very funny.'

'Almost the end of your shift, isn't it?'

'No such luck! The cloth still has to be routed for shelving.'

'What do we do with our writing-boards?'

'Give me yours, and I'll return it with mine at the main office.'

'Is that far from here?'

'It's some way, but not too bad.'

'You're senior to me. Why not let me do the walking?'

'Oh, no. They wouldn't know you at the office.'

'Then I ought to introduce myself.'

'They have their routine, and they don't like changing it.'

'Isn't that rather a nuisance?'

'Thanks for the offer, but all the same, you'd better leave it to me.'

The man seemed disconcerted. He moved away so that Bakhen couldn't see what he was recording on his board.

'Writer's cramp?' Bakhen inquired.

'No, I'm fine.'

'Just one thing: can you write?'

The lay priest turned indignantly toward Bakhen. 'Why do you ask?'

'I saw your writing-board there, on the donkey's back.'

'Nosy, aren't you?'

'Who wouldn't be, seeing how little work you've been doing? If you want, I'll fill out the records for you. Otherwise, you're going to have trouble at the office.'

'Don't pretend you don't understand, Bakhen.'

'Understand what?'

'Oh, all right. You want me to cut you in. I can understand that, but still, you're quick off the mark.'

'What do you mean?'

The foxy man came closer and spoke in a low voice. 'This temple is rich, the richest in Egypt. Priests are paid nothing. We have to manage. Karnak will never miss a length of linen here and there. Go for the quality, find regular customers, and you do very well. See?'

'Are the office staff in on it, too?'

'Just one scribe and two warehouse foremen. Since the linen we take is never recorded, there's no way of tracing it. A pretty good setup, eh?'

'Aren't you afraid of getting caught?'

'It's foolproof.'

'But the priests . . .'

'They've got other problems. They just turn a blind eye. Now tell me how much of a cut you want.'

'The same as the scribe, or whoever gets the best deal.'

'You've got a nerve! I think we can work together. In a few years we'll both have a nice little nest egg and we won't have to work here any more. How about finishing up this shipment?'

Bakhen nodded and went back to work.

Nefertari laid her head on Ramses' shoulder as the sunrise flooded their bedroom with light. Both of them venerated this daily miracle, this endlessly renewed victory of light over darkness. Celebrating the morning rites, they associated themselves with the solar barque's journey through the realms of darkness, the gods' nightly battle with the monster intent on destroying all of creation.

'I need your magic, Nefertari. This won't be an easy day.'

'So your mother agrees with me about Karnak?'

'Sometimes I have the feeling you're in league with her.'

'We see things the same way,' she admitted with a smile.

'The two of you have convinced me. Today I shall dismiss the High Priest of Amon.'

'Why did you wait so long?'

'I needed proof of mismanagement.'

'And you got it?'

'I put Bakhen on the case – my old military instructor, who's become a priest. He uncovered a ring of warehouse workers stealing linen and reselling it. That means the High Priest is corrupt himself or else he no longer knows what goes on at Karnak. In either case, he's not fit to lead the priesthood.'

'Is Bakhen trustworthy?'

'He's young, but devoted to Karnak. What he uncovered disturbed him deeply. He knew he was honour-bound to report the wrongdoing he witnessed, yet I practically had to drag it out of him. Bakhen is neither ambitious nor an informer.'

'When will you be seeing the High Priest?'

'This morning. I'm sure he'll deny any involvement and claim I'm accusing him falsely.'

'Why are you so hesitant?'

'I'm afraid he'll retaliate by crippling the temple's economic activities and interfering with food distribution, for a time at

130

least. That's the price I'll have to pay for avoiding civil war.'

Her husband's grave tone impressed Nefertari. This was no tyrant locked in a power struggle with a rival, but a pharaoh willing to take huge risks to preserve the unity of the Two Lands.

'I have a confession to make,' she said dreamily.

'Have you been making your own inquiries about Karnak?'

'No, it's nothing like that.'

'Then my mother is using you as her messenger.'

'Wrong again.'

'Is it anything to do with the High Priest's dismissal?'

'No, though it may affect the future of the kingdom.'

'How long are you going to keep me in suspense?'

'A few more months. Ramses, I'm pregnant.'

He took Nefertari gently in his strong arms. 'The best doctors in the country will be at your side every moment.'

'Don't worry.'

'How can I not worry? I hope our child will be strong and healthy, but your life and health mean even more to me.'

'I'll have the best possible care.'

'Suppose I order you to cut back on your public appearances?'

'Would you tolerate a lazy queen?'

Ramses was growing restless. The High Priest's lateness was an insult. What possible excuse could he offer? If he'd got wind of Bakhen's revelations, he was probably trying to stall the investigation, destroying evidence and discharging ringleaders and witnesses – tactics that would ultimately backfire.

As the sun reached its zenith, the Fourth Prophet of Amon requested an audience. The king admitted him at once.

'Where is the First Prophet and High Priest of Amon?' he demanded.

'He is dead, Majesty.'

24

A conclave was held by order of the pharaoh. In attendance were the Second, Third, and Fourth Prophets of Amon at Karnak, as well as the High Priests and Priestesses of the nation's other major temples. The only ones who did not attend were the prelates of Dendera and Athribis, the former being too old and infirm to travel, the latter too ill to leave his residence in the Delta. They were represented by two delegates with full voting powers.

This distinguished company met in a hall in the temple of Tuthmosis III, the pharaoh of whom it was said 'His Monument Shines like the Sun'. Here the High Priests of Amon were ordained, here they received instruction in their duties.

'I need to consult you,' declared Ramses, 'to choose the new head of this great institution.'

There was a murmur of approval. Perhaps this young pharaoh was not as impulsive as some claimed!

'I thought by rights the Second Prophet assumed his functions,' offered the High Priest of Memphis.

'I don't consider seniority a sufficient criterion.'

'May I encourage Your Majesty not to rule seniority out entirely?' chimed in the Third Prophet of Amon. 'In the secular domain, it is no doubt possible to fill high positions from the outside, but that would be a mistake where Karnak is concerned. A man of experience, a man of honour—'

'Honour! Since you bring it up, were you aware that employees have been stealing first-quality linen within these very walls?' An astonished rumble greeted the king's revelation. 'The culprits have been arrested and sentenced to work as weavers. They will never again set foot inside a temple.'

'Our late prelate . . . was he implicated in the affair?'

'Apparently not, but you can understand why I'm reluctant to choose his successor from within the temple priesthood.'

A long silence greeted Pharaoh's remarks.

'Has Your Majesty a name in mind?' asked the High Priest of Heliopolis.

'I expect this conclave to propose a serious candidate.'

'How much time do we have?'

'According to custom, it is now my duty to visit a certain number of towns and temples, accompanied by the queen and select members of the court. Upon my return, you will inform me of the outcome of your deliberations.'

Before leaving on the tour of Egypt that was a traditional part of the first year of a pharaoh's reign, Ramses visited the temple of Gurnah, on the west bank of Thebes. Here Seti's *ka* was maintained in perpetuity. Each day, specially trained mortuary priests placed offerings of meat, bread, fruit, and vegetables on the altars and recited rites to safeguard the immortal presence of the late king's soul.

The king contemplated one of the reliefs that depicted his father, for ever young, addressing the gods. Ramses implored Seti's spirit to come out of the stone, burst forth from the walls, and surround him with the power of a king who now dwelt among the stars.

With each passing day, Ramses had grown more acutely aware of Seti's absence, until it became both a trial and a summons. A trial, because he could no longer seek the

133

advice of a trusted, generous mentor; a summons, because his dead father's voice unceasingly urged him to forge ahead, no matter what obstacles lay in his path.

In plush Theban villas, under shopkeepers' awnings, on doorsteps where mothers sat nursing babies, the topic of conversation was the same: which members of the court would Ramses and Nefertari take with them as they toured the Two Lands, as the new pharaoh sealed his alliance with the pantheon of gods?

Everyone knew someone who had confidential information from someone in authority or from a palace employee. It was widely held that the royal fleet would first head south, to Aswan, then turn round and sail down the Nile to the Delta. The crews had been warned that speed was of the essence: they would have to work hard, with only short stops. There was general rejoicing that this rite of passage would be accomplished in good time, that the new king and queen would maintain harmony with Ma'at, the Eternal Rule.

As soon as the fleet was under way, Ahmeni buried Ramses in a pile of documents he was supposed to study before meeting the governors of the provinces, the temple administrators, the mayors of the major population centres. The king's private secretary provided him with a biography of each important person he would meet, outlining career, family situation, avowed ambitions, and relations with other political leaders. When the information was less than solid or had not been verified, Ahmeni pointed it out.

'This is a gold mine!' Ramses exclaimed. 'How many days and nights have you spent putting it together?'

'I don't keep track. My only concern is for accurate information. Without it, how can one govern?'

'Just skimming your masterpiece, I see that Shaanar has a network of rich, influential supporters.'

'Does that come as a surprise?'

'At this stage, yes.'

'More hearts and minds for you to win over.'

'You're an optimist.'

'You're the king and you're meant to reign. Everything else is beside the point.'

'Don't you ever rest?'

'I can rest when I'm dead. As long as I'm your sandal-bearer, it's my job to smooth the way for you. Is your chair comfortable?'

The pharaoh's folding chair consisted of a leather seat on a sturdy frame. The legs broadened into ducks' heads, encrusted with ivory. The king would be glad of it's convenience during official ceremonies and audiences.

'I've drilled your entourage,' Ahmeni assured him. 'Everything will be taken care of along the way. Your meals will be up to palace standards.'

'You're even serious about food,' teased Ramses.

'First of all, good food guarantees long life. Second, moderation in food and drink preserves energy and concentration. I've sent couriers ahead instructing the mayors and high priests in the cities where we'll be stopping to find lodging for all the members of our group. You and the queen, of course, will stay in the palaces.'

'Have you made arrangements for Nefertari?'

'Of course I have. Your wife's condition is of national concern. Her cabin is well ventilated and as quiet as we can make it. Five physicians will be on call and you'll receive daily updates. Just one small problem . . .'

'About Nefertari?'

'No, about the landing stages. I've had alarming reports that some of them are in poor condition, but I'm sceptical. I think the provincial governors are simply looking for extra money for their upkeep. Fair enough, in view of your tour, but you mustn't let them affect your judgment. You'll have to decide each case as you see it.'

'How are our relations with the two viziers?'

'Terrible, from their point of view, but excellent from ours. The Viziers of the North and South are solid public servants, but overcautious. They live in fear of being dismissed. Keep them on. They'd never dare betray you.'

'I was thinking—'

'Of appointing me vizier? I hope not. I'm of far more use to you in my present capacity. I can work behind the scenes, without a huge bureaucracy to stifle me.'

'Tell me how the courtiers feel about being invited.'

'Thrilled to be included, not too happy about Serramanna's security checks and searches. He views every one of them as a potential criminal. I listen to their complaints, then forget them straight away. Your Sard is doing an excellent job.'

'You're forgetting my dog and my lion.'

'Don't worry. They're being well looked after, and they're the best guards you could have.'

'How is Remet working out?'

'I've had glowing reports. You'd think he'd been your head steward for ages. Your household has never run more smoothly. Your instinct didn't fail you.'

'Is Nedjem having as much success?'

'He takes his role as head of the Agriculture secretariat very seriously. Spends a couple of hours every day quizzing me on administrative matters, then confers with his predecessor's technical advisers, who are helping him learn the job. He won't see much of the scenery on this trip!'

'And my beloved brother?'

'Shaanar's ship is a floating palace. He's been hosting receptions right and left, proclaiming the future glories of Ramses' Egypt.'

'Does he think I'm a naive fool?'

'It's not as simple as that,' said Ahmeni thoughtfully. 'He really seems excited about the appointment.'

'Are you saying that Shaanar is becoming an ally?'

136

'In his heart of hearts, of course not. But the man is clever and knows how far he can go. You had the foresight to indulge his taste for power and keep him in the public eye. Let's hope he enjoys it too much to make any trouble.'

'Let's *pray* he does.'

'Time for bed now. Tomorrow will be a long day: at least ten audiences and three receptions. Will your bunk be comfortable?'

Bunk? thought Ramses. He had a headrest, a mattress of plaited skeins of hemp attached to a mortise-and-tenon frame, with lion's feet on the four legs, a footrest decorated with cornflowers, and poppies and lotus blossoms to sweeten his sleep.

'You'll need more pillows,' noted the secretary.

'One is enough.'

'Heavens, no!' Ahmeni protested. 'Look at this paltry excuse for a pillow,' he said, plucking it from the head of the bed.

Then he recoiled, stiff with horror, as the black scorpion he had uncovered stirred and prepared to attack.

25

Ramses himself had to console Serramanna. The guard captain simply couldn't fathom how a scorpion had been sneaked into the pharaoh's cabin. Close questioning of the servants yielded no results.

'They're not involved,' the Sard informed Ramses. 'I need to talk to your chief steward.'

Remet had little use for Serramanna, yet did not protest when the king asked him to answer the Sard's questions frankly.

'How many of your staff have access to the royal bedchamber?'

'Five. Well, five from the permanent staff.'

'What does that mean?'

'Occasionally I take on one or two temporary workers.'

'Any at our last stop?'

'I did hire one man to take the bed linens in to the local laundry.'

'What was his name?'

'It's on the payroll register.'

'Don't bother checking,' said the king. 'He would have used an assumed name, and besides, we won't have time to turn back and track him down.'

'No one told me about this outside hiring! You've made a mockery of my security measures!'

'Has something happened?' asked Remet, staring.

'You don't need to know! In future, I want to search every single person boarding His Majesty's ship. I don't care whether it's a general, a priest or a street-sweeper.'

Remet turned to Ramses, who nodded his agreement.

'What about meals?' asked the steward.

'One of your cooks will taste every dish – under my supervision,' said the Sard.

'As you wish.'

Once Remet was out of the cabin, Serramanna slammed his fist into a beam, so hard that the wood creaked. 'That scorpion wouldn't have killed you, Majesty,' he offered, 'but it would have made you very ill.'

'And I'd have had to give up the rest of the tour – a sign of the gods' disapproval. That was the object of the exercise.'

'It won't happen again,' promised the bodyguard.

'I'm afraid it may, as long as we don't know who's behind it.'

Serramanna frowned.

'Do you suspect anyone?' asked the king.

'Men aren't always as grateful as they should be.'

'Out with it, man.'

'Remet . . . What if he lied, and he himself is the culprit?'

'It's your job to find out, isn't it?'

'You can rely on me.'

Stop after stop, the new king and queen's ritual tour was a triumph. Ramses' presence and Nefertari's charm won over every provincial governor, high priest, mayor and other notable. Ramses was careful to show he valued his older brother, in view of Shaanar's extensive contacts and the general relief at his appointment to the Foreign Affairs secretariat. In the first place, it showed that there was no serious division within the royal family; furthermore, the prince's love of country and vision for Egypt would guarantee a strong defence policy, essential for preserving civilization from barbarian attack.

In each new town, the royal pair paid homage to Tuya, who inspired reverence whenever she appeared. Frail, silent and withdrawn, Tuya embodied the continuity and tradition without which her son's reign would have seemed unlawful.

As the fleet neared Abydos, the centre of the worship of Osiris, Ramses summoned his friend Ahsha to the prow of the flagship. No matter what the hour or day, the young diplomat was always unruffled and impeccable.

'Glad you came along, Ahsha?'

'Your Majesty is winning the hearts of his subjects, which is good.'

'There's plenty of hypocrisy in some of those hearts.'

'Even if you're dealing with hypocrites, at least they acknowledge your authority.'

'What do you think of Shaanar's new position?'

'A bit unconventional.'

'In other words, it shocked you.'

'I have no right to question Pharaoh's decisions.'

'Do you consider my brother incompetent?'

'In the present circumstances, diplomacy is a highly skilled profession.'

'Who would dare to challenge Egypt's might?'

'Your personal triumph here at home mustn't blind you to reality. The Hittites realize you're going to take a hard line against them, so they'll dig in. They may even be considering direct aggression.'

'Any hard information?'

'Not yet. Just speculation on my part.'

'You see, Ahsha, my brother is a good representative, the perfect host at receptions and banquets. Foreign ambassadors will be charmed by his speeches. Who knows, he may even begin to believe his own rhetoric! But he may

140

be led astray through malice or scheming. I'm not convinced by his sudden change of heart, and that's where you come in.'

'What do you want me to do?'

'I'm appointing you head of the Secret Service of Upper and Lower Egypt. You'll be in charge of a courier network connecting the entire kingdom, including every document that leaves Shaanar's hands.'

'Are you ordering me to spy on him?'

'That will be one of your duties.'

'Won't he suspect me?'

'I've warned him that his every move will be watched. That may help keep him honest.'

'What if he finds a way round me?'

'You're too good to let that happen, my friend.'

Approaching the sacred site of Abydos, Ramses felt heartsick. Everything here spoke to him of his father, the namesake of Set, incarnation of the might of the heavens, who slew his brother Osiris. As an act of conciliation, Seti had built a magnificent sanctuary where the mysteries of Osiris's death and resurrection were celebrated. Ramses and Nefertari had been initiated into these mysteries, imprinting on their souls the certainty of eternal life, the promise of which they must in turn communicate to their people.

The banks of the canal leading to the temple landing were completely empty. Yes, this was holy ground; yes, Osiris' resurrection was a solemn celebration; all the same, the absence of a welcoming party took the royal entourage by surprise.

Serramanna was the first one off the ship, sword in hand and flanked by his fellow guardsmen. 'I smell trouble,' muttered the Sard.

Ramses was close behind. In the distance, behind a row of tall acacias, stood the Temple of Osiris.

'Careful, now,' warned Serramanna. 'Let me have a look around first.'

Sedition at Abydos? The king could hardly credit such sacrilege.

'The chariots,' he ordered. 'I'll take the lead.'

'But Majesty . . .'

He realized it would be futile to protest. Providing security for such an unreasonable monarch was virtually impossible.

The royal chariot drove briskly towards the temple enclosure. To Ramses' amazement, the outer gateway was open. Alighting, he entered the open-air forecourt.

The temple façade was covered with scaffolding. On the ground lay a statue of his father depicted as Osiris. Here and there, tools lay scattered. Not a workman was in sight.

In shock, the pharaoh entered the sanctuary. No offerings on the altars, no priest reciting the daily rites.

The temple had evidently been abandoned.

Ramses emerged and hailed Serramanna, who was waiting at the entrance gate.

'Go and find the men in charge of the construction.'

Relieved, the Sard sprang into action.

The young pharaoh's anger blazed hot as the bright blue sky over Abydos. Serramanna and his men had rounded up the priests, administrators, ritualists, and artisans who were supposed to keep the temple running and in good order. To a man, they bowed, bent their knees and touched their noses to the ground, terror-stricken by the monarch's ringing voice as he lectured them on their laziness and negligence.

Ramses accepted no excuse. It was no use blaming their scandalous behaviour on the fact that Seti's death had interrupted the temple's normal operation. That excuse would mean every crisis would make them panic and effectively shut down an important religious establishment.

Yet the harsh punishment they feared as he spoke was

not forthcoming. The new ruler merely demanded that they double their offerings to his late father's *ka*. He ordered them to lay out an orchard, plant additional trees, gild the temple doors, return to their construction work and finish the statues, and to resume the daily rites. He announced that a barque would be built for use in the celebration of the mysteries of Osiris. The farmers working on temple lands would no longer pay shares to the government, and the temple itself would receive generous grants, provided that it was never again allowed to fall into such a sorry state.

The men of Abydos filed silently out of the forecourt, thankful for the king's leniency and vowing not to provoke his anger a second time.

His fury spent, Ramses entered the central shrine, representing the heavens, where a secret light shone in the darkness. He communed with his father's soul, now one with the stars, as the barque of the sun continued its eternal voyage.

26

Shaanar was jubilant in spite of the failure of the business with the scorpion: he had never really expected Sary's latest scheme to work. The king's old tutor was too blind with hatred to think straight. Cutting Ramses down to size would be no easy task. Yet experience showed that even the strictest security measures could be breached.

Shaanar was jubilant because Ahsha, at the end of a very successful dinner party, had just told him a wonderful bit of news. In the stern of Shaanar's ship, they could have a private conversation. The few guests still on deck had been drinking heavily, and the ship's physician was attending a high government official who had become violently sick, as the rest of the party looked on.

'Head of the Secret Service . . . I must be dreaming!'

'Effective immediately.'

'And spying on me is part of your job, I suppose?'

'Exactly.'

'To all appearances, then, I'll have no real freedom of movement and only be nominally in charge.'

'That's the king's wish.'

'Let's grant it, Ahsha! I'll play my role to the hilt. And you, it seems, will become the king's principal source of information on Hittite policy?'

'Probably.'

'Does our agreement still suit you?'

'More than ever. I'm convinced that Ramses will be a tyrant. He mistrusts other people and has faith in no one but himself. His vanity will lead the country to ruin.'

'My sentiments exactly. But are you resolved to risk everything?'

'My position hasn't changed.'

'Why do you hate Ramses so much, Ahsha?'

'Because he's Ramses.'

Set in the lush green countryside, Dendera, the temple of the beautiful smiling goddess Hathor, was a hymn to the harmony of heaven and earth. Tall sycamores planted around the enclosure shaded the main temple and its outbuildings, including the famous school of music and dance. As patroness of Hathor's priestesses, and an iniate of the mysteries of the dance of the stars, Nefertari had looked forward to this stop on the tour, hoping for a few hours of meditation within the closed sanctuary. After the incident at Abydos, the royal fleet had been forced to sail southward, but the queen refused to omit Dendera from the itinerary.

Ramses seemed troubled.

'Is something on your mind?' Nefertari asked.

'I'm thinking about the new High Priest of Amon. Ahmeni prepared files on the likely candidates, but none of them is exactly what I'm looking for.'

'Have you talked to your mother?'

'She agrees with me. Seti passed them over in the first place; they're hoping I'll forget that.'

As Nefertari studied the images of Hathor's face, stunningly beautiful in stone, a strange glow suddenly illuminated her gaze.

'Nefertari . . .'

Lost in her vision, she did not respond. Ramses took her hand, fearing she would leave him for ever, transported to heaven by the sweet-faced goddess of love. But the queen, as if soothed, nestled against him.

'I was far, far away . . . In a sea of light with a voice that sang to me.'

'What did it say?'

'To forget the official candidates. We'll need to find the new High Priest all by ourselves.'

'I scarcely have time for that.'

'Listen for the voices from on high, like every pharaoh since the dawn of time.'

At the concert held in their honour, Nefertari listened blissfully as the women musicians sang and danced in the temple garden. Ramses, however, seethed with impatience. Would he have to wait for another miracle to find a High Priest of Amon untainted by personal ambition?

He wished he could return to the ship to talk it over with Ahmeni, but was obliged to tour the temple complex, workshops and warehouses. Everything was as beautiful as it was orderly.

Ramses finally found solace by the shores of the sacred lake. The serene water, the lovely beds of irises and corn-flowers, the soft tread of priestesses coming to carry water for the evening rites, would have soothed the most troubled spirit.

Nearby, an old man was pulling up weeds and tucking them into a sack. His movements were slow but precise. Kneeling on one knee, he kept his back turned to the king and queen. His irreverence could have earned him a reprimand, but so absorbed in his task was he that the king let the old man go about his work.

'Your flowers are wonderful,' Nefertari told the gardener after a while.

'I say nice things to them,' he replied gruffly. 'If I don't, they grow crooked.'

'I've noticed that, too.'

'Oh? A pretty girl like you likes working in the garden?'

'I enjoy it, when I can find the time.'

'Busy, are you?'

'My duties don't allow me much leisure.'

'Are you a priestess?'

'That's part of my work.'

'And you do other work too? Forgive me, madam. I don't mean to pry. You share my love of flowers; that's all I need to know.'

The old man grimaced in pain. 'My bad knee . . . sometimes it's hard for me to get back up.'

Ramses reached out an arm to help him.

'Thank you, Prince. You *are* a prince, aren't you?'

'Is it the High Priest of Dendera who forces a man of your years to do manual labour?'

'Yes, when it comes down to it.'

'They say he's old and cranky, in poor health, unable to travel.'

'So he is. Do you love flowers, like the pretty lady?'

'Planting trees is my favourite pastime. I'd like a word with the High Priest.'

'What about?'

'About why he isn't at the conclave at Karnak that's helping to choose a new High Priest of Amon.' By now Ramses was certain that the High Pries of Dendera was none other than this old gardener. 'I hardly think a bad knee would be enough to stop the head of Dendera from boarding a ship for Thebes.'

'There's also the frozen shoulder, the aching back, the—'

'Is the High Priest of Dendera unhappy with his lot, perchance?'

'On the contrary, Majesty. His only wish is to live out his days in peace within these temple walls.'

'What if Pharaoh asked him personally to attend the

conclave, to give his fellow prelates the benefit of his experience?'

'If our young pharaoh is already wise in the ways of men, he would spare a tired old servant. Now would Ramses be so kind as to hand me that cane on the garden wall?' The king did as he was asked. 'See for yourself, my lord, how lame poor Nebu is. Why force him out of his beautiful garden?'

'As High Priest of Dendera, will you at least consent to give your king some advice?'

'At my age, the less said the better.'

'Not according to the sage Ptah-hotep, whose maxims have guided us since the age of the pyramids. I value your wisdom. Could you please tell me whom you consider most qualified to become the new High Priest of Amon?'

'I've spent my whole life in Dendera and never set foot in Thebes. I'm really in no position to answer. Excuse me, Your Majesty, but it's almost my bedtime.'

Ramses and Nefertari spent part of the night on the flat roof of the temple. Thousands of souls glimmered in the night sky; the undying celestial bodies revolved around the Pole Star, at the axis of the Visible and the Invisible.

Then the royal couple withdrew into a palace with windows overlooking the countryside. Although their rooms were small and the furnishings rustic, for the short space before the first birdsong their chamber was a paradise. Nefertari fell asleep in Ramses' arms. They shared their dream of happiness.

After performing the morning rites, eating an ample breakfast, and bathing in the pool adjoining the palace, Ramses and Nefertari prepared to depart. The assembled clergy saluted them. But all of a sudden, Ramses veered off from the procession and slipped into the garden, skirting the sacred lake.

Nebu was on his knees, casting a critical eye over the marigolds and larkspur he had just planted.

'How did you like the queen, Nebu?'

'What do you expect me to say, Majesty? She's the soul of beauty and intelligence.'

'So her opinion would count with you.'

'Her opinion on what?'

'I hate to take you away from your garden, but you need to come to Thebes with us, at the special request of the queen.'

'But what on earth would I do there, Majesty?'

'Become the High Priest of Karnak.'

27

When the royal fleet docked at Karnak, lighting up the waters
of the Nile, all of Thebes was bubbling with excitement. What
was the meaning of the pharaoh's early return? Contradictory
rumours spread like wildfire. Some were certain the king
planned to abolish the priesthood of Amon and reduce Thebes
to the rank of a sleepy provincial capital. Others claimed Ramses
had fallen sick and was returning to die with his face towards the
Mountain of Silence. The young pharaoh's star had risen much
too fast. Now the gods were taking their revenge.

Raia, the Hittite agent, fretted and fumed. For once, he
had no reliable information. Thanks to his network of trade
contacts, including shopkeepers in the major population
centres as well as travelling merchants, he had been able
to track Ramses's progress along the Nile without ever
leaving Thebes. Yet he had no explanation for the king's
precipitate return. Ramses had stopped at Abydos according
to schedule, but then instead of continuing north he had
backtracked, stopping briefly in Dendera.

Ramses was unpredictable. He acted on the spur of the
moment, without confiding in advisers whose loose tongues
would have provided grist for the Syrian's mill. Raia was
furious. Ramses would make a formidable adversary, difficult
to control and Shaanar would be hard pressed to outmanoeuvre him. If open conflict ensued, the king might prove much

more dangerous than Raia had calculated. He could not afford to wait and see. He must move quickly and decisively to eliminate any weak links in his chain of informants.

In the Blue Crown and a long, pleated linen robe, sceptre in hand, Ramses was truly majestic. A hush fell when he entered the hall where the conclave was in progress.

'Have you a name to propose to me?' he asked.

'Majesty,' declared the High Priest of Heliopolis, 'our deliberations are still in progress.'

'As of this moment, they're finished. Here is the new High Priest of Amon.'

An old man shuffled into the hall, leaning on his cane.

'Nebu!' exclaimed the High Priest of Sais. 'I thought you were too ill to travel!'

'I am, but Ramses performed a miracle.'

'At your age,' protested the Second Prophet of Amon, 'you should be thinking about retirement. The administration of Karnak and Luxor is a daunting responsibility!'

'I quite agree, but the pharaoh's will must be done.'

'My decree is already written in stone,' revealed Ramses. 'Tablets will soon go up proclaiming Nebu's appointment. Do any of you consider him unfit to fill this position?'

There were no objections.

Ramses gave Nebu a golden ring and a staff of electrum, an alloy of gold and silver, as symbols of his office.

'I hereby name you High Priest of Amon. The treasury and granaries of this great domain are now beneath your seal. As guardian of Amon's temples and estates, be scrupulous, honest and vigilant. Work not for your own advancement but to increase the god's *ka*. Amon can fathom the human soul, read each person's mind and heart. If Amon is well satisfied, he will keep you at the head of his clergy, granting you long life and a happy old age. Do you swear to respect the Rule of Ma'at and fulfil your duties?'

'I swear on the pharaoh's life,' declared Nebu, bowing to Ramses.

The Second and Third Prophets of Amon were furious and humiliated. Not only had Ramses saddled them with a prelate who would instantly obey his every command, but he had also named a complete unknown, Bakhen, as Fourth Prophet. This young zealot would back up the doddering High Priest and become the real master of Karnak. The temple's independence would be compromised for years to come.

The two dignitaries now had no hope of one day controlling the richest domain in Egypt. Squeezed between Nebu and Bakhen, they would sooner or later be forced to resign, prematurely ending their careers. In their confusion, they cast about for an ally. Shaanar immediately came to mind, but now that the king's elder brother was a minister, he might be singing a different tune.

Since he had nothing to lose, however, the Second Prophet arranged to meet Shaanar as the representative of all Karnak's clergy members who opposed Ramses' decision. They met by a fish pond in the shade of a large awning slung between two poles. A servant offered the Second Prophet a cup of carob juice and discreetly withdrew. Shaanar rolled up the papyrus he was studying.

'Your face seems familiar.'

'My name is Doki. I'm the Second Prophet of Amon.'

The little man appealed to Shaanar. With his shaven head, narrow forehead, bulging eyes, long nose and pointed chin, he looked rather like a crocodile.

'What can I do for you?'

'You'll probably think me too forward, but I'm not used to polite society.'

'Get on with it, then.'

'An old man named Nebu has just been named High Priest and First Prophet of Amon.'

'A position you hoped would be yours, unless I'm mistaken.'

'The late High Priest made no secret of the fact that I was his chosen successor, but the king passed me over.'

'It's dangerous to question his decisions.'

'Nebu will never be able to manage Karnak.'

'Bakhen, my brother's friend, will be the one really in charge.'

'Forgive me for being blunt, but do you find this arrangement satisfactory?'

'I accept it as the pharaoh's will.'

Doki was disappointed. As he had feared, Shaanar was in Ramses' camp now. He rose to leave. 'I won't take up any more of your time.'

'Just a moment. If I understand you correctly, you refuse to accept the situation.'

'The king is trying to undermine the power of Amon's priesthood.'

'Do you have the means to oppose him?'

'I'm not alone.'

'Whom do you represent?'

'A good many in the administration, and most of the priests.'

'And are you prepared to act?'

'Lord Shanaar! We have no intention of being disloyal.'

'Make up your mind, Doki. You don't seem to know what you want.'

'I need help.'

'First prove to me that you're serious.'

'But how?'

'That's for you to determine.'

'I'm only a priest, a—'

'You're a man of action or you're a nobody. If all you're going to do is bemoan your fate, I'm not interested.'

'What if I managed to discredit the pharaoh's men?'

'Do it first, then come and see me. You understand, though, that this conversation never took place.'

Doki's spirits lifted. He left Shaanar's residence with a head full of impossible schemes. Sooner or later, he would hit on one that would work.

Shaanar was sceptical. This Second Prophet had possibilities, but he seemed indecisive and too easily influenced. Once he realized what a serious step he'd taken, he'd probably back off. But no potential ally could be discounted, and this way the prince would find out what the little priest was made of.

Ramses, Moses and Bakhen inspected the construction under way at Karnak, a project Seti had envisaged but left his son to complete: a vast Hall of Pillars. Delivery of the huge stone blocks was on schedule. The various work gangs were coordinating their efforts to raise the towering pillars, which represented papyrus stalks rising from the primordial ooze.

'How are things going with your workmen?' asked the king.

'Sary gave me some trouble, but I think I brought him back in line,' said Moses.

'What sort of trouble?'

'He's too hard on his workers. I suspect that he's also skimping on their rations and pocketing the difference.'

'Let's send him before a tribunal.'

'I don't think that will be necessary,' said Moses with amusement. 'I'd rather be able to keep an eye on him. The moment he goes too far, I'll deal with him.'

'If you press him, he may lodge a formal complaint against you.'

'Never fear, Majesty. Sary's too much of a coward for that.'

'Wasn't he your guardian?' asked Bakhen.

'Yes,' answered Ramses. 'And a good teacher, too. But

154

something came over him. After what he tried to do to me, most other men would have banished him to the desert. I'm hoping that honest work will bring him to his senses.'

'It hasn't yet,' said Moses, shaking his head.

'I know you'll get results, though it won't be here. In a few days we're leaving for the North, and you're going to come along, Moses.'

His friend looked less than pleased. 'The Hall of Pillars . . . it's not finished!'

'I'm putting Bakhen in charge as Fourth Prophet of Amon. You'll brief him before we go. He'll see to the hall's completion and also oversee my additions to Luxor. Rows of colossal statues in the forecourt, a pylon gateway, obelisks – it will be wonderful! Keep things moving, Bakhen. I may only be granted a short time to live, and I want to dedicate this masterpiece.'

'I'm honoured by the trust you place in me, Majesty.'

'I don't appoint straw men, Bakhen. Old Nebu will do his job well, and so will you. He'll run the temple and the estates, you'll do the building. Both of you will alert me to any difficulties. Now get to work and forget about everything else.'

Pharaoh and Moses left the construction site and walked down a lane of tamarisks towards the shrine of Ma'at, the goddess of truth and justice.

'This is where I come to meditate,' the king confided. 'It calms my spirit and helps me see more clearly. I envy the priests. The soul of the gods is in every stone here. Every shrine reveals their truths.'

'Why are you taking me away from Karnak?'

'You and I have work to do. Remember when we were schoolboys discussing the future with Ahsha, Ahmeni and Setau? I was convinced that only Pharaoh had true power. I was drawn to it like a moth to a flame, and it would have consumed me if my father hadn't taken me in hand.

155

Even when I'm at rest, that power moves in me, telling me to build.'

'You have a new project?'

'It's on such a gigantic scale that I can't even tell you yet. I'll need to think more during the journey. If it's possible to carry it through, there's a major role for you.'

'I have to admit you surprise me.'

'Why?'

'I was sure that, when you became king, you'd forget your old friends and concentrate on the court, matters of state and the obligations of power.'

'You misjudged me, Moses.'

'But won't power change you?'

'A man changes according to the goals he sets himself. My sole concern is the glory of Egypt, and that will never change.'

28

Sary fumed. The king's brother-in-law and former tutor reduced to being foreman of a sorry bunch of bricklayers, when he had once been head of the royal school! With another of his former students, that bully Moses, always on his back, too! Day after day, Sary found the physical hardship, the taunts, more difficult to bear. He had tried to turn the workers against the Hebrew, but Moses was so popular that the attempt failed miserably.

Yet Moses was only following orders. Sary knew he must start at the top. He wanted revenge, revenge on the cause of his downfall and unhappiness.

'I hate him, too,' admitted Dolora, nestling deeper into her pillows. 'But what you're proposing scares me half to death.'

'What have we got to lose?'

'I'm afraid, darling. Schemes like this have been known to rebound on us.'

'So? Right now you're a social outcast; I'm subjected to unspeakable brutality. How can we go on like this?'

'I understand, Sary, really I do. But would we have to go that far?'

'Are you with me, or will I have to do it alone?'

'I'm your wife.'

He helped her to her feet.

'Have you thought it over carefully?'
'I've thought of nothing else for the last month.'
'What if someone informs on us?'
'Not a chance.'
'How can you be so sure?'
'I've taken precautions.'
'Will that be enough?'
'You have my word.'
'Isn't there any way round—'
'No, Dolora. Now, are you with me?'
'Let's go.'

Inconspicuously dressed, the pair walked down a lane leading to a section of Thebes where many foreigners lived. Dolora clutched her husband's arm nervously, hesitating at every turn.

'Are we lost, Sary?'
'Of course not.'
'Are we almost there?'
'Not much farther now.'

Inquisitive stares greeted them. But Sary marched stubbornly on as his wife grew increasingly apprehensive.

'Here we are.'

He knocked at a low red door with a dead scorpion nailed to it. An old woman answered. The couple went down a wooden stairway leading to a sort of small, damp grotto ablaze with oil lamps.

'He's here,' announced the old woman. 'Sit on these stools and wait.'

Dolora preferred to remain standing. The place gave her the shivers. Black magic was against the law in Egypt, yet certain sorcerers still dared to sell their services at exorbitant prices.

The plump and obsequious Canaanite magician padded towards his clients.

'Everything is ready,' he announced. 'And the necessary consideration?'

Sary emptied a leather pouch into the man's right hand: ten chunks of perfect turquoise.

'The object you are purchasing has been placed within the grotto. Next to it you will find a shark's tooth. Use that to write the name of the person upon whom your spell is cast. Once you smash the charm, that person will fall ill.'

As the magician spoke, Dolora covered her face with her shawl. When he left, she grabbed her husband by the wrists.

'Let's leave. I can't bear it!'

'Steady. It's almost over.'

'Ramses is my brother!'

'You're wrong. He's now our worst enemy. It's up to us to act, without fear or remorse. It's quite safe – he won't even know where the attack's coming from.'

'Couldn't we—'

'It's too late to back out, Dolora.'

Deep in the grotto, on a sort of altar painted with crude designs of grotesque animals and malevolent spirits, sat a thin limestone tablet and a long tooth whittled to form a stylus. The stone was speckled with brown. The magician had probably soaked it in snake's blood to make the spell even deadlier.

Sary picked up the tooth and began to scratch the hieroglyphic symbols for Ramses' name into the limestone. His wife shut her eyes in horror.

'Now you,' he ordered.

'No, I can't.'

'The spell won't work unless it's performed by a married couple.'

'I don't want to kill my brother!'

'He won't die. The magician swears it. He'll become an invalid, Shaanar will become his regent, and we can go back to Memphis.'

'I can't.'

Sary placed the tooth in his wife's right hand and closed her fingers round it.

159

'Write "Ramses".'

He guided her trembling hand as she completed the crude inscription. Now for the last step: breaking the tablet. Sary picked it up, while Dolora again hid her face. She refused to witness such an atrocity.

Hard as he tried, Sary could not smash the tablet. The thin limestone seemed hard as granite. He groped for a rock on the floor of the grotto and angrily pounded the magic tablet, but could not even chip it.

'I don't understand. It's only limestone, it's thin . . .'

'Ramses is protected,' screamed his wife. 'Nothing can harm him, not even black magic! Let's leave here as fast as we can.'

Sary and Dolora wandered through the unfamiliar streets. With a feeling of panic in the pit of his stomach, Sary was having trouble retracing his steps. Doors slammed in their faces, eyes peered from slits in shutters. Despite the heat, Dolora still hid her face behind her shawl.

A thin man with a hawklike profile approached them, an eerie gleam in his dark green eyes.

'Might you be lost?'

'No,' replied Sary. 'Get out of the way!'

'Just trying to help.'

'We'll manage.'

'These streets can be dangerous.'

'We can take care of ourselves.'

'You wouldn't stand a chance against armed bandits. A man carrying precious stones is asking for trouble in these parts.'

'We haven't got anything like that.'

'You paid the Canaanite magician in turquoise, didn't you?'

Dolora clung more tightly to her husband.

'That's just tittle-tattle,' countered Sary.

'Both of you were careless. I believe you forgot something.' The thin man produced the limestone tablet bearing Ramses' name.

Dolora turned away and buried her head on her husband's shoulder.

'Are you aware that an act of black magic perpetrated against Pharaoh is punishable by death? Rest assured, however, I have no intention of turning you in.'

'What do you want?'

'To help, as I already told you. See the house to your left? Go inside. Your wife needs something to drink.'

The dirt-floored dwelling was humble but clean. A young blonde woman helped Sary ease his wife on to a wooden bench with a reed mat on top of it, then fetched Dolora some water.

'My name is Ofir,' said the thin man. 'And this is Lita, great-granddaughter of Akhenaton and rightful heir to the throne of Egypt.'

Sary was too amazed to speak. Dolora was slowly coming round.

'Is this some kind of joke?'

'It's the truth.'

Sary turned towards the young woman. 'Is this man lying?'

Lita shook her head, and went and sat in a corner of the room, as if uninterested in what was going on.

'Please pardon her,' Ofir advised. 'She's been through so much that the road back to normal life will be long and difficult.'

'What happened to her?'

'As a child, she was threatened with death, beaten, imprisoned, forced to renounce her faith in Aton, the One God, ordered to forget her name and her parents. In other words, they tried to destroy her soul. If I hadn't come along, she'd be no more than a poor madwoman.'

'Why are you helping her?'

161

'Because my own family was persecuted, like hers. We live only to seek our revenge, which will place Lita on the throne of Egypt and banish the false gods from Egypt.'

'Ramses isn't responsible for your suffering!'

'Of course he is. He belongs to an evil dynasty that has deceived and tyrannized the people.'

'How do you manage to live?'

'Aton still has his followers, who give us food and shelter in the hope that our prayers will be answered.'

'There can't be many left.'

'More than you'd imagine, but they have been muzzled. Even if Lita and I were the only two, we'd keep on fighting.'

'All that happened years ago,' protested Ramses' sister. 'No one cares about it any more.'

'*You* should,' Ofir said firmly.

'Let's get out of here, Sary. These people are crazy.'

'I know who you are,' revealed Ofir.

'You don't!'

'Dolora, the pharaoh's sister, and your husband, Sary, who used to be Ramses' tutor. He's mistreated you both and you want revenge.'

'That's our business.'

'I retrieved the fragment of limestone you used to cast a spell on him. If I take it to the vizier's office and testify against you . . .'

'This is blackmail!'

'Join our cause and the evidence disappears.'

'What's in it for us?' asked Sary.

'Using magic against Ramses is a good idea, but you aren't experts. The spell you tried would have made an ordinary mortal ill, but not a king. At his coronation, Pharaoh was surrounded with special protective forces. They need to be destroyed, one by one. Lita and I can see to that.'

'What do you ask in exchange?'

162

'Bed and board, a place where our followers can meet in secret.'

'Don't listen,' Dolora whispered to her husband. 'The man in dangerous. No good will come of this.'

Sary turned to face the sorcerer.

'We have a deal,' he said.

29

Ramses lit the oil lamps to reveal the *naos*, Karnak's innermost sanctuary, which he alone was allowed to enter, or the High Priest as his designate. The shadows parted to reveal the holy of holies, a pink granite shrine containing the earthly image of Amon, the Hidden One, whose true form no human being would ever know. Slow-burning incense tablets perfumed this most sacred of places, where divine energy became incarnate in both the Visible and the Invisible.

The king broke the clay seal affixed to the door of the *naos*, drew the bolt and opened the doors of the reliquary.

'Wake in peace, creator of all life. Look upon your son, whose heart is full of love for you, who comes to seek your counsel so that he may fulfil your purpose. Wake in peace and shine upon this earth, which lives only through your love. Let your divine energy flow through every living thing.'

The king shone the light on the holy statue, unwrapped the coloured bands of linen around it, purified it with water from the sacred lake, anointed it with unguents and rewrapped it with fresh, clean cloth. Then, conjuring them up with his voice, the pharaoh presented the offerings that the priests were at that moment placing on the many altars in the temple – a ritual followed each morning in every temple throughout the land.

At last came the supreme offering, in the name of Ma'at, the immortal Rule of life.

'Through her you live,' the king told Amon. 'Her fragrance invigorates you, her dew nourishes you. Your eyes are the Rule, your whole being is the Rule.'

Leaving the Divine Power with a fraternal embrace, Pharaoh closed the doors of the *naos*, bolted it shut and affixed a clay seal. Tomorrow, High Priest Nebu would perform this rite in Ramses' name.

When Ramses left the *naos*, the entire temple was astir. Priests were clearing the altars of the portion of consecrated food that was designated for human consumption; breads and cakes were coming out of the temple ovens; butchers were cutting meat for the noon meal; craftsmen began their day's work; gardeners cut flowers for the shrines. The day would be peaceful and happy.

Close behind Serramanna, Ramses' chariot headed for the Valley of the Kings. Despite the early hour, the day was already torrid. Nefertari rode serene, though she dreaded the heat. A damp cloth around her neck, as well as a parasol, helped keep her cool in the blazing valley.

Before returning to Memphis, Ramses wished to see his father's tomb once more and pray before the sarcophagus, whose name, 'Master of Life' denoted its function. Within the mystery of the golden chamber, Seti's soul lived on.

The two chariots came to a halt in front of the narrow entry to the Valley. Ramses helped Nefertari down, while Serramanna, despite the fact that the police were present, had a look around. Even here, he did not rest easy. The Sard inspected the guard detachment controlling access to the Valley and noted nothing amiss in their behaviour.

To Nefertari's surprise, Ramses did not head straight for the tombs of Seti and his father, Ramses I, which stood side by side. Instead, he veered to the right, towards a site where workmen hacked at the rock, swept up the chips, and carted them away.

A master builder from the company of Deir el-Medina had his scrolls spread over several blocks of polished stone. He bowed to the royal pair.

'This is where I'm building my tomb,' Ramses informed his wife.

'So soon?'

'In the very first year of his reign, a pharaoh must see work begun on his house of eternity.'

The veil of sadness that had fallen over Nefertari's face lifted. 'Death is our constant companion,' she agreed. 'If we prepare for it, it will be kind.'

'Does this seem like a good spot to you?'

The queen turned slowly round, as if taking possession of the place, sounding out the rock and the depths of the earth. Then she stood very still, eyes shut tight.

'It will be your resting-place,' she predicted.

Ramses held her close.

'Even though the Rule requires that your body must lie in the Valley of the Queens, the two of us will never be separated,' he told her. 'Your tomb will be the most beautiful ever created in this hallowed land. Future generations will remember it and sing of its beauty for centuries.'

The Valley's powerful spell and the solemnity of the moment forged a new link between the king and queen. The stone-carvers, quarrymen, and masterbuilder sensed its luminous intensity. They were a man and a woman in love; above and beyond that, they were a pharaoh and his consort, whose life and death bore the stamp of the eternal.

The day's work had been interrupted; the tools fell silent. Each workman felt part of the mystery of these two beings whose task was to reign, so that heaven rested on its pillars and the earth celebrated. Without them the Nile would stop flowing, no fish would leap in its currents, no birds would fly, the breath of life would desert humanity.

Ramses and Nefertari broke from their embrace, still holding each other's gaze. They had just crossed the threshold into a marriage of true minds.

As the men began to swing their picks once more, Ramses approached the masterbuilder.

'Show me your plans,' the king ordered. He studied the drawings. 'The first corridor needs to be longer. Add a forechamber with four pillars. Go deeper into the rock here and open out the Hall of Ma'at.'

Taking the brush the masterbuilder held out to him, the king sketched his modifications in red, specifying the dimensions he wanted.

'Starting from the Hall of Ma'at, we'll angle right into a short, narrow passageway leading to the House of Gold, with eight pillars. The sarcophagus will lie in the centre. Put in several shrines for the funerary furnishings, leading off it. What do you think?'

'Technically, it's quite feasible, Majesty.'

'Let me know immediately if you run into problems during the construction.'

'My job is to solve them.'

The royal couple and their escort left the Valley of the Kings and turned back towards the Nile. Since the king had not informed Serramanna of their destination, the bodyguard scanned the surrounding hilltops carefully. Ramses was indifferent to danger, so keeping him safe was virtually impossible. One day his luck was bound to run out.

At the edge of the cultivation, the royal chariot turned right, passing in front of the nobility's necropolis and the funerary temple of Tuthmosis III, the illustrious pharaoh who had pacified Asia and spread the Egyptian civilization throughout the Near East and beyond.

Ramses stopped at an empty spot at the edge of the desert, not far from the workmen's settlement. Serramanna immediately ordered his men to fan out; a potential attacker might be lurking in the wheat fields to their rear.

'What do you think of this place, Nefertari?'

The lithe and elegant young queen had taken off her sandals, the better to gauge the energy coming from the earth. Her bare feet trod lightly on the burning sand as she paced, circled and came to rest on a flat stone in the shade of a palm tree.

'Power dwells here, exactly like the power within your heart.'

Ramses knelt and gently massaged his queen's delicate feet.

'Yesterday,' she confessed, 'I had a strange, almost frightening, sensation.'

'Can you describe it?'

'You were lying inside a sort of protective stone shell. Someone was trying to break the stone, to remove the protection and destroy you.'

'Did it work?'

'My spirit fought with the dark force and drove it off. The stone remained intact.'

'A bad dream?'

'No, I was awake. I *saw* it in my mind's eye, far away, but real, so real . . .'

'Are you better now?'

'Not completely. I still feel uneasy, as if someone were hiding in the shadows, out of reach, intent on hurting you.'

'I have countless enemies, Nefertari. Is it any wonder? They'd stoop to anything. My choice is between never doing anything that would put me in danger – meaning nothing at all – and going forward without worrying about them. I choose to go forward.'

'Then it's my duty to protect you.'

'Serramanna takes care of that.'

'He'll counter any physical attacks on you, but what about the invisible ones? That will be my role, Ramses. My love will surround you with a wall the demons cannot climb over. But it's not enough. We need more.'

'What do you have in mind?'

'A being who does not yet exist, and who will preserve your name and your life.'

'It will be born here, on the soil your bare feet have trodden. I know you've seen it, a massive guardian with a body of stone, a soul made of everything that endures. On this spot I'll build my Temple of a Million Years. I want us to conceive it together, like our child.'

30

Serramanna groomed his whiskers, put on perfumed oils, dressed in a purple tunic with a flared collar, and checked his haircut in a mirror. Given what he planned to say to Ramses, he needed to look respectable, like someone whose opinion counted. He had hesitated long enough. His suspicions had grown so strong that he had to get them off his chest.

He approached the king in his dressing-room. Ramses would be receptive when it was bright and early.

'You're looking smart,' said Ramses. 'Don't tell me you're resigning as captain of my bodyguard to become a haberdasher!'

'I thought—'

'You thought that, in view of delicate nature of your business, you'd better look as sophisticated as possible.'

'Who told you?'

'No one, I promise. Your secret is safe.'

'I'm right, Majesty!' blurted the Sard.

'Well, that's a good start. What about?'

'The scorpion that was supposed to put you out of commission – someone planted it in your room.'

'Obviously. Go on.'

'It bothered me to have that happen, so I investigated.'

'And you don't like what you found.'

'Majesty, I . . .'

'Are you afraid, Serramanna?'

The colour drained from the Sard's broad face. Anyone but the Pharaoh of Egypt would have earned a punch in the mouth for such an insult.

'I'm responsible for your security, Majesty. You don't always make it easy.'

'Are you saying I'm unpredictable?'

'If you could slow down a bit . . .'

'You'd be bored.'

'Even though I used to be a pirate, I like to do a good job.'

'What's stopping you?'

'Passive protection is no problem, but am I allowed to go any further?'

'Out with it, man.'

'I suspect someone close to you. Whoever sneaked the scorpion in had to know the location of your cabin.'

'That could be any number of people.'

'Possibly, but my instincts tell me I'm close to identifying the culprit.'

'How?'

'Well, I have my methods.'

'Justice is the basis of Egyptian society, my friend. As the first servant of the Rule of Ma'at, Pharaoh is not above the law.'

'In other words, I'll receive no official order to proceed.'

'Wouldn't it only get in the way?'

'I understand.'

'I'm not sure you do, Serramanna. Follow your instincts, but take care. I won't have you using brute force. Official order or no, I consider myself responsible for your actions.'

'No one will get hurt.'

'Give me your word.'

'Do you trust a pirate?'

'A man of courage knows how to keep his word.'

'When I say "hurt", I mean—'

'Your word, Serramanna.'
'All right, Majesty. You have it.'

A spotless palace was one of Remet's obsessions. As Ramses' new head steward, he was responsible for the king's personal comfort. The sweeps, floor-scrubbers, and other cleaners were busy as bees under the direction of a finicky scribe who hoped to bolster his position by pleasing Remet. He checked every job and was quick to threaten salary cuts for substandard performance.

Night was falling when the scribe left the sparkling clean palace. Tired and thirsty, he made haste towards a tavern where they served his favourite beer. As he passed through a narrow street packed with laden donkeys, strong hands grabbed the collar of his tunic and dragged him backwards into a darkened shop, the door slamming shut behind him. Frightened out of his wits, the scribe did not even cry out.

Two enormous hands gripped his neck.

'You're going to talk, scum!'

'Let go! You're choking me.'

Serramanna loosened his grip. 'You follow the boss's orders, eh?'

'Boss?'

'Remet, the head steward?'

'You can't fault my work.'

'Remet hates Ramses, doesn't he?'

'I don't know. No, no, I don't think so. And I'm the king's faithful servant!'

'Remet is a scorpion-fancier, I hear.'

'Scorpions? He's scared to death of them.'

'You're lying.'

'No, it's the truth, I swear!'

'You've seen him handle scorpions.'

'Never!'

The Sard began to have doubts. Usually, this method

yielded excellent results. The man did appear to be telling the truth.

'Are you looking for someone who likes scorpions?' the scribe ventured.

'You know of someone?'

'A friend of the king's called Setau . . . he lives for his snakes and scorpions. They say he even speaks their language and they obey him.'

'Where can I find this Setau?'

'He has a laboratory in the desert outside Memphis. His wife is a Nubian sorceress, as frightening as he is.'

Serramanna released his captive, who rubbed his neck and breathed deeply.

'Can I go now?'

The Sard shooed him away. 'Wait,' he said suddenly. 'I didn't hurt you, did I?'

'No, not at all.'

'Go, but never tell anyone we spoke. If you do, my arms will turn into snakes and choke you to death.'

The scribe bolted into the darkness. Serramanna walked calmly out of the shop and headed in the opposite direction.

His instincts had pointed towards Remet. After his sudden promotion, the steward was in the ideal position to harm the king. He was also the type of man Serramanna mistrusted; a jovial façade often cloaked ruthless ambition. Still, he might as well admit his mistake – a profitable mistake, though, since the scribe had perhaps put him on to a good trail, one that led to Setau, one of the king's friends.

He grimaced. Ramses held friendship sacred. Going after Setau would be risky, especially considering his daunting defence. Nevertheless, Serramanna was honour-bound to follow every lead. As soon as they returned to Memphis, he would pay very special attention to the unconventional couple who lived on such easy terms with reptiles.

'I've received no complaints about you,' noted Ramses.

'I've kept my promise, Majesty,' Serramanna asserted.

'Are you quite sure?'

'Sure as can be.'

'Any results?'

'Not yet.'

'Nothing at all?'

'Only one false lead.'

'But you haven't given up, I take it.'

'My job is to protect you – within the limits of the law, of course.'

'Are you hiding anything from me, Serramanna?'

'Do you think I'd be able to, Majesty?'

'Who knows what a pirate might do?'

'A *former* pirate. I like my new life too much to take needless risks.'

Ramses' eyes narrowed. 'Your prime suspect wasn't the right one, but you want to keep trying.'

Serramanna nodded evasively.

'For the time being, you'll have to call off the investigation.'

The Sard was crestfallen. 'I was careful, just as I promised . . .'

'Not because of anything you've done – because tomorrow we're leaving for Memphis.'

31

Remet didn't know whether he was coming or going, so fraught with difficulty were the preparations for moving the court from Thebes to Memphis. Not a single society lady must miss her pot of rouge, not a single gentleman must be wanting a comfortable chair. Meals on board ship must be of the same high quality as on land. Ramses' dog and lion must enjoy a plentiful and varied diet. Then there was the cook who had fallen ill, the washerman who was late, the weaver who had mixed up the towel order . . .

But Ramses had spoken, and Remet would obey. He had expected to spend his life refining his prize recipes. Now he was struck with admiration for this demanding and ambitious young pharaoh. Yes, Ramses was hard on his entourage, could appear intolerant, burned with a fire that might singe those who ventured too near. But he was as fascinating as the falcon arching high in the sky. Remet wanted to prove himself to his king, even at the expense of his own peace of mind.

The steward, carrying a basket of fresh figs, arrived at the gangway to the royal flagship.

Serramanna blocked his path. 'Mandatory search.'

'I'm His Majesty's steward!'

'Mandatory search,' repeated the bodyguard.

'Are you trying to cause trouble?'

'Are you trying to hide something?'

Remet looked shaken. 'What do you mean?'

'Are you or aren't you?' growled Serramanna.

'I think you've finally gone mad, Sard. All right, if you're so suspicious, take this basket to the king yourself. I have a thousand other things to do.'

Serramanna lifted the white cloth covering the basket. The figs were gorgeous, but what evil might they conceal? One by one, he gingerly lifted them out and set them aside, fully expecting to see a scorpion's deadly tail menacing him.

When the basket was empty, there was nothing to do but refill it, taking care not to bruise the perfectly ripened fruit.

Iset the Fair was lovelier than ever.

She bowed to Ramses, like a young noblewoman meeting the king for the first time and in danger of fainting.

Firmly and tenderly, he helped her up.

'You weren't always such a fragile flower.'

'No, Majesty,' she acquiesced. Her face was grave, almost anxious, but her eyes were smiling.

'Is something worrying you?'

'May I speak confidentially?'

They sat side by side on low chairs. 'I can spare a few minutes,' said the king.

'That's all?'

'My time is no longer my own, Iset. I have more work than there are hours in the day, which is as it should be.'

'You're moving the court to Memphis.'

'Correct.'

'I've received no instructions. Am I to go with you or stay here in Thebes?'

'Do you understand the reason for my silence?'

'I've been trying to.'

'The decision is up to you, Iset.'

'Why?'

'I love Nefertari.'

'You love me too, don't you?'

'You ought to hate me.'

'You rule an empire, but can you see into a woman's heart? Nefertari is special, unique, and I am not. But no one can stop me loving you – not you, not your wife, not even the gods – no matter what place you give me in your life. Why shouldn't a lesser wife glean every scrap of happiness she can? Seeing you, talking to you, sharing a few stolen moments of your day, are precious joys, which I wouldn't exchange for any others.'

'What is your decision.'

'I'm leaving for Memphis with the court.'

Forty or more boats sailed from Thebes, to the cheers of the huge crowd Ramses and Nefertari attracted. The new High Priest had assumed control without incident, the mayor and vizier remained in their positions. The court had thrown elaborate banquets. The people rejoiced because the Nile had risen sufficiently to guarantee their continued prosperity.

Remet allowed himself a brief rest. Everything on board the flagship was perfectly under control, unless you counted Serramanna. The Sard seemed to have some grudge against him. An unannounced search of every cabin and each crew member was his latest move. Some day the foreigner would be cut down to size, and no one would mind. His lack of respect for eminent persons had already earned him an impressive number of enemies. Only the king's support kept him in his job. But would that last?

The steward smoothed the already perfect bedlinen, steadied the armchairs, rechecked the table settings, and bustled up to the bridge with a skin of cool water for the king's pets to share as they lay on their shaded platform.

From one of the windows of Nefertari's spacious cabin, Ramses observed the steward, amused and pleased.

'I've finally found a steward who's more concerned with his work than with his privileges. A pleasant surprise, isn't it?'

A hint of fatigue dulled his wife's habitual glow. Ramses sat down on the bed and held her to him.

'Serramanna would hardly agree with you,' she said. 'He and Remet have taken a dislike to each other.'

The king was astounded. 'Why on earth—'

'Serramanna is suspicious, always on the alert.'

'Suspecting Remet doesn't make sense.'

'Let's hope not.'

'Don't you trust him, either?'

'He hasn't been with us long,' said Nefertari.

'But I've given him his chance to shine.'

'After a while, he'll forget that.'

'You're pessimistic today,' he told her.

'I hope Remet proves me wrong.'

'Have you any reason to doubt his loyalty?'

'Nothing but Serramanna's animosity.'

'You know how I count on your opinion . . .'

She laid her head on his shoulder. 'No one can be indifferent to you, Ramses. They're either for you or against you. Your power is too much for some people.'

The king stretched out on his back. Nefertari snuggled against him.

'My father's power was greater than mine.'

'You're the same, but different. Seti imposed his authority without having to say a single word. His force was hidden. You're like a fire, a raging river. You blaze a trail without a thought for the difficulties ahead.'

'I have a plan, Nefertari, an important new plan.'

'Only one?'

'This one is truly immense. Ever since the coronation, I've had a vision. It can't be denied, and if my plan succeeds, it will change the face of Egypt.'

Nefertari stroked her husband's forehead. 'Has this project taken shape, or is it still a dream?'

'I can make my dream a reality, but I'm waiting for a sign.'

'Why this hesitation?'

'Because heaven must approve of what I'm doing. No one can break a pact with the gods.'

'Do you want to keep it a secret?'

'Just putting it into words seems daring at this stage, but as Great Royal Wife, you have a right to know everything.'

Ramses explained and Nefertari listened. Yes, the plan was indeed immense.

'You're wise to look for a sign,' she concluded. 'I'll help you look for it.'

'If it doesn't come?'

'A sign will come, if we know how to read it properly.'

Ramses sat up and looked at his queen. 'Fairest of the Fair' was her coronation title, and throughout the land people repeated it. She was the womanly ideal of ancient love songs, with limbs of porcelain and turquoise, her slender body restful and deep as heavenly waters.

The king gently laid his ear on his wife's stomach.

'Do you feel our child growing?'

'This one will be strong, I promise you.'

One of the straps of Nefertari's dress had slipped off a shoulder to reveal the swell of her bosom. Ramses bit the gauzy linen, baring his wife's sublime breasts. In her eyes he saw the flow of the celestial Nile, the well of desire, the magic of two bodies joined in a love without limits.

32

For the first time since his coronation, Ramses set foot in his father's office in Memphis. Bare white walls, three barred windows, one large table, a straight-backed armchair for the king and chairs with woven seats for visitors, a chest for papyrus.

Intense emotion choked him.

Seti's spirit still moved in this austere study where he had spent so many days and nights at work, governing Egypt, keeping his country secure and happy. The room spoke to him not of death, but of an undying, invincible spirit.

Tradition dictated that each new pharaoh should build his own home, create his own surroundings. Ramses was expected to order this building pulled down. And such had been his intention, until he had stepped inside the huge chamber again.

From one of the windows, Ramses could see the inner courtyard where the royal chariot was housed. Then he touched the desk, opened the chest containing blank papyrus, and sat on the straight-backed chair.

Seti's soul did not turn him away.

The son had succeeded the father, the father accepted the son as Lord of the Two Lands. Ramses would keep the office intact and work here whenever he was residing in Memphis. It would stay as plain as he found it; it would be an invaluable help when he had to reach a judgment.

On the table sat two springy twigs from an acacia tree, lashed together at the bottom. This was the diviner's rod Seti had used to find water when their expedition was lost in the desert. It had marked a turning-point in Ramses' education in the art of kingship. Seti had shown him that Pharaoh must master the elements, the very mystery of creation. Pharaoh must go to the heart of all matter and draw on its hidden powers.

For a pharaoh was more than a head of state. He was also a conduit to the Invisible.

With his age-stiffened fingers, Homer packed his mixture of sage leaves into the bowl of his pipe, an oversized snail shell that was finally seasoned to his satisfaction. Between two puffs, he treated himself to a sip of full-bodied wine, flavoured with anise and coriander. Thus was the old Greek poet enjoying the cool of evening, in a comfortable armchair beneath his beloved lemon tree, when the maid announced that the king had come to see him.

As Ramses came closer, Homer was astonished at how regal he had become. The poet struggled to his feet.

'Please don't get up.'

'Majesty, how you've changed!'

'Majesty? Are you becoming reverential?'

'You're a king now. A monarch of your bearing commands respect. I can tell that you're not the hot-headed adolescent I used to lecture – though I hope Pharaoh still listens to me.'

'I'm happy to see that you're well. Is everything to your liking?'

'The maid is finally used to me, the gardener is quiet, the cook is a treasure, and the scribe who takes down my verses seems to approve of them. What more could I ask?'

Hector, the black and white cat, jumped into the poet's lap and began to purr.

As was his habit, Homer had rubbed his whole body with olive oil. Nothing could be more healthy or smell better, according to him.

'Making progress with your poem?'

'I'm not unhappy with the words Zeus addresses to the gods: "Attach a golden cord to the sky. If I pull hard on it, I shall drag up the land and the sea; I shall tie it to Olympus, and this world will remain hanging in the winds."'

'In other words, I'm new on the throne and my kingdom is being buffeted by the wind.'

'How would I know, sitting here in my garden?'

'Your muse and the servants' gossip should keep you well enough informed.'

Homer scratched his white beard. 'Could be . . . The reclusive life is not without its convenient aspects. It was time you returned to Memphis, Ramses.'

'I had a tricky situation to resolve first.'

'Finding a High Priest of Amon who won't work against your interests? Difficult, but you accomplished it. Choosing an old and unworldly man showed unusual political finesse for one so young.'

'I chose him on merit.'

'Why not? The main thing is that he obeys you.'

'If conflict between the North and South broke out, Egypt would be ruined.'

'A strange country, but very endearing. I'm getting so used to your customs I've even started to drink my wine plain on occasion.'

'Are you taking care of yourself ?'

'There must be two doctors for every Egyptian, I swear! A dentist, an eye doctor, and a physician have all come to see me. They've given me so many potions that I've given up taking them all. Though I admit the eyedrops have helped a

bit with my vision. If I'd had them in Greece, I might not have
lost my sight. I won't go home now – too much fighting, too
many factions, too many tribal chiefs and princelings mired
in their rivalries. To write, I need peace and quiet. Concentrate
on building one great nation, Majesty.'

'My father had begun doing so.'

'Here are some words of mine: "What good are tears which
shake the soul, since this is the fate the gods have decreed
for mortals, condemned to live in sorrow?" You can't escape
the common lot, and yet your role is to be placed beyond the
suffering mass of humanity. The fact that there is a pharaoh,
that there has been for centuries, allows your people to believe
in happiness, experience it, even share it.'

Ramses smiled. 'You're beginning to undertand the mysteries of Egypt.'

'Don't waste time pining for your father, and don't try to
imitate him. Become what he was: irreplaceable.'

Ramses and Nefertari had celebrated rites in every temple
in Memphis and praised the High Priest for his excellent
administration of the city's famous art schools, where the
finest sculptors in Egypt trained and worked.

The dreaded moment had now arrived when the king and
queen must pose for these same sculptors. Enthroned, with
their heavy crowns and sceptres, they were required to sit
motionless for hours on end while the sculptors 'Those Who
Give Life', captured the royal couple in stone, for ever young.
Nefertari bore the ordeal with dignity, while Ramses grew
increasingly restless. On the second day, unable to spend a
moment more away from work, he called for Ahmeni.

'The inundation?'

'Fair,' answered his private secretary. 'The farmers were
hoping for more, but the reservoir foremen are hopeful. The
water supply will be adequate.'

'How is my agriculture minister getting on?'

'He leaves the administrative details to me and never sets foot in his office. He travels from field to field, farm to farm, solving all kinds of practical problems day in and day out. It's not what you'd expect from the head of a secretariat, but—'

'He's on the right track. Are the farm workers complaining?'

'The harvest was good, the granaries are full.'

'Livestock?'

'Numbers on the rise, according to the latest tallies. No reports from the animal doctors of any new diseases.'

'And my beloved brother?'

'Shaanar is a model of responsibility. He met his staff, praised you to the skies, and told them all to serve Egypt with dedication and efficiency. He's taking his position very seriously, starts early in the morning, consults his advisers, and defers to Ahsha. Your brother is becoming a credit to your government!'

'Are you serious, Ahmeni?'

'The Foreign Affairs secretariat is no laughing matter.'

'Have you talked to him?'

'Of course.'

'How did he treat you?'

'Courteously. He didn't object in the least when I asked him to furnish me with a weekly report on his activities.'

'Surprising. He should have shown you the door.'

'He's putting on an act. But insofar as you control him, don't worry.'

'Keep him in line for me, will you?'

'I've already seen to that, Majesty.'

Ramses got up, set the sceptres and crown on his throne, and dismissed the sculptor in mid-sketch. Relieved, Nefertari followed his lead.

'Posing is torture,' the king confessed. 'If anyone had

told me how awful it was, I would never have consented. Fortunately, this likeness will be the only one we sit for.'

'Every station in life has its share of hardships. Your Majesty must never shirk your duties.'

'Watch out, Ahmeni. They may raise a statue to you if you become a sage.'

'No chance of that, with the life you make me lead.'

Ramses drew closer to his friend. 'What do you think of Remet, my new head steward?'

'A good man, but tormented.'

'Tormented?'

'He's obsessed with the smallest detail in his quest for perfection.'

'He's like you, then.'

Annoyed, Ahmeni crossed his arms. 'Anything wrong with that?'

'I want to know if Remet's behaviour puzzles you.'

'Quite the opposite. If all officials behaved like him, I could rest easy. Is there some problem with him?'

'Not yet.'

'You have nothing to fear from Remet. If Your Majesty is finished with me, I'll go back to my office.'

Nefertari tenderly took her husband's arm. 'Ahmeni is a rock.'

'He's a one-man government.'

'You spoke of a sign. Have you seen it?'

'No, Nefertari.'

'I feel it coming.'

'What form will it take?'

'I'm not sure, but it's heading for us like a horse at full gallop.'

33

In early September, the floodwaters spread until Egypt resembled an immense lake from which the occasional hilltop village emerged. Those who did not seek work on one of Pharaoh's building-sites devoted their time to relaxation and boat travel. Well-sheltered on hillocks, livestock fattened on forage. On estates the labourers fished in the fields they had lately tilled.

At the southern tip of the Delta, just above Memphis, the Nile was so wide that one couldn't see one bank from the other. On the northern fringe, it was ten times wider, pushing out into the sea.

Papyrus and lotus grew dense, as if the country were reverting to primeval times, before man walked the earth. The water's benediction purified the earth, drowned vermin and spread the fertile silt that gave the land its fertility and prosperity.

Every morning since mid-May a technician had descended the stairs to the Memphis river-gauge. The cubit ruler carved into its walls provided accurate records of the yearly inundation and a means of calculating the rate of the river's rise. At this time of year, the waters began to recede almost imperceptibly until the level dropped markedly towards the end of September.

The river-gauge was a kind of square well, built of stone

blocks. The technician climbed down the steps carefully, afraid of slipping. In his left hand, he carried a wooden tablet and the fish bone he used as a writing instrument. With his right, he braced himself against the wall.

His foot touched water.

Amazed, he stopped dead and studied the marks on the wall. His eyes must be playing tricks on him! He checked, checked again, then turned and ran up the steps.

The canal district supervisor for the Memphis region looked at the technician in astonishment. 'These figures can't be right.'

'That's what I thought at first, but I checked again today. There's no doubt about it.'

'Are you sure what date it is?'

'Of course! Early September.'

'You've been a reliable worker, set to move up a grade at your next evaluation. Because of your record, I'll agree to forget this incident, provided that you resubmit the report after correcting your mistake.'

'It isn't a mistake.'

'Are you going to make me take disciplinary measures?'

'Check for yourself, sir, please.'

The technician's steady confidence unnerved his superior.

'You know as well as I do that these measurements are impossible!'

'I don't understand it, but it's true. The same measurement, recorded two days in a row.'

The two men went together to check the gauge.

Afterwards, the district supervisor could no longer deny that something extraordinary was happening: instead of receding, the Nile was rising.

Sixteen cubits, the ideal water level. Sixteen cubits, or 'Perfect Joy'.

The news swept the country as fast as a speeding jackal,

187

causing an uproar. Ramses, in the first year of his reign, had performed a miracle! The reservoirs would be filled to the brim, the next season's crops irrigated throughout the dry months. The Two Lands would know a time of plenty, thanks to this royal magic.

Thus Ramses took Seti's place in his subject's hearts. The new pharaoh was beneficent, endowed with supernatural powers, able to control the inundation, banish the spectre of famine and fill people's bellies.

Shaanar was enraged. How could one deal with a people so stupid that they insisted on attributing a natural phenomenon to magic? This damned return of the inundation, which no river-gauge inspector had ever seen before, was strange, of course, even incredible. But Ramses had nothing to do with it! Even so, in every town and village the new pharaoh was being fêted and his name praised to the heavens. He was destined one day to equal the gods.

The king's elder brother cancelled his appointments and gave his entire secretariat a day off in celebration, following the lead of his fellow ministers. Doing otherwise would be a tactical error.

Why did Ramses have all the luck? In the space of a few hours, his popularity had surpassed Seti's. A number of his adversaries caved in, deciding it would be hopeless to oppose him. Instead of forging ahead, Shaanar must proceed more cautiously than ever, slowly weaving his web.

His persistence would pay off in the long run. Fortune was notoriously fickle, and in the end always deserted her followers. When Ramses' luck ran out, Shaanar would make his move. Until then, he would choose his weapons. He would have to strike accurately and hard.

Cries rose from the street. Shaanar thought there must be a scuffle, but the noise grew louder until it was almost deafening. The whole city was cheering! The minister climbed the few steps to his building's roof terrace.

The spectacle that greeted him, along with thousands of his countrymen, turned him to stone.

A huge blue bird, something like a heron, was circling the skies above Memphis.

The phoenix, thought Shaanar. It can't be . . . The phoenix is back?

He struggled in vain to rid himself of the foolish notion, eyes fixed on the soaring bird. Legend had it that the phoenix returned from the underworld to announce a glorious reign and herald a new era.

A bedtime story, a priestly fantasy, a tall tale for the simple folk! Yet there it was, a splendid blue creature circling wide over Memphis, as if surveying the city before choosing a new direction.

If he'd been an archer, Shaanar would have shot the bird down to prove that it was only a migrating waterfowl, confused and disorientated. Order a soldier to do it? None of them would obey him and people would think he was mad. The entire city breathed as one, watching the phoenix. Suddenly, a hush fell.

Shaanar took heart. They knew, of course! If the blue bird really was the phoenix, it would do more than circle over Memphis. According to legend, it would have a specific destination. When the bird departed, it would take the crowd's delusion along with it. The people would stop believing in his brother's second miracle and perhaps even reassess the first one.

The crowd became even quieter. Hah! Ramses' luck was already deserting him! The odd baby cried. Then there was silence.

The huge blue bird continued to circle. In the clear air, the graceful movement of its wings could be heard, like the rustling of cloth. The people's joy seemed to give way to disappointment. This couldn't after all be the phoenix, which appeared only once every fifteen centuries. It must

189

be some poor dazed heron separated from its flock and hopelessly lost.

Relieved, Shaanar went back to his office. This showed how right he was never to heed old wives' tales designed to addle feeble minds. No bird, no man, could live for thousands of years. No phoenix flew in to mark a pharaoh with greatness. Still, there was a lesson to be learned from the incident: knowing how to manipulate the crowd was crucial. People craved dreams in the same way they needed food. If a ruler wasn't popular, it was advisable to manufacture popularity, using rumour and hearsay.

Shouts rang out once more.

No doubt, thought Shaanar, the anger of a crowd balked of the miracle it had expected. He heard the name of Ramses – whose defeat threatened to be more and more bitter.

He hurried back to the terrace, and was astonished to see the crowd exploding as the huge bird landed on top of the city's greatest monument, the sacred obelisk. It *was* the phoenix!

Insane with rage, Shaanar conceded that the gods were indeed proclaiming a new era: the age of Ramses.

'Not one sign, but two,' Nefertari concluded. 'The second inundation, and now the phoenix. Could there be a better beginning?'

Ramses was reading the stack of reports that had just reached him. The Nile's unprecedented return to the ideal water level was a blessing for Egypt. And the entire population of Memphis had beheld the huge blue bird perching on the tip of the great obelisk at the temple of Heliopolis, a ray of sun preserved in sacred stone. There the phoenix remained, contemplating the land the gods loved.

'You look puzzled,' observed the queen.

'Such powerful omens – it's enough to make anyone wonder.'

'You think they're a warning?'

190

'No, Nefertari. I think they mean I should go ahead and not concern myself with doubters, hindrances or difficulties.'

'Then it's time to launch your great project.'

He took her in his arms. 'According to the Nile and the phoenix.'

A breathless Ahmeni burst into the audience chamber.

'The superior . . . of the House of Life . . . He wants to talk to you.'

'Show him in.'

'Serramanna is trying to search him . . . he'll cause a scandal!'

Ramses hurried towards the antechamber, where a robust man of sixty, with a priest's shaven head and white robe, was trying to stand up to the colossal Sard decked out in helmet and breastplate, sword in hand.

The superior bowed to Pharaoh. Serramanna noted that Ramses seemed less than pleased.

'No exceptions,' grumbled the giant. 'Otherwise I can't vouch for your security.'

'What brings you here?' the king inquired of the priest.

'An urgent request from the House of Life, Majesty. You're needed there.'

34

When Seti had first brought Ramses to Heliopolis, it was to undergo an ordeal on which his future hinged. Today he entered as a pharaoh, passing through the gateway to the great temple of Ra, as vast as that of Amon at Karnak.

On this holy ground, with its own canal, stood a complex of buildings: the temple of the primordial stone, the sanctuary of Atum, the creator, in the shade of a sycamore; the shrine of the willow with the king list carved into its trunk; the memorial shrine of Djeser, builder of the step pyramid at Saqqara.

Heliopolis was a place of enchantment. Garden paths, lined with wayside stone altars holding statues of the gods, led through stands of acacia, willows, and tamarisks. Orchards and olive groves thrived. Beekeepers harvested rich loads of honey, the cowsheds housed cows with well-filled udders, craftsmen trained in the temple workshops, the estates included a hundred villages contributing to the upkeep of Heliopolis and protected in turn by the temple.

Here the lore of the ancients had been handed down and codified in rituals. A long oral tradition of mythology continued. Scholars, ritualists and magicians transmitted their knowledge in silence and secretly.

The superior of the House of Life at Heliopolis, which served as the model for all other institutions of religious learning in Egypt, had grown unaccustomed to the world outside. Dedicated to meditation and learning, he rarely left his domain.

'Your father often spent time among us,' he revealed to Ramses. 'His fondest wish was to enter a religious order, although he knew it could never come true. You, Majesty, are young, and innumerable plans are jostling in your head and heart. But will you live up to the name you bear?'

Ramses controlled his anger with some difficulty. 'Have you any cause to doubt it?'

'Heaven will answer in my place. Follow me.'

'Is that an order?'

'You're lord of this land, and I am your servant.'

The superior of the House of Life did not lower his eyes. Ramses had faced tough adversaries since becoming pharaoh, but none as formidable as this.

'Follow me, please.'

'Show me the way.'

The superior walked at a measured pace towards the sanctuary of the primordial stone, from which an obelisk covered with hieroglyphs rose. On top of it sat the phoenix, perfectly still.

'If Your Majesty will raise your head and fix your eyes on that bird.'

The midday sun was so dazzling that the phoenix was lost in a blur.

'Is your intention to blind me?'

'That is for you to judge, Majesty.'

'Do you expect a king to act on a dare?'

'If it's in his nature.'

'Explain the reason for your attitude.'

'The name you bear, Majesty, is what gives your reign legitimacy. Until now, it's been only an ideal. Will it remain so, or will you dare to make it a reality, no matter what risk that entails?'

Ramses looked straight at the sun.

The golden disc did not burn his eyes. He saw the phoenix rise, flap its wings, and move heavenward. Still the young monarch's gaze remained fastened on the shining orb that lit up the firmament and created the day.

'You are truly Ramses, Ra-Begot-Him, Son of the Light and Child of the Sun. May your reign proclaim victory over darkness.'

The young king understood that he would never have anything to fear from the sun whose earthly incarnation he was. Communing with it, he would be fed by its energy.

Without another word, the superior made his way towards an oblong building with high, thick walls. Ramses followed him and entered the House of Life. In its centre was the mound where the sacred stone lay hidden, covered with a ram's fleece. Alchemists used it to perform transmutations, and pieces of it were buried with the initiates to aid in their passage from death to resurrection.

The superior showed the king into a huge library where works on astronomy and astrology, prophecies and the royal annals were preserved.

'According to our annals,' declared the superior, 'the phoenix was last seen in Heliopolis fourteen hundred and sixty-one years ago. Its appearance in Year One of your reign coincides with the intersection of two astronomical calendars: the fixed-year calendar, which loses a day every four years, and the real-year calendar, which loses a quarter of a day a year. At the precise moment you ascended the throne, these two cosmic cycles came together. A stele will be erected to mark the event, if you so desire.'

'What lesson am I to draw from your revelations?'

'That chance does not exist, Majesty, and that your destiny belongs to the gods.'

A miraculous inundation, the return of the phoenix, a new era . . . It was all too much for Shaanar. Dazed and forlorn, he put up a brave front at the ceremonies organized in honour of Ramses, whose reign, begun under such auspices, promised to be remarkable. The gods had clearly chosen him to govern the Two Lands, preserve their union and increase their prestige.

Only Serramanna was out of sorts. Maintaining security for the king seemed to get harder every day. Dignitaries travelled in packs to shake his hand, it seemed. Even worse, Pharaoh rode in his open chariot through the main streets of Memphis, to the cheers of his people. Intoxicated by his own popularity, he refused the safety measures his guard captain recommended.

As if exposing himself to urban dangers were not enough, the king also ventured into the countryside, most of which lay under the floodwaters. Peasants repaired their tools and ploughs, and stocked granaries, while children learned to swim using floats. Overhead flew cranes with red and black beaks. Herds of belligerent hippos lazed in the muddy river. Allowing himself only two or three hours of sleep a night, Ramses visited a staggering number of villages. He earned the loyalty of provincial administrators and mayors, and gained the trust of the common folk.

When he returned to Memphis, the inundation was beginning to recede and the farmers were preparing for sowing.

'You don't even look tired,' remarked Nefertari.

'What could be tiring about mingling with my people? But you . . . you don't look very well.'

'There's nothing I can put my finger on . . .'

'What do the doctors say?'

'That I must stay in bed if I want a normal delivery.'

'Then why aren't you in your bed?'

'With you away, I had to—'

'I won't leave Memphis again until you give birth.'

'And your great project?'

Ramses frowned. 'Perhaps just one short trip, with your permission.'

The queen smiled. 'Your wish is my command.'

'Egypt is so beautiful, Nefertari. My travels have made me realize that it is a miracle, the child of water and sunlight, the epitome of Horus' strength and Hathor's beauty. We must devote our every waking moment to this country. You and I are meant not to govern but to serve her.'

'I believed that once.'

'What do you mean?'

'Service is the noblest of human achievements. Only by serving a higher goal can we find fulfilment. *Hem*, "the servant", is such a lovely word. It encompasses everyone from the humblest – the seasonal building worker or toiler in the fields – to Pharoah, the most powerful man in the land, the servant of the gods and of his people. Since the coronation, though, I have come to see things differently. Neither one of us can simply serve. We must also direct, guide, ply the helm that keeps the ship of state on a steady course. No one else can do it for us.'

The king grew sombre.

'I felt the weight of that responsibility when my father died. I was so used to having someone who could guide, give advice and orders. Thanks to him, no difficulty was insurmountable, no misfortune without remedy.'

'And that's what your people expect from you.'

'I have looked into the sun and it didn't burn my cycs.'

'The sun is within you, Ramses. It gives life, it makes plants, animals and people grow, but it can also wither and kill if it's too strong.'

'The desert sun is strong, but there's life in the desert.'

'The desert is the underworld on earth. It's not for human habitation, except for houses of eternity that will outlast the ages. A pharaoh's greatest temptation is to immerse his thought in the desert, and forget the world of men.'

'My father was a man of the desert.'

'Every pharaoh should be, but he must also look towards the Valley and see it flourish.'

Then Ramses and Nefertari fell silent in the still of the evening as the sunset gilded the single obelisk towering over Heliopolis.

35

Once the windows in Ramses' bedchamber went dark, Serramanna left the palace, first making sure that his hand-picked guards were at their posts. Jumping on the back of a superb black horse, he galloped through Memphis in the direction of the desert.

Egyptians did not like to go abroad at night. In the absence of the sun, demons were likely to creep out of their lairs and attack unwary travellers. The huge Sardinian scoffed at these superstitions. He could hold his own against a horde of monsters. When his mind was made up, he was unstoppable.

Serramanna had hoped Setau would come to the court and join in the celebrations in Ramses' honour, but, true to his eccentric reputation, the snake-handler stayed at home. In the course of his continuing investigation of the scorpion incident, the Sard had questioned many people. He had learned that no one liked Setau. They feared his evil spells and loathed his reptilian companions, while forced to acknowledge that he was doing a booming business. By selling venom to people who prepared remedies for use in treating serious illnesses, he was beginning to make his fortune.

Though he was still suspicious of Remet, Serramanna had to admit that Setau made an excellent suspect. Suppose he was staying out of sight because he didn't dare face Ramses since planting the scorpion? His reclusiveness was practically an admission of guilt.

Serramanna needed to face Setau in person. The ex-pirate was used to sizing up his opponents, and owed his survival to his ability to read them. Before he could make his move, he needed a good look at Setau. And, since the man was hiding, he would have to flush him out.

As cropland gave way to desert, Serramanna dismounted and tethered his horse to the trunk of a fig tree, whispering a few words of reassurance in the animal's ear. Then he walked noiselessly towards Setau's laboratory. There was barely a crescent of moon, but the night was clear. The laughter of a hyena troubled him not in the least. He felt much as he had when boarding a ship in a surprise attack.

There were lights on in the laboratory. What if Setau took some extra persuading? He'd promised Ramses that he would not use brute force – but necessity made its own rules . . . He cautiously hunched down, skirted a rise and approached the building from the rear.

His back to the wall, the Sard listened.

Low moans issued from the laboratory. Was the snake-charmer torturing some poor wretch? Serramanna edged along to a slit in the wall and peeked inside. Pots, jars, filters, caged snakes and scorpions, knives of various sizes, baskets – all kinds of equipment littered the shelves and workbenches.

On the floor lay a man and a woman, naked and intertwined. A beautiful black woman groaned in pleasure, her slender body arching. Her swarthy, square-jawed partner was stocky and virile.

The Sard looked away. While he freely indulged his own taste for women, he was no voyeur. Yet this woman's beauty had stirred him. Interrupting such passionate lovemaking would be criminal, so he resigned himself to waiting. Spent, Setau would be easier to interrogate.

He smiled to himself thinking of the Memphis beauty he'd be meeting for dinner the following evening. According to her best friend, she liked big, strong men. Serramanna waited.

There was a strange sound to his left.

The Sard looked round to see a huge cobra, its head raised ready to strike – one opponent he'd rather not face. He backed away, bumped into the wall and froze. A second cobra barred his way.

'Get away, you filthy creatures!'

The giant's dagger didn't frighten the snakes. If he did kill one of them, the other one would attack him.

'What's going on here?'

Naked, carrying a torch, Setau inspected the intruder. 'You came to rob my laboratory. Good thing my watchdogs are always on the alert. Unfortunately for you, their bite is definitely worse than my bark.'

'You're not going to commit murder, Setau!'

'So you know my name. No matter, you're a burglar caught red-handed, waving a dagger. The judge will rule that it was self-defence.'

'I'm Serramanna, the captain of Ramses' bodyguard.'

'I thought I recognized you. Why are you trying to rob me?'

'I wanted to see you, have a look at your place, that's all.'

'At this time of night? Not only are you stopping me making love to Lotus, but you're lying through your teeth.'

'It's the truth.'

'Why this sudden wish to see me?'

'Security reasons.'

'What does that mean?'

'My job is to protect the king.'

'You think I'm a threat to Ramses?'

'I didn't say that.'

'But you think it – why else spy on me?'

'I can't afford to make a mistake.'

The two cobras inched closer to the Sard. Setau's eyes blazed with fury.

'Are pirates afraid to die?'

'That way, yes.'

'Get away from here, Serramanna, and don't ever bother me again. Next time I'll let them at you.'

At a signal from Setau, the cobras wriggled aside. The Sard, drenched in sweat, walked straight between them, heading back to his horse.

One thing was clear in his mind: Setau had the soul of a criminal.

'What are they doing?' asked little Kha, watching some peasants herd a flock of sheep through a sodden field.

'After the sowing, the sheep help work the seeds into the soil,' explained Nedjem, the agriculture minister. 'The inundation leaves a huge amount of silt on the banks and fields. That helps us grow strong, plentiful wheat.'

'And the sheep are helpers?'

'Just like cows and every other animal in creation.'

The inundation had begun to recede, and the sowers were out in the fields, glad to trample in the fertile mud that the river had brought in abundance. They began early in the morning, having only a limited number of days while the soil was moist and easily worked. After hoeing to break up the waterlogged clumps of soil, they scattered the seeds and covered the furrows. Livestock followed to help pack down the soil.

'The country is nice,' said Kha, 'but I still like my scrolls and hieroglyphs better.'

'Would you like to visit a farm?'

'All right.'

Nedjem took the little boy by the hand. Even his walk was serious, extraordinary for his age, like his academic gifts. Kind-hearted Nedjem was so concerned for the child, with his lack of interest in toys and playmates, that he'd begged Iset the Fair to let him act as Kha's tutor. He thought it essential to take the little prince outside his gilded cage and introduce him to the wonders of nature.

Kha took in everything around him – not as a surprised and delighted child, however, but as a fully fledged scribe mentally compiling a report.

The farm had granaries, barns, cowsheds, a farmyard, bread ovens and a kitchen garden. At the gate, Nedjem and Kha were invited to wash their hands and feet. Then the owner welcomed them, delighted to have such important visitors. He showed off his best milch-cows, which were fed and tendered with loving care.

'My secret,' he confessed, 'is finding the right pasture, where they don't get too hot and have plenty of grass.'

'The cow is the animal of the goddess Hathor,' ventured the little boy. 'That's why cows are kind and gentle.'

The farmer's eyes widened. 'How do you know that, Prince?'

'I read it in a story.'

'You can already read?'

'Will you do something for me?'

'Anything.'

'Bring me a piece of limestone and a reed-tip.'

'Yes, right away.'

The farmer glanced at Nedjem, who winked his approval. Writing implements in hand, the little boy began to walk round the farmyard, then the cowsheds, much to the farmhands' astonishment.

An hour later, when he returned it to his host, the slab of limestone was covered with writing.

'I've counted carefully,' Kha told him. 'You own a hundred and twelve cows.'

The child rubbed his eyes and clung to Nedjem.

'Now I'm sleepy,' he confessed.

By the time the old man had settled Kha in his arms, the boy was asleep. 'Another of Ramses' miracles,' Nedjem said to himself.

36

Athletic as Ramses, broad-shouldered, with a high forehead, flowing dark hair, and bearded, weather-beaten face, Moses walked casually into the King of Egypt's office.

Ramses rose and the two men embraced.

'This is where Seti worked, isn't it?'

'Yes. I haven't changed a thing. His thought lives on in these walls. I want it to be my inspiration.'

Light filtered through the three barred windows designed to keep air circulating through the room. The late-summer heat was agreeable.

Ramses abandoned his straight-backed royal armchair and sat on a plain seat of woven straw, facing his friend.

'How are you, Moses?'

'Fine, but I don't have enough to do.'

'We never see each other these days. I'm afraid that's my fault.'

'You know that being idle, even in luxury, gets on my nerves. Why did you bring me to Memphis? I was better off working at Karnak.'

'You're not enjoying high society?'

'The courtiers bore me. They never stop singing your praises. They'll be making a god of you soon. It's stupid and pointless.'

'Have I done something wrong?'

'The miraculous inundation, the phoenix, the new era . . . The facts are undeniable, and they explain your popularity. Have you got supernatural powers? Are you one of the Predestined? The people think so.'

'And you don't agree?'

'It may be true. But you're not the True God.'

'Have I ever claimed to be?'

'Be careful, Ramses, or your courtiers' flattery may make you abominably vain.'

'You don't seem to understand the role and the function of a pharaoh. You don't give me much credit, either!'

'I'm only trying to help you.'

'I'm going to give you the chance to do that.'

Moses' eyes shone with curiosity. 'You're sending me back to Karnak?'

'I have a much more important undertaking to entrust to you, if you accept.'

'More important than Karnak?'

The king rose and leaned his back against the window frame.

'I have a tremendous project. So far I've shared it only with Nefertari. We agreed it would be best to look for a sign before I went ahead. The second inundation and the phoenix – in the end the gods gave me two signs. The House of Life confirmed that a new era really has begun, according to the laws of astronomy. Of course I'll continue the work my father began, in Karnak, in Abydos and elsewhere. But this new era should be marked with new creations. Is that vanity, Moses?'

'Every pharaoh must build, according to tradition.'

Ramses looked concerned. 'The world is changing. The Hittites constitute a permanent threat; Egypt is a rich and coveted prize. Those are the truths that led me to conceive my project.'

'To increase your military strength?'

'No, Moses. To move the strategic centre of the country.'

'Do you mean—'

'To build a new capital.'

The Hebrew was astounded. 'What? How will—'

'The northern border is where Egypt's fate will be decided. Therefore, my government should have its seat in the Delta to keep up with the latest developments in Canaan, Syria and our protectorates under threat from the Hittites. Thebes will remain the city of Amon, the home of great Karnak and wonderful Luxor. I'll make sure they're grander and more beautiful than ever. On the west bank, the Mountain of Silence reigns over the Valley of the Kings, the Valley of the Queens and the mortuary temples on the plain.'

'But what about Memphis?'

'Memphis is the fulcrum of the Two Lands, where the Delta joins the Nile Valley. It will remain our economic and administrative capital. But we must go farther to the north and east, Moses, not believe we exist in splendid isolation, nor forget we've been invaded before. Remember that Egypt is a tempting prey.'

'Isn't the line of fortresses enough of a deterrent?'

'In case of danger, I'll have to move quickly. The closer I am to the northern border, the less time it will take information to reach me.'

'Building a capital is a perilous undertaking. Look what happened to Akhenaton.'

'Akhenaton made some unforgivable errors. The site he chose, in Middle Egypt, was doomed from the start. He forgot about the good of his people and pursued his mystical fantasies.'

'He challenged the priesthood of Amon, and so have you.'

'If the High Priest of Amon is faithful to the Rule and loyal to the king, I'll have no quarrel with him.'

'Akhenaton believed in a single god and built a new city to glorify him.'

'His father, the great Amenhotep, left him a prosperous country. He almost ruined it. Akhenaton was weak and indecisive, lost in his prayers. Under his reign, hostile powers seized Egyptian territory. Are you trying to defend him?'

Moses hesitated. 'Today his capital lies abandoned.'

'Mine will be built to last for generations.'

'You almost frighten me, Ramses.'

'Take heart, my friend.'

'How many years does it take to raise a city starting from nothing?'

Ramses smiled. 'It won't start from nothing.'

'What do you mean?'

'While I was Seti's co-regent, he took me to all the most important places. On each journey, he taught me something – though I didn't always understand it then. Today I'm beginning to make more sense of our travels. One of the places we visited was Avaris.'

'The capital of the Hyskos invaders? But the place is cursed.'

'Seti was the namesake of Set, who murdered his brother Osiris. My father had the strength to dominate the forces of destruction, draw out their hidden light and use it to build.'

'And now you want to make Avaris the city of Ramses?'

'Yes, and that's what I plan to call it. *Pi-Ramses*, "the City of Ramses", the capital of Egypt.'

'It's madness!'

'Pi-Ramses will be magnificent and welcoming. Poets will sing of its beauty.'

'How long will it take to build?'

'I haven't forgotten your question. In fact, it's why I called you here.'

'Does this mean what I'm afraid it does?'

'I need someone I can trust to supervise the work and keep the project on schedule. I need Avaris turned into Pi-Ramses as quickly as possible.'

206

'How long have you allowed?'

'Less than a year.'

'That's impossible!'

'No, it isn't, thanks to you.'

'You think I can move stone with the speed of a falcon and put blocks together through sheer force of will?'

'Stone, no. Bricks, yes.'

'I'm beginning to see . . .'

'Your fellow Hebrews make up most of the brickmaking companies around the country. If we bring them all together, you'll form a group of highly skilled workmen capable of taking on such a gigantic project.'

'Aren't temples supposed to be made of stone?'

'I'll enlarge the temples already there. That can be done over several years. We'll use brick to build the palaces, government offices, villas for the nobles, and large and small houses. In less than a year, Pi-Ramses will be habitable and become a working capital.'

Moses seemed unconvinced. 'I still say it's impossible. The plans alone—'

'The plans are in my head! I'll sketch them myself on papyrus and you'll take personal charge of their execution.'

'The Hebrews are a fairly unruly lot. Each tribe has its own chief.'

'I'm not asking you to become ruler of a nation, only a project leader.'

'Keeping them in order won't be easy.'

'I have faith in you.'

'As soon as the news is out, other Hebrews will try to take my place.'

'Will they be able to?'

Now Moses smiled. 'No one will be able to meet your deadline.'

'We'll build Pi-Ramses to shine under the Delta sun and cast a glow over all Egypt with its beauty. Get to work, Moses.'

37

Abner the brickmaker could stand it no longer. Just because Sary was Ramses' brother-in-law, he thought he could treat his workers like dirt. He reduced their overtime pay, cut their rations and denied them time off, claiming their work had been done badly.

As long as Moses was in Thebes, he had kept Sary in line. Now that he was gone, the situation was worse than ever. Yesterday evening the foreman had caned a fifteen-year-old boy, accusing him of not getting the bricks to the boat fast enough.

It was the last straw.

When Sary arrived at the brickyard, the Hebrews were seated in a circle. Only Abner was standing in front of the empty baskets.

'Get up and go to work!' snarled Sary, who grew thinner by the day.

'We demand an apology,' Abner said calmly.

'What did you say?'

'The boy you beat last night is confined to bed. He did nothing wrong. You owe him and all of us an apology.'

'Have you lost your mind, Abner?'

'We won't go back to work until you agree.'

'Abner, you're a fool.' Sary laughed fiercely.

'All right. We'll file a complaint instead.'

'You're pathetic as well as a fool. I've already called the police in to investigate. They ruled that the boy was injured in an accident, entirely through his own fault.'

'That's a lie!'

'A scribe took his sworn statement in my presence. If the boy goes back on his word, he'll be accused of perjury.'

'How dare you twist the truth so!'

'If you men don't get back to work at once, you'll face stiff penalties. You're supposed to deliver bricks for the mayor's new mansion, and he doesn't like delays.'

'But the law—'

'Don't talk to me about the law, Hebrew. It's over your head. If you file a complaint, your family and friends will suffer the consequences.'

Abner was afraid of Sary. He and the rest of the brickmakers went back to work.

Dolora was more and more fascinated by the strange personality of Ofir, the Libyan sorcerer. His hawklike face was unsettling, yet his voice mesmerized, and when the subject was Aton, the solar disc, his enthusiasm was catching. A discreet house guest, he had agreed to meet a number of the princess' friends and speak about the unjust persecution Akhenaton had suffered, and the need to promote the cult of a single god.

Ofir cast a spell over people. No one walked away from these sessions unchanged. Some were upset by his views, others persuaded. He slowly entangled some worthwhile connections in his web, attracting more support for Aton – and Lita – with each passing week. Even though the throne of Egypt remained only a remote possibility, a movement was beginning to form.

Lita attended these talks without joining in. The young woman's dignity, bearing and reserve were the deciding factor for quite a few notables. She clearly belonged to a royal line that deserved to be taken into consideration. Sooner or later, she must surely regain her rank at the court.

Ofir never criticized, and made no demands. In a low, persuasive voice, he evoked Akhenaton's profound convictions, the beauty of his poetry in honour of Aton, his love of truth. Love and peace: was that not the message of the persecuted king and his descendant, Lita? And this message heralded a magnificent future, a future worthy of Egypt and her civilization.

When Dolora introduced the sorcerer to the former minister for foreign affairs, Meba, she was proud of herself. Proud that she had snapped out of her habitual apathy, proud to be serving a noble cause. Ramses had abandoned her; the sorcerer gave meaning to her existence.

The old diplomat, with his broad, reassuring face and stately manner, made no attempt to hide his distrust.

'I'm only doing this as a favour to you,' he told Dolora.

'I'm grateful, Meba. You won't regret it.' She led him to where the sorcerer sat beneath a persea tree, weaving two strands of linen into a thin cord that would hold an amulet.

He rose and bowed.

'It's a very great honour for me to receive a minister.'

'I'm nothing now,' Meba said bitterly.

'Injustice can strike anyone at any time.'

'That's small consolation.'

Ramses' sister chimed in: 'I explained everything to our friend Meba. Perhaps he'll agree to help us.'

'Let's not fool ourselves, my dear. Ramses has shut me up in a gilded retirement-cell.'

'You want revenge,' said the sorcerer evenly.

'That's going too far,' protested Meba. 'I still have some influential friends who—'

'They're out to protect their own interests, not yours. I have another goal in mind: proving Lita's legitimacy.'

'You're dreaming. Ramses has an extraordinarily forceful

210

personality. He's not about to step aside. What's more, the miraculous happenings of late have made him very popular. Believe me, it's a lost cause.'

'It's a challenge. I agree we can't fight him on his own ground.'

'What's your plan, then?'

'Interested?'

'Well . . .' Meba fiddled with the amulet around his neck.

'With that gesture you've just given one of the answers: magic. I know how to break through the spells protecting Ramses. It will be long and difficult, but I can do it.'

The diplomat recoiled. 'I can't offer you my assistance.'

'I'm not asking for it, Meba. But there's another area where we must attack Ramses: ideas.'

'I don't follow you.'

'Aton's believers need a respected and respectable leader. When Aton has destroyed the other gods, that leader will play a leading role in overthrowing a pharaoh who's weakened and unable to act.'

'It's . . . It's very risky!'

'Akhenaton was disgraced, but never Aton. His cult has never been banned, and he has many followers, who are determined to impose his worship. Where Akhenaton failed, we'll succeed.'

Meba's hands trembled. 'I'll have to think about it.'

'Isn't it exciting?' asked Dolora. 'A new world is opening up to us, a world where we'll take our rightful place!'

'Yes, of course. Let me think it over.'

A most satisfactory meeting, Ofir thought afterwards. A cautious, faint-hearted diplomat, Meba did not really have the makings of a leader. But he hated Ramses and dreamed of regaining his former rank. Unable to make up his mind, he would turn to his confidant, Shaanar, the man Ofir really

211

hoped to attract. Dolora had told him a great deal about the new minister for foreign affairs and his old rivalry with Ramses. Unless he'd changed completely, Shaanar was proceeding stealthily, his desire to destroy his brother intact. The sorcerer felt sure that Meba would put him in touch with this powerful figure, who was destined to become their most valuable ally.

After a long and exhausting day of work, Sary's right big toe was red and swollen, twisted with arthritis. Standing on it was so painful that he could barely drive his official chariot. His only satisfaction had been taking disciplinary measures against the Hebrews, who had finally understood that it was useless to challenge his authority. Thanks to his connections in the Theban police and the support of the mayor, he was free to vent his frustrations on the brickyard riffraff.

Having Ofir and his silent muse as house guests was beginning to grate on his nerves. They tried to stay out of his way, of course, but their influence over Dolora was getting out of hand. Her new-found devotion to Aton was exasperating. With all the time she spent in prayer or lapping up the Libyan's words as if they were spring water, she was neglecting her conjugal duties.

Tall, dark and languid, she was waiting for him on the doorstep to their villa.

'Go and get the liniment and rub my feet,' he barked at her. 'The pain is unbearable.'

'A hard day at the brickyard?'

'Don't make fun of me! You can't imagine what it's like. Those Hebrews are hopeless.'

Dolora took his arm and led him gently to their bed-chamber. Sary reclined against a heap of pillows as his wife washed and oiled his feet, massaging liniment into his sore toe.

'Is your sorcerer still hanging around?' he asked irritably.

'Meba called on him today.'

'Your father's minister for foreign affairs?'

'He was interested in what Ofir had to say.'

'Meba, a follower of Aton? He's too craven-hearted.'

'He's still an important and well-respected man. Attracting him would really help our cause.'

'Aren't you attaching too much importance to those two lunatics?'

'Sary! How dare you talk like that!'

'All right, forget it.'

'This is our only chance to reclaim our rank. And then this faith is so pure, so appealing. Aren't you moved when Ofir talks about Aton?'

'Who means more to you, your husband or that Libyan sorcerer?'

'What? There's absolutely no comparison.'

'He's with you all day long, while I have to oversee a bunch of lazy Hebrews. A blonde and a brunette to choose from . . . Your Ofir is one lucky fellow.'

Dolora stopped rubbing his inflamed toe.

'You're raving, Sary! Ofir is a sage and a man of prayer. It must be ages since he's thought of—'

'But I'll bet *you* do.'

'You're disgusting!'

'Take off your dress, Dolora, and keep on massaging me. I don't give a damn for prayers.'

'Wait, I forgot to tell you something.'

'What?'

'A royal courier delivered a letter for you.'

'Let me see it.'

Dolora went to fetch the letter. Sary's toe felt better already. What could this official business be? Perhaps an appointment to an office job, where he wouldn't have any Hebrews to supervise?

His wife returned with the scroll. Sary broke the seal on the papyrus, unrolled it and read.

He winced, the colour draining from his face.

'Bad news?'

'I'm to report to Memphis with my team of brickmakers.'

'That sounds like a promotion!'

'Yes, but the letter is signed by Moses, head of royal construction.'

38

Every Hebrew brickmaker in the country answered the summons. When Moses' letters reached the various work sites, the response was enthusiastic. Moses' reputation had spread throughout the land during his tenure at Karnak. Everyone knew he championed the rights of his fellow Hebrews and permitted no ill-treatment. Being Ramses' friend gave him a remarkable advantage, and now he had been named to oversee all royal construction projects. For many, new hope stirred: surely Moses would improve their salaries and working conditions?

Moses was frankly surprised by this success. A few tribal chiefs were upset, but there was no questioning Pharaoh's orders. They yielded to Moses' authority, welcoming him when he toured the tent city north of Memphis, checking on the workers' comfort and sanitary conditions.

Suddenly Sary barred his way. 'What's the meaning of this summons?'

'You'll soon find out.'

'I'm not one of these Hebrews.'

'There are several other Egyptian foremen.'

'Are you forgetting that my wife is the king's sister?'

'And I am head of his building projects. In other words, you must obey my orders.'

Sary chewed his lips. 'My lot of Hebrews are unruly. I

cane them when I need to, and I don't plan to stop.'

'Judicious use of physical discipline can make men listen with their third ear, the one on their back. But anyone who uses the cane without reason should be punished in kind. In fact, I'll see to it personally.'

'Don't try to bully me.'

'Watch yourself, Sary. I can have you demoted. By now you should be an excellent brickmaker yourself.'

'You wouldn't dare.'

'Ramses has given me full authority. Keep that in mind.'

Moses brushed past Sary, who spat in the young Hebrew's footsteps.

The return to Memphis, about which Dolora had been so happy, threatened to become a nightmare. Ramses had been officially informed of her sister's return, along with her husband, but nothing had come of it. They had taken a modest villa, passing Ofir and Lita off as servants. The trio, despite Sary's half-hearted objections, had every intention of continuing to proselytize as they had in Thebes. Given the number of foreigners living in Memphis, the country's economic capital, their work would be easier here. The South was more traditional and resistant to new religious concepts. Dolora considered the summons to Memphis a favourable sign.

Sary remained sceptical and preoccupied with his own fate, pondering what announcement Moses was about to make to the thousands of excited Hebrews.

Guarding the entrance to the Foreign Affairs secretariat was a statue of the god Thoth in the form of an enormous pink granite baboon. Thoth, the scribe god, had created all the world's languages, and members of the secretariat sought his patronage. Learning several foreign tongues was a requirement for diplomats, since the knowledge of hieroglyphs was not for export. When serving abroad, ambassadors and couriers used the local language.

Like other high-ranking officials in the secretariat, Ahsha often meditated in the shrine to the left of the entrance and laid narcissi on the altar of Thoth. Before addressing delicate issues of national security, it was wise to seek the favour of the scribe god.

His offering made, the rising star of Egyptian diplomacy passed through several busy rooms where officials were hard at work, to Shaanar's spacious upstairs office.

'There you are, Ahsha. What kept you?'

'I'm afraid I overslept; I was making rather merry last night. I do hope I haven't inconvenienced you, sir.'

Shaanar's face was red and puffy; he was obviously worked up about something.

'Tell me,' Ahsha said soothingly.

'Have you heard about the Hebrew brickmakers gathering north of town?'

'Yes, but I didn't take much notice.'

'Neither did I, but we should have!'

'What have these people to do with us?' Ahsha felt nothing but disdain for manual labourers, although he hardly knew any.

'You'll never guess who's behind it. The new head of royal construction – Moses!'

'Is that so surprising? He supervised Seti's additions to Karnak; it's a logical promotion.'

'If only that were all. Yesterday Moses called an assembly and told them about Ramses' project: he's going to build a new capital in the Delta!'

A long silence followed this revelation as Ahsha, ordinarily unflappable, registered the shock.

'Are you quite certain?'

'Absolutely certain. Moses is carrying out my brother's orders.'

'A new capital . . . It's impossible!'

'Not for Ramses!'

'How ambitious a project is it?'

'Pharaoh himself drew the plans and chose the site. And what a site – Avaris, the shameful city of the Hyskos invaders we had so much trouble getting rid of !' Shaanar's moon face suddenly brightened. 'What if Ramses has gone mad? A project on this scale can only lead to ruin. Men of sound mind will have to take over eventually . . .'

'I wouldn't be too optimistic. It's true that Ramses takes enormous risks, but his instinct is solid. It's actually the smartest thing he can do. Moving the capital so far north-east and so close to the border, he's sending the Hittites a clear warning signal. They'll see that Egypt is taking nothing for granted, is aware of the danger and won't give up a single cubit of land. The king will have good access to information about enemy actions and will react quickly.'

Shaanar sat down, disheartened. 'It's a catastrophe. Our strategy is falling apart.'

'I wouldn't be too pessimistic, either,' Ahsha advised. 'On the one hand, Ramses' dream may never become reality, and on the other, why should we change our plans?'

'But my brother is obviously taking foreign policy in hand . . .'

'That comes as no surprise, but his policy will still be based on the intelligence he receives, on the basis of which he'll appraise the situation. We may as well let him think he's in charge.'

Shaanar's confidence returned. 'You're right, Ahsha. We won't let a new capital get in our way.'

Queen Tuya had missed the gardens of her Memphis palace. The times she had strolled there with Seti seemed too few and far between, the years she had spent with him too brief. She remembered his every word, his every glance, and had often imagined a peaceful old age at his side, enjoying shared memories. But now Seti roamed through paradise

218

and she walked alone in this marvellous garden, shaded by pomegranates, tamarisks, jojoba trees. On either side of the path bloomed cornflowers, anemones, lupins, ranunculi. Tuya sat pensively by the lotus pond, beneath a wisteria arbour.

When she saw Ramses approaching, her sadness fled.

In less than a year as Pharaoh, her son had grown so self-assured that it was hard to believe he had ever doubted his capabilities. He ruled with the same vigour his father had, with seemingly inexhaustible reserves of energy.

Tenderly and respectfully, Ramses kissed his mother, then he sat down beside her. 'I need to talk to you.'

'That's what I'm here for, my son.'

'Do you approve of the men I've chosen for my government?'

'Do you recall Seti's advice to you?'

'I did my best to follow it: "Look deep in the souls of men. Look for advisers who are upright and firm, able to give an impartial opinion yet ever mindful of their oath of obedience." Have I succeeded? Only the next few years will tell.'

'Do you fear opposition so soon?'

'It's inevitable, at the rate I've been going. I know I'll run up against proud hearts and vested interests. When the idea for this new capital came to me, it was like a lightning bolt. I saw it and knew it was true.'

'The *sia*,' nodded his mother, 'direct intuition, without reasoning or analysis. It was the source of many of Seti's decisions. He believed it was handed down from pharaoh to pharaoh.'

'Has my new capital your blessing?'

'Since the *sia* spoke your heart, why do you need my approval?'

'Because my father's spirit is in this garden, and both of us hear his voice.'

'The signs are clear, Ramses. Your reign opens a new era, and Pi-Ramses will be your capital.'

The pharaoh took his mother's hands in his own.

'You'll see my city, Mother, and be glad.'

'I'm concerned about your protection.'

'Serramanna is ever watchful.'

'I'm talking about your magical protection. Have you thought about building your Temple of a Million Years?'

'I've picked the site, but for now Pi-Ramses is my priority.'

'Don't forget your temple. If the forces of darkness are unleashed upon you, it will be your strongest ally.'

39

The setting was magnificent.

Fertile land, broad fields, thick grass, flower-lined foot-paths, apple orchards full of honeyed fruit, a flourishing olive grove, teeming ponds, salt marshes, dense thickets: here sat Avaris, once so despised, now reduced to a handful of houses and a temple to the god Set.

This was where Seti had taught his son the meaning of true power. This was where Ramses would build his capital.

The Hebrews and their Egyptian foremen were part of the expedition Ramses had led in person, accompanied by his lion and dog. Serramanna, on high alert, had ridden ahead with a scouting party of ten.

The little town of Avaris dozed in the sun. Its only inhabitants were government workers in dead-end jobs, slow-moving peasants and papyrus-gatherers. The place seemed suspended in time.

The expedition had made a stop in Heliopolis, where Ramses made an offering to his protector, Ra, and had then headed towards Bubastis (home to the goddess of gentleness and love, Bastet, who had been incarnated as a cat) and along the Pelusiac branch of the Nile, dubbed 'the Waters of Ra'. Near Lake Menezaleh, Avaris was at the western end of the 'Road of Horus', leading across the Sinai coastline towards Palestine and Syria.

The beauty and lushness of the countryside surprised Moses. 'A strategic location,' he commented, as he studied the map Ramses had shown him.

'Do you understand the reasons for my choice now? With the aid of a canal, the "Waters of Ra" will give us access to the lakes around the isthmus of el-Qantara. In an emergency, we can quickly reach the fortress of Sileh by boat, and the smaller frontier outposts as well. I'll be reinforcing the eastern side of the Delta, which commands the invasion routes, and I'll hear immediately of any trouble in our protectorates. The summers are milder here. Our garrisons won't suffer from the heat and so will remain more alert.'

'You're a man of vision,' said Moses admiringly.

'How are your workers?'

'They seem happy to work under me, but the increased wages you're offering probably have a lot to do with that.'

'If I'm generous, they'll give me their best. I want a splendid city.'

Moses bent to study the map again. Four major temples were planned: to the west, one to Amon, 'The Hidden'; to the south, the temple of Set, the local deity; to the east, a shrine to Astarte, the Syrian goddess; and to the north the temple of Wadjet, 'The Verdant', guarantor of the place's prosperity. Near the temple of Set would be the river port. This was at the meeting point of two broad canals, linking the 'Waters of Ra' and the 'Waters of Avaris', which surrounded the city and supplied drinking water. Close to the port lay warehouses, granaries and workshops. Farther north, in the centre of town, were the palace, government buildings, noblemen's villas, and residential neighbourhoods where grand and humble dwellings stood side by side. The main street led away from the palace towards the temple of Ptah, the Creator, with two side roads leading to the temples of Amon and Ra. Set's temple was set apart, on the opposite side of the canal connecting the 'Ra' and 'Avaris' branches.

222

There were also four military barracks, one between the Pelusiac branch and the government buildings, the three others along the 'Waters of Avaris' – the first behind the temple of Ptah, the second adjoining the residential neighbourhoods, the last near the temples of Ra and Astarte.

'Production of ceramic tiles is ready to start tomorrow,' revealed Ramses. 'From the smallest house to the palace reception hall, Pi-Ramses will sparkle with colour. But first everything has to be built, and that's where you come in, Moses.'

With his right index finger, Moses indicated where the various buildings in the monarch's plan would be situated.

'It's ambitious. I like the way you think on a grand scale. Still . . .'

'Yes, Moses?'

'No offence, Majesty, but one temple is missing. It could easily go in the space between the temples of Amon and Ptah.'

'Which god would it honour?'

'The god who created the institution of pharaoh. Won't it be in this temple that your rededication is celebrated?'

'For that to happen, a pharaoh must have reigned for thirty years. To build it now would be tempting fate.'

'You've left room for it, though.'

'Leaving it out of my plans would also be tempting fate. If I do reach Year Thirty of my reign, at that celebration you'll be in the first rank of dignitaries, together with our other old friends.'

'Thirty years . . . Who knows what God has in store for us?'

'For the moment, he's telling us to build the capital of Egypt together.'

'I've divided the Hebrews into two groups. The first will transport blocks of stone to the temple sites and work under Egyptian supervisors. The second will manufacture the thousands of bricks to be used in your palace and government buildings. Coordinating the two groups will be awkward; I'm afraid my new-found popularity won't last. Do you know what the men call me? *Masha*, "Rescued from Drowning".'

'Is this some miracle I haven't heard about?'

'No, an old Babylonian legend they're fond of repeating. It's a pun on my name, which means "He Who is Born". In their eyes, the gods have blessed me. A Hebrew, educated at the royal school and friend to Pharaoh! God saved me from drowning in poverty and misfortune. A man with my luck is worth following. That's why the brickmakers trust me.'

'Treat them well. You have my permission to use the royal granaries if you lack provisions.'

'I'll build your capital, Ramses.'

The Hebrew brickmakers tied white headbands around the black wigs that stopped above their ears. Many wore moustaches or short beards. A narrow forehead and a thick lower lip were common features. They also shared a pride in their expertise. Syrian and Egyptian brickmakers tried to compete with them, but the Hebrews remained the best and most sought-after in the trade. The work was hard and closely supervised by Egyptian foremen, but the pay was decent and the leave days liberal. Here in Egypt, the food was good and lodgings fairly easy to find. The hardier souls among them even built themselves comfortable homes with salvaged materials.

Moses had made no secret of the fact that at Pi-Ramses the pace would be hotter than usual, but promised bonuses in compensation. Many a Hebrew would prosper here, provided they spared no effort. Under normal conditions, three workmen could produce eight to nine hundred small bricks a day. At Pi-Ramses, they would have to manufacture different sizes: larger bricks for foundations, then a multitude of smaller ones. Usually foremen and stonemasons were responsible for the foundations.

By the end of the first day, the Hebrews realized that Moses would be as stern a taskmaster as he had promised. Any hope of spending their afternoons asleep in the shade of a tree quickly vanished. Like his co-workers, Abner threw himself into his work: mixing mud from the Nile with chopped straw. Finding the right consistency was the trick. Several huge flat areas had been set aside and trenches dug to a canal for water to moisten the river silt. Then, keeping time to songs, the men worked the mixture with picks and hoes, a technique that resulted in stronger bricks.

Abner performed his tasks quickly and well. As soon as the mixture felt right to him, he loaded it into a basket, which a labourer hauled to the workshop, where it was poured into a rectangular wooden mould. Turning out the moulds was a delicate operation; occasionally Moses supervised it in person. The bricks were left to dry for some four hours, then stacked and transported to the various worksites, beginning with the best-cured and therefore lightest-coloured ones.

Humble as it was, the well-made mud brick proved to be a remarkably solid building material. Correctly laid, it could literally last for ages.

A competitive spirit awakened among the Hebrews. The higher salary and bonuses played a part, of course, but so did their pride in being part of such a colossal undertaking and their determination to rise to the occasion. If their enthusiasm waned, Moses got them fired up again. Thousands of perfect bricks were being produced each day.

Pi-Ramses was coming to life, springing out of the pharaoh's dream to become reality. Foremen and stone-cutters, following the king's plans, laid solid foundations; labourers tirelessly carted load after load of the Hebrews' bricks.

Beneath the Delta sun, a city was taking shape.

At the close of each day, Abner admired Moses more. The Hebrew leader moved from group to group, checking the quality of the food, sending those who were sick or overworked off to rest. Contrary to his expectations, his popularity continued to grow.

Abner had already earned enough bonus money to build his family a fine new house right here in the new capital and—

'Pleased with yourself, Abner?' Sary's hollow face wore an evil grin.

'What do you want with me?'

'I'm your foreman. Have you forgotten that?'

'I do my job.'

'Badly.'

'What?'

'Your bricks are below the standard.'

'That can't be!'

'Two building foremen found bad bricks in the loads you sent them. They've written a report. If I pass it on to Moses, you'll be fired, maybe even put in jail.'

'What's this all about? Why are you lying?'

'You have one alternative: buying my silence. Hand your pay over to me and the report will disappear.'

'You're a jackal, Sary!'

'You have no choice, Abner.'

'Why do you hate me?'

'You're a Hebrew, one among many. Let's say you're paying for all the rest.'

'You have no right!'

'I need an answer. Now.'

Abner hung his head. Sary had beaten him again.

40

In Memphis, Ofir felt more at ease than in Thebes. The northern capital was home to many foreigners, who seemed for the most part to fit in perfectly. Some adhered to Akhenaton's doctrine. The sorcerer revived their flagging faith, promising that it would bring them happiness and prosperity in the near future.

Those who were privileged to see Lita, silent as ever, were greatly impressed. None of them doubted that royal blood flowed in her veins, nor that she was the ill-fated pharaoh's rightful heir. The sorcerer's patient, well-reasoned arguments for the existence of a single god worked wonders, and Dolora's Memphis villa was the setting for productive meetings that netted a daily increase in the number of believers.

Ofir was not the first foreigner to propagate original ideas, but he was the only one to revive the heresy quashed by Akhenaton's successors. His capital and burial place had been abandoned; no person of rank had been entombed nearby in the necropolis. Everyone knew that Ramses, after bringing Karnak under his control, would stand for no religious trouble. Therefore, Ofir took care to be sparing in his criticism of the king and his policies, so as not to invite disapproval.

The sorcerer was finally getting somewhere.

Dolora brought him a drink of cool carob juice.

'You seem tired, Ofir.'

'Our work demands constant effort. How is your husband doing on his project?'

'He's very unhappy. According to his last letter, he spends his days scolding lazy, dishonest Hebrews.'

'I've heard the work is going very quickly, though.'

'Everyone says it will be splendid.'

'But dedicated to Set, the evil lord of the powers of darkness! Ramses wants to snuff out the light and hide the sun. We must stop him.'

'I'm convinced of it, Ofir.'

'Your support is essential, as you know. Will you consent to let me use all the resources of my art to keep the pharaoh from destroying Egypt?'

The tall, languid woman bit her lips. 'Ramses is my brother!'

Ofir gently took Dolora's hands.

'He's already done us so much harm. Of course, I'll abide by your decision, but why wait any longer? Ramses isn't waiting for anything! And the further he goes, the stronger his magical defences become. I'm not sure I'll be able to break through them if we delay much longer.'

'It's such a big step . . .'

'Be aware of your responsibilities, Dolora. I can still act, but soon it will be too late.'

Dolora was still unwilling to attack her brother. Ofir let go of her hands.

'There may be another way,' he said after a moment's pause.

'What are you thinking?'

'Queen Nefertari is rumoured to be pregnant.'

'It's no rumour. You've only to look at her.'

'Have you any affection for her?'

'Not in the least.'

228

'I'll ask one of my compatriots to bring what I need tonight.'

'I'll stay in my room!' cried Dolora, retreating hastily.

The man arrived in the middle of the night. The house was quiet; Dolora and Lita were asleep. Ofir opened the door to the merchant, took the sack from him and paid with two linen sheets Dolora had donated.

The transaction took only a few moments.

Ofir shut himself up in a small room to which he had blocked all the openings. A single oil lamp gave off a dim light.

On a low table, the sorcerer laid out the contents of the bundle: a statuette of an ape, an ivory hand, a crude figurine of a naked woman, a miniature pillar, and another figurine of a woman, this one holding snakes in her hands. The ape would supply him with the power of the god Thoth. The hand was for action. The naked woman gave him power over the queen's reproductive organs. The pillar represented the lasting effect of his spell. The snake woman would poison Nefertari's body with black magic.

Ofir's task would not be easy. The queen possessed great personal strength, and, like her husband, had been endowed with protective forces at the time of her coronation. But pregnancy weakened those defences. The new life inside her sapped Nefertari's own life force.

It would take at least three days and nights for the spell to take hold. Ofir was slightly disappointed not to be attacking Ramses directly, but without his sister's consent that would be impossible. When he had Dolora completely in his sway, he would pursue a more ambitious goal. For now, he could begin to weaken the enemy.

Leaving the daily business of governing in the hands of Ahmeni and his ministers, Ramses made frequent visits to

Pi-Ramses. Thanks to Moses' leadership and organization, as well as a strict schedule, the work was progressing by leaps and bounds.

The atmosphere was lively and bustling. The men were happy with the quality and quantity of their rations. On top of that, generous bonuses were paid as promised, on the merit system. The hardest workers would make a tidy packet and be able to set themselves up either in the new capital or in another city, even to buy a plot of land. There was also a well-equipped infirmary to provide free care for the sick and injured. Unlike other construction sites, Pi-Ramses was not plagued with workers feigning illness in order to go on leave.

The king was safety-conscious; several foremen were permanently assigned to site safety. All but a few minor injuries had been avoided when the Temple of Amon's granite blocks were set in place. Thanks to a scrupulously observed rotation of work gangs, the men never reached the point of exhaustion. Two days off after every six working days allowed them to rest and recuperate.

The only person Moses allowed no rest was himself. He checked all work, resolved conflicts, took urgent decisions, reorganized substandard work crews, ordered materials and supplies, wrote reports, slept for an hour after lunch and three hours each night. Their leader's energy impressed the Hebrew brick workers so deeply that they gave him instant, unquestioning obedience. No supervisor in their experience had ever defended their interests as he did.

Abner could have spoken to Moses about Sary's extortion, but he was afraid of how his foreman might retaliate, given his strong police connections. If he was labelled a trouble-maker, Abner would be deported and never see his wife and children again. Once Sary'd started receiving payments, the foreman had stopped harassing him and had been almost pleasant. It seemed the worst was over. The Hebrew retreated

230

into silence and moulded his bricks with the usual care and speed.

That morning, Ramses was touring the worksite. As soon as his visit was announced, the Hebrews washed, trimmed their beards and moustaches, tied fresh white bands round their best wigs and lined up their bricks in perfect order.

The first chariot that stopped in front of the brickyard discharged a glowering giant with sword and shield in hand. Was one of the workers about to be disciplined? The presence of twenty archers did little to lighten the mood.

Serramanna passed silently along the tense and motionless rows of Hebrew brickmakers. When his inspection was finished, the Sard signalled one of the soldiers to let the royal chariot advance.

The brickmakers bowed to Pharaoh, who congratulated them on their work one by one, addressing each man by name. Cheers greeted his announcement that new wigs and white Delta wine were to be distributed; but what touched the men most deeply was the attention the king paid to the freshly moulded bricks. He picked up several, weighing them in his hands.

'Perfect,' he declared. 'Double rations for a week and an extra day off. Where is your foreman?'

Sary stepped forward.

Ramses' old teacher was the only one who was not glad to see the monarch. He was afraid of meeting the king against whom he had plotted.

'Satisfied with your new duties, Sary?'

'I thank Your Majesty for awarding them to me.'

'If my mother and Nefertari hadn't interceded, your punishment would have been much stiffer, believe me.'

'I'm aware of that, Majesty, and hope my new attitude will persuade you to forgive my past transgressions.'

'They're unforgivable, Sary.'

'The remorse that gnaws at my heart is more painful than acid.'

'It can't be too bad; it's quite some time since your crime, and you're still around.'

'Is it too much to hope for Your Majesty's pardon?'

'I am not familiar with that notion, Sary. One lives within or outside the Rule of Ma'at. You've flouted it, and your soul is for ever stained. Make sure you cause Moses no trouble. This is the last chance I'm giving you.'

'I swear to Your Majesty that—'

'Enough said, Sary. Be glad of the chance to take part in creating Pi-Ramses.'

When the king climbed back in his chariot, cheers rose again, even louder this time. Reluctantly, Sary joined in.

41

As planned, work proceeded more slowly on the temples than on secular edifices. Nevertheless, immediate shipments of granite began, and expert stone-haulers, including a number of Hebrews, made regular deliveries to the work site.

Thanks to the brickmakers' industriousness, the royal palace was rising quickly from its stone foundations, and already dominated the centre of the capital. Shipping was under way, the warehouses were open, carpenters were turning out fine furniture, ceramic tiles were being mass-produced. Villa walls seemed to spring up out of the ground, the residential areas of the city took shape, and the barracks would soon be ready to house their first troops.

'The palace lake will be splendid,' announced Moses. 'It ought to be dug by the middle of next month. Your capital is going to be beautiful, Ramses. It's built with love.'

'You can take credit for that, Moses.'

'All I've done is execute your plans.'

The king detected a slight reproach in his friend's tone of voice. Just as he was about to ask why, a courier from Memphis galloped up. Serramanna made him stop at a respectable distance. The messenger jumped down and approached his sovereign, panting.

'Your Majesty's presence is urgently requested in Memphis. The queen has been taken ill.'

Ramses collided with Dr Pariamaku, head of the palace medical staff, a learned and commanding man of fifty with long, expressive hands. An experienced surgeon, he had the reputation of being an excellent doctor, though strict with his patients.

'I want to see the queen,' demanded Ramses. He was cursing himself for not having honoured his promise to Nefertari to be with her until the birth.

'The queen is sleeping, Majesty. The nurses applied a massage oil mixed with a sleeping-draught.'

'What's wrong with her?'

'There are signs of a premature delivery.'

'Isn't that dangerous?'

'Very, I'm afraid.'

'I order you to save Nefertari.'

'I still predict a favourable outcome.'

'What makes you say that?'

'My staff performed the usual tests, Majesty, placing barley and wheat in two cloth sacks that were sprinkled with the queen's urine for several days in a row. Both grains sprouted, indicating she will give birth successfully. Since the wheat sprouted first, she will have a girl.'

'I've heard the opposite.'

Dr Pariamaku gave him an icy stare. 'Your Majesty must be referring to another technique, in which the grains are covered with soil. In any case, we must hope that the seed of your heart, implanted in the queen's heart, is firmly fixed in the infant's spine and bones. High-quality sperm gives an excellent spinal cord and perfect bone marrow. Need I remind you that the bones and tendons come from the father, the flesh and blood from the mother?'

The doctor was rather pleased with his lecture. And to such an illustrious student!

'Need I remind you that I studied anatomy and physiology at the royal school, Doctor?'

'Of course not, Majesty.'

'Nothing led you to expect complications?'

'My learning has certain limits, Majesty . . .'

'My power has none, Doctor, and I demand a safe delivery.'

'Majesty . . .'

'Yes, Doctor?'

'Your own health must be closely monitored. I have not yet had the honour of examining you, which is among my foremost responsibilities.'

'No need. I've never had a day's illness in my life. Call me the moment the queen wakes up.'

The sun was low in the sky when Serramanna granted Dr Pariamaku entry into the king's office.

The physician was ill at ease. 'The queen has awakened, Majesty.'

Ramses rose.

'However . . .'

'Out with it, Doctor!'

Pariamaku, who had boasted that he would be able to handle Ramses, was beginning to miss Seti, taciturn and uncooperative though he had been. Ramses was like a raging storm – best to stay out of his way.

'The queen has just been taken to the delivery room.'

'I demanded to see her immediately!'

'The midwives decided there wasn't a second to lose.'

Ramses snapped the reed pen in his hand. If Nefertari died, would he have the strength to go on?

Six midwives from the House of Life, wearing long tunics and turquoise necklaces, helped Nefertari to the delivery room, an airy, flower-filled pavilion. Like all Egyptian women, the queen would give birth naked, straight-backed, squatting over stones with a bed of reeds on top of them. This symbolized each newborn's destiny, its life span determined by Thoth.

The first midwife would support the queen from behind, the second would ease her through each stage of labour, the third would catch the baby, the fourth would attend to its first needs, the fifth was the wet-nurse, and the sixth would hold two *ankh* amulets – the 'Keys of Life' – for the queen until the infant's first cry was heard. Though aware of the dangers facing them, the six women moved serenely.

After thoroughly massaging Nefertari, the head midwife had applied poultices over her lower abdomen. Judging it necessary to hasten what promised to be a painful labour, she inserted a paste of turpentine resin, onion, milk, fennel, and salt into the vagina. To ease the labour pains, she prepared dried earth to be mixed with warm oil and rubbed on the genital area.

The six midwives knew that Nefertari's labour would be long and its outcome uncertain.

'May the goddess Hathor grant the queen a child,' chanted one of the women. 'May no sickness touch it. Begone, demon of darkness, who enters slyly, with your face turned backwards. You will never embrace this infant, put it to sleep, harm it or carry it off. May the spirit move in the child, may no evil spell touch it, may the stars be favourable.'

As night fell, the contractions came closer together. Bean paste was packed around the queen's teeth so that she could clench them without hurting herself.

Professional, focused, reciting ancient incantations to banish pain, the six midwives helped the Queen of Egypt bring forth new life.

Ramses couldn't stand it a moment longer. When Dr Pariamaku reappeared for the tenth time, he thought the king might fly at his throat.

'Is it finally over?'

'Yes, Majesty.'

'Nefertari?'

'The queen is alive and well and you have a daughter.'

'How is the baby?'

'Too soon to tell . . .'

The king pushed past the physician and charged into the delivery room, where one of the midwives was cleaning up.

'Where are they? The queen and my daughter?'

'In a palace bedchamber, Majesty.'

'Tell me the truth!'

'The baby is very weak.'

'I demand to see them.'

Relieved, radiant, but exhausted, Nefertari was asleep. The head midwife had given her a sedative.

The baby was remarkably beautiful. Fresh, her eyes at once astonished and curious, the child of their love greeted life like the miracle it was.

The king held her. 'She's perfect! Why do you think something's wrong?'

'The cord broke on the amulet we were putting around her neck. A bad omen, Majesty, a very bad omen.'

'Have the signs been read?'

'We're waiting for the prophetess.'

The prophetess appeared a few minutes later. With the six midwives, she formed the circle of the seven Hathors, foreseeing the newborn's destiny. Huddled round the infant, they went into a trance.

Their meditation seemed to last longer than usual.

Grim-faced, the prophetess broke away from the circle and approached the king.

'The time isn't propitious, Majesty. We cannot—'

'Don't lie to me.'

'We may be wrong.'

'Just tell me what you see.'

'The child's fate will be decided within the next twenty-four hours. If we don't find a way to dispel the demons eating away at her heart, your daughter won't live until tomorrow night.'

42

The royal infant's blooming wet-nurse had been personally checked by Dr Pariamaku. Her milk had the pleasant odour of carob flour. To ensure a good milk supply, the nurse had been drinking fig sap and eating roasted fish spines ground up in oil.

Much to the distress of the doctor and wet-nurse, the baby would not take the breast. Another nurse was called in, with the same result. The final remedy, a special reserve of milk kept in a hippopotamus-shaped vessel, worked no better. The child would not take the thick milk flowing from the animal's teats.

The doctor moistened his tiny patient's lips and was preparing to wrap her in damp clothes when Ramses took her in his arms.

'She's becoming dehydrated, Majesty!'

'Your science can't help her. My strength will keep her alive.'

Holding his tiny daughter to his chest, the king went to Nefertari's bedside. Despite her exhaustion, the queen was radiant as ever.

'I'm so happy, Ramses! Nothing can harm her now.'

'How do you feel?'

'Don't worry about me. Have you thought of a name for our baby?'

'That's up to the mother.'

238

'We'll call her Meritamon, "Beloved of Amon". She'll see your Temple of a Million Years finished. While I was in labour, I had the strangest sensation . . . You must start work on it right away. It will be your best defence against the forces of evil and keep us united against adversity.'

'You'll have your wish, I promise.'

'Why are you holding her so tight?'

Nefertari's gaze was so clear, so trusting, that Ramses was unable to keep the truth from her.

'Meritamon isn't well.'

'What's wrong with her?'

'She won't take the breast, but I'll make her better.'

The queen sank back into the bed. 'I've already lost one child, and now death is trying to take our daughter. It's dark, dark . . .'

Nefertari swooned.

'Your diagnosis, Doctor?' asked Ramses.

'The queen is very weak,' Pariamaku replied.

'Can you save her?'

'I don't know, Majesty. If she survives, she mustn't have any more children. Another pregnancy would be fatal.'

'And our daughter?'

'I've never seen anything like it. She seems so peaceful, now that you're holding her. The midwives may be right, although I find their theory absurd.'

'What is it, then?'

'They think she's under some sort of magic spell.'

'A spell, here, in my palace?'

'That's why I didn't take it seriously. Still, it might be a good idea to consult the court magicians.'

'But what if one of them is involved? No, there's only one thing left to do.'

Meritamon slept in her father's powerful arms.

The court buzzed with rumours: Nefertari's child had been stillborn; the queen was near death; Ramses was mad with despair. While not daring to believe them, Shaanar hoped there might be some truth to these excellent reports.

On the way to the palace with Dolora, Shaanar put on a grave and tearful face. His sister seemed genuinely grief-stricken.

'Been taking acting lessons, sister dear?'

'Can't you see that I'm upset?'

'You don't care about Ramses or Nefertari.'

'No, but the baby . . . the baby isn't responsible.'

'So what? I had no idea you were so sentimental. If the rumours are true, things are looking up for us.'

Dolora could never tell Shaanar what was really upsetting her: Ofir's successful spell. To break through the royal couple's defences and shatter their lives, the Libyan must have extraordinary power over the forces of darkness.

Ahmeni, paler than usual, received Dolora and her brother.

'Given the circumstances,' said Shaanar, 'we thought the king might like his family nearby.'

'Sorry, he'd rather be alone.'

'How is Nefertari?'

'The queen is resting.'

'The baby?' asked Dolora.

'Dr Pariamaku is attending her.'

'Can you tell us anything more definite?'

'You'll have to be patient, I'm afraid.'

As Shaanar and Dolora left the palace, they saw Serramanna and his guard detail escorting a scruffy-looking, bare-headed man, dressed in a strange antelope-skin tunic studded with pockets. They were walking briskly towards the royal couple's private apartments.

'Setau! You're my last hope.'

The snake-charmer went up to the king and gazed at the baby in his arms.

'I don't care for babies, but that one's a beauty. The mother's looks, of course.'

'Meet our daughter, Meritamon. She's dying, Setau.'

'She's . . . ?'

'She's under a spell.'

'Has it come from inside the palace?'

'I'm not sure.'

'What has it done to her?'

'She won't take the breast.'

'Nefertari?'

'Sinking fast.'

'I suppose good old Pariamaku has given up?'

'He doesn't know what to do.'

'As usual. Put your daughter in her cradle. Gently, now.'

Ramses did as he was told. The moment he let go of Meritamon, her breathing grew laboured.

'Your strength is all that's keeping her alive. Just as I feared. What's this now? The baby isn't even wearing an amulet! Don't they know anything in this palace?'

Setau dug a scarab amulet out of a pocket, strung it on a fine cord with seven knots, and put it round Meritamon's neck. The scarab bore the inscription: 'Ravenous death will not take me. The divine light will preserve me.'

'Pick her up again,' ordered Setau, 'and show me the palace laboratory.'

'Do you think you'll be able to —'

'We'll discuss it later. Every minute counts now.'

There were several sections to the palace laboratory. Setau shut himself up in the room where male hippopotamus tusks were stored. He selected one over a cubit in length, and carved it into an elongated crescent moon. He smoothed the surface without damaging the ivory, then carved several symbols with the power to repel the forces of darkness that were trying to kill mother and child. A winged griffin with

241

a lion's body and falcon's head, a female hippo brandishing a knife, a frog, a shining sun, a bearded dwarf with his fists full of snakes – these, he considered, were best suited to the situation. Describing his magical helpers aloud as he carved, he ordered them to cut the throats of all demons, male and female, in their path, to trample them underfoot, to lacerate them and put them to flight. Next, he prepared a potion based on viper venom to clear the opening to Meritamon's stomach, though even the minutest of doses might be too much for a newborn.

When Setau emerged, Dr Pariamaku came running frantically towards him.

'Hurry! The baby is almost dead.'

Looking out at the sunset, Ramses held his daughter, trustfully slumbering against him. Despite his magnetism, her breathing was growing ragged. Nefertari's baby, the only child of their union who might survive . . . If Meritamon died, Nefertari would not survive. Anger welled up in the king's heart, an anger that would repel the creeping shadows and save his daughter from their evil spell.

Setau entered the chamber, holding the newly carved tusk.

'It ought to break the spell,' he explained. 'But it's not enough. We can't reverse the damage to her internal organs unless she swallows this potion.'

When he told them what it was made of, Dr Pariamaku said indignantly, 'I can't recommend this, Majesty!'

'Are you sure it will work, Setau?'

'I admit it's dangerous. It's up to you to decide.'

'Let's go ahead,' said Ramses.

43

Setau laid the carved tusk on Meritamon's chest. Snug in the cradle, her huge eyes inquisitive, the infant breathed peacefully.

Ramses, Setau, and Dr Pariamaku remained silent. The talisman seemed to be working, but would it last?

Ten minutes later, Meritamon began to struggle and cry.

'Have them bring a statue of the goddess Opet,' ordered Setau. 'I'm going back to the laboratory. Doctor, moisten the baby's lips, and make sure that's all you do.'

Opet, the female hippopotamus, was the patroness of midwives and wet-nurses. In the heavens, she took the form of a constellation separating the Great Bear (linked to Set, and therefore potentially destructive) from the reborn Osiris. Magicians from the House of Life had charged the statue with positive energy. Filled with mother's milk, it was placed at the head of the cradle.

Meritamon stopped crying and dozed off again.

Setau reappeared, holding a crudely carved tusk in each hand. 'Not pretty,' he said, 'but they ought to do what's necessary.'

He laid one tusk on the baby's stomach and the other at her feet. Meritamon did not stir.

'A field of positive forces is protecting her now. The spell has been broken, the evil undone.'

'Is she out of danger?' asked the king.

'Not unless she takes the breast. The passage to her stomach has to open, or she'll die.'

'Give her your potion.'

'No, you do it.'

Ramses gently parted his sleeping daughter's lips and poured the amber liquid into her tiny mouth. Dr Pariamaku turned his head away.

Moments later, Meritamon opened her eyes and squalled.

'Quick!' said Setau. 'The statue's breast!'

Ramses picked up his daughter, Setau removed the thin metal stopper in the statue's nipple, and the king brought the baby's mouth to meet it.

Meritamon gulped the life-giving liquid, barely stopping to catch her breath, and gurgled with contentment.

'What can I do to thank you, Setau?'

'Nothing, Ramses.'

'I'll appoint you director of the palace magicians.'

'They can get along without me. How's Nefertari doing?'

'She's amazing. She's going to walk in the garden tomorrow.'

'And the baby?'

'She has an unslakable thirst for life.'

'What were the seven Hathors' predictions?'

'The black cloud over Meritamon's destiny has lifted. They saw a priestess' vestments, a woman of great nobility, the stones of a temple.'

'An austere life.'

'You deserve a fortune, Setau.'

'My snakes, my desert creatures and Lotus are enough for me.'

'You'll have unlimited funds for your research. As for your venom production, the palace will pay top price for it and distribute it to the hospitals.'

'I don't want any favours.'

'It's no favour. Since your pharmaceuticals are the best in Egypt, your salary must be raised and your work encouraged.'

'There *is* one thing . . .'

'Anything.'

'Have you still got any of that red Faiyum wine from Year Three of your father's reign?'

'I'll have several jars of it sent your way tomorrow.'

'Let me know how many vials of venom I'll owe you.'

'It's a present.'

'I don't like presents, especially coming from the king.'

'It's your friend, not your king, who asks you to accept it. Tell me, where did you learn the technique you used to save Meritamon?'

'My snakes teach me almost everything, and Lotus knows the rest. Nubian sorcerers are peerless, believe me. The amulet I put around your daughter's neck will do her a world of good, provided you have its magic renewed every year.'

'I'm giving you and Lotus an official residence.'

'In town? You can't be serious. How would we do our work? We need the desert, the darkness and the danger. Speaking of danger, that was an unusual spell they cast on Meritamon.'

'What do you mean?'

'I had to use extreme measures because the spell was so strong. There was some foreign wizardry at work – Syrian, Libyan or Hebrew. Without three magic tusks, I'd never have been able to break the negative forces. Not to mention the fact that it takes an exceptionally twisted mind to go after a newborn baby.'

'A palace magician, do you think?'

'That would surprise me. No, a familiar of the forces of evil.'

'Then he'll try again.'

'Of that you can be sure.'

'How can we find him and put a stop to his wickedness?'

'I've no idea. A fiend that powerful is sure to be a master of deception. It could even be someone you've met, who seemed friendly and harmless. Or he could be hiding in some inaccessible lair.'

'How can I keep my wife and my daughter safe?'

'Stick to the proven methods: amulets and ritual invocations to the forces of good.'

'What if that's not enough?'

'You'll need to surround yourself with energy more powerful than black magic.'

'A source of such energy,' mused Ramses.

The Temple of a Million Years – that would be his best hope.

Pi-Ramses was growing.

It wasn't a city yet, but buildings and houses were taking shape in the imposing shadow of the palace, whose stone foundations rivalled those of its Thebes or Memphis counterparts. The work was proceeding at a lightning pace. Moses seemed tireless and continued to run a model worksite. Seeing results so quickly made everyone, from masterbuilders to rough labourers, eager to see the project reach completion. Some planned to live in the capital their own hands were helping to build.

Two Hebrew tribal chiefs, resentful of Moses's growing authority, had tried to challenge him. Before he could even respond, the brickmakers had unanimously demanded that he remain their leader. From that moment on, Moses became the uncrowned king of a people without a homeland. Building the new capital took so much energy that his mental turmoil abated. He no longer wondered about the One God and concentrated only on organising the worksites efficiently.

The announcement that Ramses had arrived made him happy. The sighting of certain birds of ill omen had made the men uneasy about the queen and her baby. For days, their spirits were low. Moses had told them not to worry, predicting that Ramses would be back before they knew it – and Ramses was proving him right.

Try as he might, Serramanna could not stop the workers lining up on both sides of the royal chariot's route through town. The men wanted to touch their pharaoh, so that some of his magic would rub off on them. The Sard muttered curses. What if one of them had a dagger? Why wouldn't Ramses listen?

The king went straight to Moses' temporary quarters. When he alighted, Moses bowed, but once they were inside, out of public view, the friends embraced.

'If we can keep going at this rate, we may just meet your ridiculous deadline.'

'Let me guess: you're ahead of schedule!'

'We certainly are.'

'This time I want to see everything.'

'I think you'll be pleased. May I ask after Nefertari?'

'The queen is very well indeed. So is our daughter. Meritamon will be a beauty, like her mother.'

'I heard that they came within a hair's-breadth of death.'

'Setau saved them.'

'With his snake venom?'

'No, he's become quite adept at magic. He broke an evil spell someone cast on my wife and daughter.'

Moses was aghast. 'Who'd dare try such a thing?'

'We don't know yet.'

'You'd have to be beneath contempt to attack a mother and child. And insane, to make an attempt on the royal family.'

'I wonder if there's a connection between this vile attack and the building of Pi-Ramses. I've ruffled the feathers of a lot of important people.'

'I don't think so. It's too big a jump from discontent to murder.'

'If it turned out a Hebrew was guilty, how would you feel?'

'A criminal is a criminal, no matter what his race. But I think you're on the wrong track.'

'If you learn anything at all, don't keep it from me.'

'What? Don't you trust me?'

'Would I talk to you this way if I didn't?'

'No Hebrew would stoop so low.'

'I have to be away for several weeks, Moses. Take good care of my capital.'

'The next time you come, you'll hardly recognize it. Don't wait too long, though. We wouldn't want to postpone the opening ceremonies.'

44

The beginning of June brought stifling heat and a round of festivities marking the beginning of Ramses' second year on the throne. Already more than a year since Seti's departure for the kingdom of the stars!

The royal couple's boat moored at Gebel el-Silsila, where the great river narrowed. According to tradition, the spirit of the Nile resided here. Pharaoh must reawaken him so that he would become the father of life and make the waters of the inundation rise.

After making the offering of milk and wine and saying the ritual prayers, the royal pair entered a shrine carved into the river bluffs. Inside, it was pleasantly cool.

'Did Dr Pariamaku speak to you?' Ramses asked Nefertari.

'He prescribed something new to give me back my energy.'

'Nothing else?'

'Is he hiding the truth about Meritamon?'

'No, you can rest easy on her account.'

'Then what was he supposed to tell me?'

'Courage is not the good doctor's greatest virtue.'

'What was he afraid of?'

'It's a miracle you survived childbirth this time.'

A shadow passed over Nefertari's face. 'You're telling me I can't have any more children, aren't you? I'll never give you a son.'

249

'Kha and Meritamon are the legitimate heirs to the throne.'

'Ramses should have more children and more sons. If you want me to step aside, to join a religious order . . .'

The King clasped his wife to him. 'I love you, Nefertari. You're the light of my life. You are Queen of Egypt. Our souls are joined for eternity. Nothing and no one can come between us.'

'Iset will bear you sons.'

'Nefertari . . .'

'It's necessary, Ramses. You're no ordinary man, you're Pharaoh.'

As soon as they arrived in Thebes, the royal couple proceeded to the site where Ramses was to raise his Temple of a Million Years. The location had grandeur and pulsed with the energy that flowed from the looming Peak of the West and the fertile Theban plain.

'I shouldn't have neglected this project for the benefit of Pi-Ramses,' the king admitted. 'My mother's warning and the threat of black magic opened my eyes. Only a Temple of a Million Years can shield us from the forces of darkness.'

Noble and resplendent, Nefertari paced the vast stretch of rock and sand, which looked doomed to barrenness. Like Ramses, she was a child of the sun, her skin never burning, only glowing from its touch. Time froze. She was the founding goddess. Each place her feet touched became holy ground.

The Great Royal Wife sprang from eternity, and she etched it into this sun-baked land, which was already marked with Ramses' seal.

The two men collided on the gangway to the pharaoh's ship and stopped dead, face to face. Setau was shorter than Serramanna but just as broad of shoulder. Their eyes locked.

'I was hoping not to find you anywhere near the king, Setau.'

'I'm not sorry to disappoint you.'

'There's talk of black magic nearly killing the queen and her baby.'

'Still no idea who was behind it? Some security Ramses has here.'

'Do you want me to shut your mouth?' the Sard growled.

'You're welcome to try. But watch out for my snakes.'

'Is that a threat?'

'Take it any way you want. To me, a pirate is a pirate, no matter how you dress him up.'

'It would save me a lot of time if you'd just confess.'

'For someone in your position, you're not very well informed. Haven't you heard that I saved the princess' life?'

'To cover your tracks. You're a sly bastard, Setau.'

'You've got a warped mind.'

'Make the slightest move in the king's direction and I'll crush you skull.'

'You talk big, Serramanna.'

'Try me.'

'An unprovoked attack on a friend of the king's would land you in jail.'

'That's where you'll end up.'

'You'll beat me to it, Sard. Now get out of my way.'

'Where are you going?'

'To meet Ramses and, at his request, drive the snakes away from his future temple.'

'I'm watching you, sorcerer.'

Setau shoved past Serramanna. 'Stop spouting foolishness and get back to guarding the king.'

Ramses spent several hours at the Temple of Gurnah, on the west bank of Thebes, meditating in the shrine dedicated to his father's perpetual memory. He had brought an offering of grapes, figs, juniper berries and pine cones. Here Seti's soul could rest in peace, nourished by the subtle essences of the offerings.

It was here that Seti had first announced that Ramses would be his successor. At the time, the young prince had not understood the full import of his father's words. He moved in a dream, safe in his father's giant shadow, lost in admiration of a mind that moved like the divine barque through the celestial reaches.

When the Red Crown and the White Crown had been placed on his head, Ramses had left behind for ever the peaceful life of the heir to the throne, and had been thrust into a world whose harshness he had never suspected. On these temple walls, grave and smiling gods sanctified life. Within these walls, a pharaoh's eternal spirit honoured the gods and communed with the Invisible. On the outside were men. Humanity – courageous and craven, upright and hypocritical, generous and greedy. And caught in the middle of these opposing forces was Ramses, entrusted with maintaining the link between gods and men, no matter what his own desires and failings might be.

He had reigned for only a year, but he had long since ceased to live for himself.

When Ramses climbed into the chariot with Serramanna at the reins, the sun was low in the sky.

'Where to, Majesty?'

'The Valley of the Kings.'

'I had every boat in the fleet searched.'

'Anything suspicious?'

'Nothing.' The Sard was edgy.

'Is that really all you have to report, Serramanna?'

'It is, Majesty.'

'Are you sure?'

'To accuse someone without evidence is a serious offence.'

'Do you think you've identified the sorcerer?'

'What I think isn't important. Only facts count.'

'Let's get moving, then.'

The horses galloped towards the Valley, the entrance to which was guarded night and day. In the late summer afternoon, the rocky walls radiated heat absorbed during the day. It was stifling.

Dripping sweat and red with effort, the ranking officer of the guard detachment bowed to the pharaoh and assured him that no robbers would find their way into Seti's tomb.

Ramses directed the chariot not towards his father's final resting place, but to his own. Their working day finished, the stone-carvers were cleaning their tools and arranging them in their baskets. At the unexpected sight of the sovereign, a hush fell. The workmen huddled together behind their foreman, who was finishing his daily report.

'We've finished the corridor into the Chamber of Ma'at. May I show you, Majesty?'

'I'll go alone.'

Ramses went through the entrance to his tomb and descended a short flight of stairs carved into the rock, symbolizing the sun's nightly descent into the darkness. The walls of the corridor below were carved with vertical columns of hieroglyphs, prayers that a pharaoh, depicted as youthful for all eternity, was addressing to the power of light, whose secret names he was reciting. Next came the hours of darkness, the ordeal of the hidden chamber which the old sun must undergo before it could be reborn with the morning.

Passing through this realm of darkness, Ramses next encountered his likeness worshipping the gods, alive in the next world as they were on earth. Skilfully drawn, brightly painted, these images preserved the king's spirit through all eternity.

On the right was the chariot chamber with its four pillars. The shaft, bodywork, wheels and other parts of Ramses' ritual chariot would be stored here, that it might be reassembled in the other world and enable him to travel about as he did battle with the forces of darkness.

From here, the passage narrowed. The walls were decorated with scenes and texts relating to the ritual opening of the mouth and the eyes, carried out on the statue of the risen, transfigured king.

Then all was rock, rough-hewn by the stone-carvers' chisels. It would take them several more months to finish the Hall of Ma'at and the House of Gold where the sarcophagus would be laid to rest.

Ramses' death rose up before him, calm and mysterious. No word would be missing from the ritual texts, no scene from the tableau of the afterlife. The young king felt himself move beyond his earthly body, into a world whose laws were beyond any human understanding.

When the pharaoh emerged from his tomb, a peaceful night had fallen on the Valley of his ancestors.

45

The Second Prophet of Amon, Doki, hurried from the Temple of Amon to the royal palace. The king was here in Thebes and had summoned Karnak's highest officials. Stunted, with a shaven head, narrow face, pointed nose and jutting chin, Doki looked like a crocodile. He rushed on, cursing his idiot of a secretary. Knee-deep in livestock tallies, the fool had neglected to pass on the pharaoh's message. He'd be sent to a farm, far from the comfort of the temple offices.

Serramanna searched Doki and showed him to the pharaoh's audience chamber. Across from him, in a chair with arm-rests, sat old Nebu, the High Priest and First Prophet of Amon. Wizened and slouching, his bad leg propped on a cushion, Nebu sniffed a bottle of flower essences.

'Please forgive me, Majesty,' panted Doki. 'I'm only late because—'

'Don't fret, Doki. Where's the Third Prophet?'

'He's in charge of the rites of purification at the House of Life and wishes to remain in seclusion.'

'Very well. What about Bakhen, the Fourth Prophet?'

'He's at the Luxor worksite.'

'Surely he could take the afternoon off !'

'They're raising the obelisks, a delicate operation, I understand. If you want me to send to Luxor—'

'No matter. The High Priest is in satisfactory health, I hope?'

'No,' replied Nebu wearily. 'I can barely get around. Most of my time is spent in the archives. My predecessor didn't pay much attention to older rituals, and I hope to revive them.'

'And you, Doki? More concerned with affairs of this world?'

'Someone has to be! Bakhen and I run the temple and its estates – under the guidance of our revered leader, of course.'

'I may be lame, but there's nothing wrong with my eyesight,' barked Nebu. 'My young subordinates have come to understand that. The mission the king has given me will be carried out to the last detail. I'll tolerate no carelessness or laziness.'

The firmness in his voice startled Ramses. Weary as he might seem, Nebu was clearly in firm control.

'We rejoice in your visit, Majesty. It shows that the creation of your new capital doesn't mean you're abandoning Thebes.'

'That was never my intention, Nebu. What pharaoh worthy of the role would turn his back on the city of Amon, god of victories?'

'Then why stay away so long?' he asked, almost accusingly.

'It's not the High Priest of Amon's place to question government policy.'

'I agree completely, Majesty, but it *is* his place, I believe, to concern himself with the future of his temple.'

'Put your mind at ease, Nebu. The Hall of Pillars at Karnak has the biggest and most beautiful colonnade ever built, has it not?'

'And I give thanks to Your Majesty for it; but would you permit an old and unworldly man to inquire as to the true reason for your visit?'

Ramses smiled. 'Which of us is more impatient, Nebu?'

'You feel the fire of youth, I hear the call of heaven. I can't waste what little time I have left in idle chatter.'

The clash left Doki speechless. If Nebu continued to challenge the king like this, Ramses was bound to lose his temper.

'The royal family is in danger,' explained Ramses. 'I've come in search of stronger magic to protect us.'

'Why Thebes?' asked the High Priest.

'Because this is where I'll build my Temple of a Million Years.'

Nebu gripped his cane. 'Excellent. But first I suggest you increase your *ka*, the special power with which you are endowed.'

'How is that?'

'By finishing work on the temple at Luxor, where your *ka* is paramount.'

'Pleading the cause of your own temple, Nebu?'

'Under different circumstances, I might have done so, but not after what you've just told us. Luxor is Karnak's direct connection to divine power and might – the power you need in order to reign.'

'I'll make note of your advice, High Priest. For now, prepare to officiate at the ground-breaking of my Temple of a Million Years on the west bank of Thebes.'

To ease his feverish excitement, Doki downed several cups of strong beer. His hands shook and cold sweat ran down his back. He'd suffered so much injustice, but his luck was finally changing!

He was only Second Prophet of Amon, condemned to grow old in this subordinate position, yet he had just been entrusted with a state secret of the highest importance. Ramses had made a serious error of judgment, and if Doki played his cards right he might become High Priest after all.

The Temple of a Million Years – an unexpected opportunity, the solution he thought he'd never find. But he had to calm himself, move slowly and cautiously, not waste

257

one precious second, know what to say and when to say nothing.

His position at Karnak would allow him to steal goods which he could then turn into money. It was simply a matter of removing a line here and there from the inventories. Since he was in charge of the scribes who kept the records, the risk was negligible.

Perhaps he was being too optimistic. Was he really capable of embezzlement on such a scale? The High Priest and the pharaoh were no fools. One unwise move and he'd be done for. Still, it was the chance of a lifetime. A pharaoh built only one Temple of a Million Years.

From Karnak to Luxor it was half an hour's walk down an avenue of sphinxes. Consulting the archives of the House of Life, where all the secrets of heaven and earth were stored, and reading the books of Thoth, Bakhen had drawn up a plan to enlarge Luxor according to Ramses' wishes. Thanks to Nebu's support, the work had proceeded at a rapid pace. A spacious courtyard adorned with statues of Ramses would be added on to the original temple of Amenhotep III. In front of the elegant pylon gateway, six colossal statues of the new pharaoh would guard the entry to this temple of *ka*, while two towering obelisks rose towards the heavens, warding off evil forces.

The richly coloured sandstone, of matchless beauty, the walls covered with electrum, the silver flooring, would combine to make Luxor the finest achievement of Ramses' reign. The poles with their banners affirming the presence of the gods would reach to the stars.

But the strange events of the last hour had plunged Bakhen into despair. An oversized barge hauling the first obelisk from the Aswan quarries was whirling madly in the middle of the Nile, trapped in an uncharted whirlpool. The captain, busy taking soundings from the bow to check for sandbanks, had seen the danger too late. Panic-stricken, the helmsman had lost his grip and fallen into the water. At that moment, one of the rudders broke. The other jammed and was useless.

The barge's chaotic movements had unbalanced the cargo. The shifting obelisk – two hundred tons of solid pink granite – had already snapped several of the ropes that secured it. Soon the rest would give way and the monolith would be flung into the river.

Bakhen clenched his fists and wept.

The accident would be the end of his career. He would and should be held responsible for the wreck, the loss of the obelisk, the deaths of several men. In his haste to see Luxor finished, he, Bakhen, had ordered the barge to sail north before the inundation, ignoring the danger to the crew. What had made him think he could defy the laws of nature?

The Fourth Prophet of Amon would gladly have given his life to undo this disaster. But the boat spun faster and faster, and ominous creakings showed that the hull could not last much longer. The obelisk was a work of art, complete except for the gilding on the pyramidion, to make it glitter in the sunlight. Now its splendour would vanish at the bottom of the river.

On the far shore, a man was gesticulating – a bewhiskered giant with sword and helmet. His shouts were lost in the whipping wind.

He was yelling at a swimmer, Bakhen realized, begging him to turn back. Instead, the man's rapid strokes brought him closer and closer to the spinning barge. At the risk of drowning in the current or being hit by an oar, the swimmer managed to reach the prow and pull himself along the hull, using a dangling rope.

Then he gripped the jammed rudder, struggling with both hands to free it. With a superhuman effort, braced against his heels, the muscles of his arms and chest popping, he dislodged the huge block of wood.

The boat righted itself and was still for a few seconds, parallel to the shore. Taking advantage of a favourable gust of wind, the helmsman steered it out of the whirlpool. Soon the oarsmen were able to help.

The moment the barge reached the shore dozens of stone-carvers and labourers ran up to unload the giant pillar.

The daring swimmer appeared at the top of the gangway, and Bakhen knew him at once. Ramses, King of Egypt, had risked his life to save the obelisk which would reach to heaven.

46

On six meals a day, Shaanar was getting fatter by the day. Whenever he lost all hope of winning the throne and finally taking revenge on Ramses, he ate. Food made him feel better, helped him forget about his brother's burgeoning new capital and flagrant popularity. Even Ahsha failed to raise his spirits, convincing as his arguments seemed. Power would take its toll on Ramses, he argued; the popularity of the first months of his reign would unravel, and his path would be strewn with obstacles . . . Yet Ahsha had nothing concrete to back up his claims. The Hittites were inactive, daunted by what they'd heard of the young monarch's miracles.

In short, things were going from bad to worse.

Shaanar was gnawing on a plump goose drumstick when his steward announced Meba, the former minister for Foreign Affairs.

'I don't want to see him.'

'He's insisting.'

'Send him away.'

'He claims he has important information concerning you.'

The former minister was not one to exaggerate; his entire career had been built on proceeding with caution.

'All right, then.'

Meba was the same as ever: a broad, reassuring face, a

self-important manner, a droning voice. A high government official who had felt he was set for life and could never understand the real reasons for his dismissal.

'Thank you for seeing me, Shaanar.'

'Always a pleasure, old friend. May I offer you anything to eat or drink?'

'Water would do very nicely.'

'Have you given up wine and beer?'

'Since I lost my job, I've suffered from dreadful head-aches.'

'I'm so sorry to have benefited from this injustice to you. Perhaps in time I can find a place for you.'

'Ramses isn't the type to go back on his decisions. And look how far he's come in one short year!'

Shaanar bit into a goose wing.

'I was quite resigned,' the former diplomat admitted, 'until your sister, Dolora, introduced me to a most uncanny man.'

'Do I know him?'

'A Libyan named Ofir.'

'Never heard of the fellow.'

'He's in hiding.'

'Why is that?'

'Because he's protecting a girl by the name of Lita.'

'What sort of squalid story is this?'

'According to Ofir, Lita is a descendant of Akhenaton.'

'But all his descendants are dead!'

'And what if this claim is true?'

'Ramses would banish her on the spot.'

'Your sister has fallen in with them and other believers in Aton, the One God, who will expel all others. In Thebes there is quite an extensive membership.'

'I hope you're not joining! No good can come of this foolishness. Ramses belongs to the dynasty that put an end to Akhenaton's experiment.'

'I'm well aware of that and simply meeting Ofir made me nervous. But on reflection, I think he could be a valuable ally against Ramses.'

'A Libyan who lives in hiding?'

'Ofir has a certain advantage: he's a sorcerer.'

'There are hundreds in Egypt.'

'How many of them could endanger the lives of Nefertari and her baby daughter?'

'Whatever do you mean?'

'Dolora is convinced that Ofir is a wise man and that Lita is destined to be queen. Since she is relying on me to unite the followers of Aton, she tells me everything. Ofir is a master of black magic, determined to break through the royal couple's magical defences.'

'Are you quite certain?'

'Once you've seen him, you'll believe it. But that's not all, Shaanar. Have you given any thought to Moses?'

'No. Why Moses?'

'Akhenaton's beliefs are not that different from those of the Hebrews. I've heard rumours that the pharaoh's oldest friend is tormented by the idea of a single god, and that he's disenchanted with our civilization.'

Shaanar studied Meba attentively. 'What are you getting at?'

'I think you should encourage Ofir to practise his magic, and introduce him to Moses.'

'This girl, Akhenaton's heir, bothers me.'

'Me too, but never mind,' Meba countered. 'Let's convince Ofir that we believe in Aton and back his Lita. Once the sorcerer has undermined Ramses' health and recruited Moses, we'll get rid of the Libyan and his princess.'

'An interesting plan, old friend.'

'I'm counting on you to improve it.'

'What's in this for you?'

'I want my job back. Foreign Affairs was my life. I miss receiving ambassadors, hosting state banquets, holding secret talks with foreign dignitaries, nurturing relationships, setting traps, juggling protocol . . . It's hard to understand unless you've been part of it. When you become king, appoint me to my old position.'

'Your suggestions all deserve serious attention, Meba.'

The old diplomat beamed. 'If it's not too much trouble, I might take some of that wine you offered me. My headache is gone.'

Bakhen, the Fourth Prophet of Amon, prostrated himself before his pharaoh.

'I have no excuse to offer, Majesty. I take complete responsibility for this catastrophe.'

'What catastrophe?'

'The obelisk could have sunk, we almost lost the crew.'

'Your nightmares are foolish, Bakhen. Only reality counts.'

'That doesn't excuse my carelessness.'

'It's not like you, I agree. What were you thinking?'

'I wanted Luxor to be the jewel of your reign.'

'Did you think I'd settle for only one jewel? Rise, Bakhen.'

The former soldier was burly as ever. He looked more like an athlete than a holy man.

'You were fortunate, Bakhen, and I like the men around me to be lucky. There's magic in knowing how to stay out of harm's way.'

'If you hadn't been there . . .'

'You were even able to make Pharaoh appear! Nice trick – in fact, it's one for the royal annals.'

Bakhen was afraid some terrible punishment would be pronounced after these ironic remarks. Instead, Ramses turned his piercing gaze towards the barge. The gigantic pillar was being unloaded without further incident.

264

'It really is a splendid obelisk. When will the other one be ready?'

'By the end of September, I hope.'

'The hieroglyph-carvers had better get busy!'

'Aswan is hotter than here, and in the quarries—'

'Excuses, excuses! Go to Aswan yourself and see that the work's done on schedule. And what about the colossal statues?'

'The sculptors have found the perfect sandstone at Gebel el-Silsila.'

'Get them moving, too. Send someone today to make sure they're not wasting a minute. Why isn't the courtyard finished?'

'We're going as fast as we can, Majesty!'

'Wrong, Bakhen. When you're building a home for the pharaoh's *ka*, a resting-place for the force that continuously creates the universe, you can't behave like a humble foreman, quibbling over technique, unsure of your materials. Your mind has to meet the stone like a bolt of lightning for the temple to rise from the ground. You've been slow and lazy: that's your real mistake.'

Astonished, Bakhen was unable to protest.

'When Luxor is finished, my *ka* will prosper. I need its energy as soon as possible. Find more workmen – the best available.'

'Some of them were assigned to your House of Eternity in the Valley of the Kings.'

'Bring them back here. My tomb can wait. And there's another urgent matter for you to see to: the building of my Temple of a Million Years on the west bank. Its existence will guard the kingdom against many evils.'

'You're planning—'

'A colossal complex, a temple so powerful that its magic will repel adversity. We'll start on it tomorrow.'

'But there's Luxor, Majesty.'

'There's also Pi-Ramses, an entire new city. Call forth the sculptors from every province and weed out all but the best.'

'Majesty, there are only so many hours in a day!'

'Make time, Bakhen.'

47

Doki met the sculptor in a tavern in Thebes where neither of them was known. They sat in the darkest corner, near a noisy bunch of Libyan labourers.

'I got your message and here I am,' said the sculptor. 'Why all the mystery?'

Wearing a wig that came low on his forehead and covered his ears, Doki was unrecognizable.

'Have you mentioned this meeting to anyone?'

'No.'

'Not even your wife?'

'I'm single.'

'Your girlfriend, then?'

'I shan't see her until tomorrow night.'

'Give me back my letter.'

The sculptor handed the papyrus scroll to Doki, who tore it to shreds.

'In case we can't reach an agreement,' he explained, 'there should be no evidence that we were ever in contact.'

The sculptor, a broad-backed and forthright fellow, took a dim view of this.

'I've worked for Karnak before with no complaints, but no one ever made me sneak into a tavern and listen to mumbo-jumbo.'

'I'll get to the point, then. Would you like to be rich?'

267

'Who wouldn't?'

'I can offer you a quick way to make a fortune, but it does involve risk.'

'What kind of risk?'

'Before I tell you, we have to agree on something.'

'What is it?'

'If you turn me down, you get out of town for good.'

'And if I don't?'

'Perhaps we should leave it at that,' said Doki, rising.

'All right, I agree. Don't go.'

'Do you swear on the pharaoh's life and in the presence of the goddess of silence who strikes down oath-breakers?'

'I do.'

Giving one's word was a magic act, which, committed one's entire being. Breaking it caused a person's *ka* to flee, weakening the spirit.

'All I'm asking is for you to carve hieroglyphs on a stele,' Doki said.

'That's what I do for a living! Why all the mystery?'

'You'll see when the time comes.'

'About the payment . . .'

'Thirty dairy cows, a hundred sheep, ten fattened steers, a light boat, twenty pairs of sandals, furniture and a horse.'

The sculptor was stunned. 'All that for a simple stele?'

'Yes.'

'Only a fool would say no. You're on!' The two men shook hands. 'When do I start?'

'Tomorrow at dawn, on the west bank.'

Meba had invited Shaanar to a country villa belonging to one of his former staff. The two men arrived by different routes, two hours apart. Shaanar had thought it best not to inform Ahsha of the meeting.

'Your sorcerer is late,' complained Shaanar.

'He promised he'd be here.'

268

'I'm not used to waiting. If he doesn't show up soon . . .'

Ofir made his entrance, accompanied by Lita.

Shaanar's irritation vanished. He stared in fascination at this disturbing stranger. Gaunt, with high cheekbones, a hooked nose, and thin lips, the Libyan was like a vulture about to devour its prey. The girl had a blank, hangdog look about her.

'You do us great honour,' declared Ofir in a deep voice that sent a chill down Shaanar's spine. 'We hardly dared to hope for such a favour.'

'My friend Meba told me about you.'

'Aton will be grateful to him.'

'That's a name I wish you wouldn't mention.'

'I've devoted my life to pursuing Lita's claim to the throne. The fact that you're willing to meet me must mean that you agree with what I'm doing.'

'Quite right, Ofir, but aren't you ignoring one major obstacle – Ramses himself ?'

'On the contrary. The pharaoh is endowed with exceptional calibre and breadth of vision, a formidable adversary. Breaching his defences will be difficult. However, I have a few secret weapons.'

'If you're caught practising black magic, you face the death penalty.'

'Ramses and his dynasty have tried to wipe out the memory of Akhenaton. The fight between him and me will be to the finish.'

'Then it's no use preaching moderation.'

'No,' Ofir said firmly.

'I know my brother well. He's a stubborn, violent man, who will not tolerate any challenge to his authority. If he finds followers of the One God standing in his way, he'll crush them.'

'That's why we need to attack him from behind.'

'A good plan, but hard to execute.'

'My magic will eat away at him like acid.'

'What if we had an ally in his inner circle.'

The sorcerer's eyes narrowed to inscrutable slits, like a cat's.

Yes, thought Shaanar. I've hooked him.

'Who is it?'

'Moses. A boyhood friend of Ramses, a Hebrew he put in charge of building Pi-Ramses. If you can persuade him to help you, I'll join you, too.'

For the commanding general at the southern outpost of Elephantine, it was a good life. Since the raid that Seti had led a few years earlier, the Nubian provinces under Egyptian control were quiet as well as profitable.

The southern frontier of the Two Lands was well guarded. For decades, no Nubian tribe had dreamed of attacking or even protesting against the line of fortifications. Nubia belonged to Egypt for good. Tribal chieftains sent their sons north to be educated, and they returned as loyal subjects of the pharaoh, under the guidance of the Viceroy of Nubia, who was appointed by the king. Although the thought of living abroad was painful to Egyptians, the post was highly sought-after because of the considerable privileges attached to it.

Still, the general wouldn't want to trade places. Elephantine was tranquil, the climate was wonderful and, besides, he'd been born here. The garrison trained at dawn, then reported to the quarry, overseeing the docks where granite was loaded on to northbound barges. His fighting days were far behind him – the farther the better.

Since his appointment, the general had become a customs official. His men inspected shipments from the Far South and levied taxes on a sliding scale worked out by the Finance secretariat. His headquarters were cluttered with government documents, but he'd rather fight documents than a formidable band of Nubian warriors.

In a little while he'd take a fast boat down the Nile to check the fortifications from the river. He always enjoyed the soft breeze and feasting his eyes on the beauty of the lush banks and scenic cliffs. Smiling, he thought ahead to his dinner engagement with the young widow he was tenderly consoling.

A strange sound startled him: footsteps, running.

'Urgent message, sir,' panted his orderly.

'Where is it from?'

'Desert patrol in Nubia, sir.'

'The gold mines?'

'Yes, sir.'

'What did the courier say?'

'That it's very serious.'

In other words, the scroll couldn't be tossed into a chest and forgotten. He broke the seal, unrolled it and skimmed it with growing alarm.

'It's a fake. A joke!'

'No, sir. You can talk to the messenger.'

'Attack,' he read, incredulously. 'Nubian rebels have attacked a convoy carrying gold to Egypt!'

48

The new moon had just risen.

Bare-chested, Ramses wore a wig and kilt in the style of those worn by the pharaohs of the Old Kingdom. The queen was dressed in a long, close-fitting white dress. In place of a crown, she wore the seven-pointed star of the goddess Sechat, whom she represented in the evening's ritual. The cornerstone of the pharaoh's Temple of a Million Years, was being laid.

Ramses thought of the time he had spent in the quarries of Gebel el-Silsila, working with mallet and chisel alongside the stone-cutters. He had wanted to stay there, but his father had woken him from that dream.

Twenty ritualists from the temple of Karnak assisted the royal couple, with three of the Four Prophets presiding: Nebu, Doki and Bakhen. The next day two architects would descend on the site with their work gangs.

The complex would be vast – twelve acres, Ramses had decreed. Room for the temple itself, as well as numerous annexes, including a library, storerooms and a garden. This holy city, economically self-sufficient, would be dedicated to the supernatural power present within the pharaoh.

Stunned by the scope of the project, Bakhen refused to dwell on what lay ahead, focusing his attention on the rites performed by the king and queen. After marking the symbolic corners of the future temple, they pounded in stakes and stretched a cord around them, invoking the memory of Imhotep, father of architecture, builder of the first pyramid and exemplar of architects.

Then Pharaoh dug a section of the foundation with a hoe and laid down small bars of gold and silver, amulets and miniature tools, which he covered with sand. With a sure hand, he laid the first cornerstone with a lever, then moulded a brick. His act of creation would make the temple, its floors, walls and ceilings rise fast. Next came the ritual purification: Ramses walked round the temple site scattering incense, whose hieroglyphic name, *sonter,* meant 'That Which Makes Divine'.

Bakhen held up a wooden model of the monumental entrance. In blessing it, the king opened the mouth of his Temple of a Million Years, bringing it to life. Henceforth the Word was in it. Ramses struck the door twelve times with the white club called 'She Who Illuminates', summoning the gods. He lit a lamp, showing the way to the inner sanctuary where the Invisible would reside.

He concluded with the ancient words affirming that this temple was built not for him but for his true master, the Rule – the beginning and end of every temple in Egypt.

Bakhen had the sensation that he was witnessing a miracle. What had happened here, before the eyes of a privileged few, was beyond human understanding. In this empty space, which already belonged to the gods, the power of Ramses' *ka* was beginning to manifest itself.

'The foundation stele is ready,' declared Doki.

'Let it be embedded,' ordered the king.

The sculptor Doki had hired appeared with a small stone tablet covered with hieroglyphs. The text consecrated for ever the site of the temple. The magical symbols transformed the earth into heaven.

Setau came forward, holding a blank papyrus and a flask

of fresh ink. Doki jumped. This rough-looking character had been given no role in the ceremony!

Setau wrote on the papyrus, in horizontal lines from right to left, then read his text aloud.

'May any living mouth be sealed which would speak ill of the pharaoh or so intend, either night or day. May this Temple of a Million Years be the magical haven protecting the royal person and shielding him from evil.'

Doki was sweating profusely. No one had mentioned this magical incantation. Fortunately, it would not affect the working-out of his plan.

Setau rolled up the papyrus and presented the scroll to Ramses. The king affixed his seal to it and placed it at the foot of the stele, where it would be buried. By letting his gaze rest on the hieroglyphs, the king would bring them into existence.

He whirled round. 'Who carved these hieroglyphs?'

The sculptor stepped forward. 'I did, Majesty.'

'Who gave you the text to inscribe on the tablet?'

'The High Priest of Amon himself, Majesty.'

The man prostrated himself, partly out of respect and partly to avoid Ramses' rising fury. The traditional inscription for the foundation of a Temple of a Million Years had been modified and distorted, destroying its protective powers.

Nebu! The High Priest must be in league with the forces of darkness. He'd sold out to Ramses' enemies. The pharaoh felt like smashing the old man's head with the ceremonial mallet. But then a strange force seemed to emanate from the newly consecrated ground, a wave of soothing warmth rising up his spine, the 'tree of life'. A door opened within his heart. Violence was not the answer. Out of the corner of his eye, he saw Nebu make a gesture that confirmed his opinion.

'Rise, sculptor.'

The man obeyed.

'Now go to the High Priest and bring him to me.'

Doki gloated. His plan was working perfectly. The old man's protests would be ineffectual, the punishment merciless, and the office of High Priest vacant. This time, the king would call on a man who knew how to run Karnak. He, Doki, was that man.

The sculptor was well rehearsed. He stopped in front of an old man who held a gilded staff in his right hand and wore a golden ring on his middle finger, the two symbols associated with the High Priest of Amon.

'You're sure that's the man who gave you the text for the stele?'

'I am.'

'Then you're a liar.'

'No, Majesty! I swear it was the High Priest in person who —'

'Sculptor, you've never laid eyes on him.'

Nebu retrieved his cane and staff from the elderly ritualist to whom he had handed them when the sculptor, who had turned away from him, began to make his accusation.

Frantic, the sculptor began to cry out, 'Doki! Where are you, Doki? Help me! It wasn't my idea! You were the one who told me to say the High Priest of Amon wanted to destroy the temple's magic!'

Doki made a run for it.

The sculptor went after him, blind with rage, fists flying.

Doki succumbed to his injuries. The sculptor, accused of a crime of blood, debasing hieroglyphs, bribe-taking and perjury, would appear before the vizier's tribunal and be sentenced either to death by suicide or else to forced labour in a remote desert prison.

The day after the incident, at sunset, Ramses embedded the correctly reworded commemorative stele with his own hands.

The foundation was complete. The Temple of a Million Years was born.

'Did you suspect Doki?' Ramses asked Nebu.

'It's human nature,' replied the High Priest. 'Satisfaction with one's lot in life is the exception, unfortunately, not the rule. As the sages so aptly put it, envy is a fatal disease, which no physician can cure.'

'We'll have to find another Second Prophet.'

'Are you thinking of Bakhen, Majesty?'

'Of course.'

'I won't oppose your decision, but I'm not sure it's time yet. You've put Bakhen in charge of both the renovations at Luxor and the construction of your Temple of a Million Years, and that was wise of you. He's worthy of your trust in him. But don't overburden him, don't pull him in too many directions at once. When the time is right, he can move up through the hierarchy.'

'What do you suggest?'

'Replace Doki with an old man like me, preoccupied with meditation and priestly duties. That way the Temple of Amon at Karnak will no longer be a source of worry for you.'

'Good idea. You can choose him yourself. Have you taken a look at the plans for the temple?'

'My life has been a long and happy one, with only one regret: that I won't live long enough to see your temple finished.'

'Who knows, Nebu?'

'My bones ache, Majesty, my eyes are growing dim, I'm hard of hearing and I have trouble staying awake these days. The end is near – I can feel it.'

'I thought sages lived to be a hundred and ten.'

'I've been blessed in my life. I don't mind if death wants to take me and share my good fortune with others.'

'You see pretty clearly, I'd say. If you hadn't handed

your staff and your ring to the ritualist, what would have happened?'

'Needless to speculate, Majesty. The Rule of Ma'at protected us.'

Ramses looked out over the expanse where his Temple of a Million Years would be built.

'I see a magnificent building, Nebu, a temple of granite, sandstone and basalt. The pylons will reach to the sky. The doors will be gilded bronze. Trees will shade pools of pure water. The granaries will be full of wheat, the treasury full of gold and silver, precious stones and rare vases. Living statues will fill the courtyards and shrines. A rampart will protect all these wonders. At sunrise and sunset, the two of us will go up to the roof terrace and survey this slice of eternity. Three spirits will live for ever in this temple: my father's, my mother's and my wife Nefertari's.'

'You're forgetting the fourth one, which should be the first: yourself, Ramses.'

The Great Royal Wife approached the king, carrying an acacia seedling.

Ramses knelt and planted the seedling, and Nefertari watered it carefully.

'Take care of this tree for us, Nebu. It will grow with my temple. Let us pray that the gods let me come to rest one day in its kindly shade, forgetting the world of men. That the Lady of the West will show herself in its leafy branches, then bend down and take me by the hand.'

49

Moses stretched out on his sycamore bed.

It had been an exhausting day. Fifty minor incidents, two slight injuries at the palace worksite, rations delivered late to the third barracks site, a thousand reject bricks to destroy. Nothing out of the ordinary, just an accumulation of headaches that slowly wore him down.

The old questions began to plague him. Building this new capital was a joy, but wasn't raising temples to several different divinities, including the evil Set, an offence to the One God? His work on Pi-Ramses meant contributing to the greater glory of a pharaoh who was perpetuating the old ways.

In a corner of the room, near the window, someone moved.

'Who's there?'

'A friend.'

A gaunt figure with a hawklike face stepped out of the shadows and moved through the flickering lamplight.

'Ofir!'

'I need to talk to you.'

Moses sat up. 'I'm tired and I want to sleep. Come and see me on the site tomorrow. I'll try to find time for you.'

'I'm in danger, my friend.

'Why?'

'You know why! Because I believe in the One God, the saviour of humanity. The god your people worship in secret, the god who will one day reign supreme, destroying false idols. And his conquest must begin with Egypt.'

'Are you forgetting that Ramses is the pharaoh?'

'Ramses is a tyrant, obsessed with his own power. He cares nothing for religion.'

'You'd better not discount his power. Ramses is my friend, and I'm building his capital.'

'I respect your loyalty, but you're being torn in two, Moses, and you know it. In your heart, you reject this pharaoh's supremacy and long for the rule of the One True God.'

'You're raving, Ofir.'

The Libyan stared hard into his eyes. 'Be honest, Moses. Stop lying to yourself.'

'Do you think you know me better than I know myself ?'

'Why not? We reject the same errors and share the same ideal. If we join forces, we can transform this country and the future of its inhabitants. Like it or not, Moses, you've become the leader of the Hebrews. With you in charge, the faction fighting has ceased. Without you realizing it, they've become a people.'

'The Hebrews are subject to Pharaoh's authority, not mine.'

'That tyranny! I reject it, and so do you.'

'You're wrong. I know my place.'

'Your place is at the head of your people, guiding them towards the truth. Mine is to place Lita, the legitimate heir of Akhenaton, on the throne and reinstate the supremacy of the One True God.'

'Stop your ranting, Ofir. Inciting a revolt against Pharaoh will only lead to disaster.'

'Do you know of any other means to our end? Or don't you think the truth is worth fighting for?'

279

'You and Lita . . . Two lunatics! It's laughable.'

'It's not just the two of us any more.'

Moses raised an eyebrow. 'No?'

'Since the last time we met,' Ofir informed him, 'the situation has changed considerably. The movement is larger and far more determined than you imagine. Ramses' power is nothing but an illusion, which will lead him into a trap of his own making. A good part of the country's elite will follow us once you blaze the trail, Moses.'

'But why me?'

'Because you have the ability to guide us, and to become leader of the movement when the time is ripe. Lita must remain in the background until it's time for her to take the throne. I'm the keeper of the flame, not a man of influence. We need your voice to make our ideas heard.'

'Who are you really, Ofir?'

'A simple believer, like Akhenaton, convinced that the One God will rule all nations, once proud Egypt bends to his will.'

Moses knew he should have shown this madman the door long since, but . . . What he said was compelling. Ofir gave voice to Moses' own repressed and highly subversive thoughts.

'Your plan is crazy. You have no chance of succeeding.'

'Time is on our side,' Ofir reassured him. 'Take charge of the Hebrews, give them a country, let them acknowledge the supreme being. Lita will govern Egypt and we'll be your ally. Our alliance will foster the truth that will sweep the world.'

'It's only a dream.'

'I'm no dreamer, and neither are you.'

'Ramses is my friend, I tell you, and he rules with an iron fist.'

'No, Moses, he's not your friend but your worst enemy – the man who wants to snuff out the truth.'

280

'Get out, Ofir.'

'Think over what I've said and prepare for action. We'll meet again soon.'

'Don't count on it.'

'I'll be seeing you, Moses.'

The Hebrew spent a sleepless night. Ofir's words swept through his mind like a wave, washing away all his fears and objections.

Whether or not he was ready to admit it, this meeting was what he'd been waiting for.

Side by side, the pharaoh's dog and pet lion were licking chicken carcasses clean as Ramses and Nefertari sat entwined beneath a palm tree, admiring the scenery. With some difficulty, the king had persuaded Serramanna to let them leave Thebes for a day in the country, taking Invincible and Wideawake as bodyguards.

The news from Memphis was excellent. Little Meritamon was thriving on her wet-nurse's milk. Her brother Kha flourished under Nedjem's watchful eye. Iset the Fair had been delighted to learn of the princess' safe birth and sent warm congratulations to Nefertari.

The late-evening sun shone gold on Nefertari's silken skin. A flute tune drifted through the soft air. Cowherds sang as they rounded up their cattle; heavily laden donkeys lumbered homeward. In the west, the sun glowed orange, while above Thebes the Peak turned red.

The hard day gave way to the tender night. How beautiful Egypt was, resplendent in her golds and greens, the silver of the Nile and the blaze of sunset. How beautiful Nefertari was, in her sheer linen dress. An intoxicating scent wafted from her recumbent body. Her expression was grave and peaceful, a noble window on her luminous soul.

'Am I worthy of you?' asked Ramses.

'What a strange question.'

'Sometimes you seem so far from this world and its vileness, from the court and its pettiness, from all the temporal duties we have to carry out.'

'Have I failed in my duties?'

'Quite the contrary: you do everything perfectly, as if you'd been a queen all your life. I love you and admire you, Nefertari.'

Their lips met, warm and vibrant.

'I'd made up my mind not to marry,' she confessed, 'and to live secluded in a temple. It wasn't that I didn't like men, but they all seemed driven by ambition which in the end made them small and weak. But you were beyond ambition, for fate had chosen your path in life. I admire you and love you, Ramses.'

They both knew that they thought as one and that nothing would ever come between them. Conceiving the plan for the Temple of a Million Years had been their first magical act as royal couple, the source of an adventure that only death would end, and then only outwardly.

'But I'll have to keep reminding you of your duty,' she added.

'Which one?'

'To have sons.'

'I already have one.'

'You need more. If your life is long, you may outlive some of them.'

'Why couldn't our daughter succeed me?'

'According to the astrologers, her nature will have a contemplative bent, just like Kha's.'

'That might be a good attribute in a ruler.'

'Depending on circumstances. Tonight our country is perfectly serene, but what will tomorrow bring?'

The sound of a galloping horse shattered the quiet. Serramanna leaped to the ground in a cloud of dust.

'Forgive the disturbance, Majesty. Emergency dispatch.'

282

Ramses skimmed the papyrus the Sard handed him.

'A report from the commander at Elephantine,' he explained to the queen. 'Nubian rebels have attacked a convoy carrying gold for our principal temples.'

'Any dead?'

'More than twenty, and there are injured.'

'Was it just robbery or the start of an uprising?'

'No one knows yet.'

Shaken, Ramses began to pace. The lion and dog, sensing their master's mood, came and licked his hands.

The king said the words the Great Royal Wife had been dreading: 'I'll leave at once. Pharaoh must set his house in order. In my absence, Nefertari, you will govern Egypt.'

50

Pharaoh's war fleet was made up of roughly twenty boats. Their hulls were crescent-shaped, with bow and stern curving upward from the water. A large sail was rigged on the single sturdy mast. In the centre was a huge cabin for crew and troops. The smaller forward cabin housed the captain.

Aboard the flagship, Ramses had personally checked the port and starboard rudders. A covered pen had been built for his pets. The dog snuggled up between the lion's front paws; both were replete from their daily feed.

As on his previous voyage, Ramses was fascinated by the barren, green-flecked hills, the bright blue sky and the thin band of lush growth the river carved through the desert. It was a land of fire, unforgiving and yet beyond all conflict, like his soul.

Swallows, crested cranes and pink flamingoes flew over the fleet, while high in the palm trees baboons whooped at their passage. The soldiers spent their time gambling, drinking palm wine and dozing in shady corners, as if they were on a pleasure cruise.

Their arrival in the land of Kush, beyond the Second Cataract, was a rude awakening. The boats moored alongside a dreary shore, and the men disembarked in silence. After pitching their tents on the desolate shore and building a palisade, they awaited Pharaoh's orders.

A few hours later, the Viceroy of Nubia and his military escort reported to the monarch, who was seated on his travelling throne of gilded cedar.

'What have you to say for yourself ?' asked Ramses.

'We have the situation well in hand, Majesty.'

'I asked for an explanation.'

The Viceroy of Nubia had grown very stout. He mopped at his brow with a white cloth. 'A deplorable incident, to be sure, but we mustn't blow things out of proportion.'

'An entire shipment of gold lost, soldiers and miners slaughtered – doesn't that justify the presence of Pharaoh and an armed force?'

'The message that was sent to you may have been somewhat alarmist, but of course we rejoice that Your Majesty has come.'

'My father pacified Nubia and entrusted you with preserving the peace. Now your laxness and dawdling have compromised it once again.'

'It was fate, Majesty, fate!'

'You're the Viceroy of Nubia, royal standard-bearer, superintendent of the southern desert region, head of a royal cavalry division, and you dare speak to me of fate! You are presumptuous!'

'My performance has been flawless, I can assure you, Majesty. But it's too big a job for one man: meeting village mayors, making sure the granaries are stocked, checking the—'

'What about gold production?'

'Mining and shipping are under my close supervision, Majesty.'

'Is that why you let the convoy go unescorted?'

'How could I know that a handful of madmen was on the loose?'

'I thought that was part of your job.'

'Majesty, fate—'

'Take me to the scene of the attack.'

'It's on the gold route, a barren and lonely spot. It won't tell you anything.'

'Who are these rebels?'

'Some miserable tribe. They probably primed themselves with drink.'

'Have you searched for them?'

'Nubia is a very large province, Majesty, and my troop levels have been cut.'

'In other words, no serious investigation has been attempted.'

'Only Your Majesty could order a military sweep.'

'That's all, Viceroy.'

'Shall I help Your Majesty hunt down the rebels?'

'Just tell me the truth: is Nubia prepared to rise up in support of them?'

'Well, it's unlikely, but—'

'Is a rebellion already under way, then?'

'No, Majesty, but there does seem to be some unrest. That's why we were hoping you'd come to help us.'

'Drink up,' Setau told Ramses.

'Can't I get along without it?'

'Yes, but I'd rather err on the side of caution. Serramanna can't guard you from snakes.'

The king drank the dangerous brew made from nettle extracts and diluted cobra blood. Setau gave him regular doses to build up his immunity to snakebite. At least he could eliminate one risk along the gold route.

'Thanks for bringing us along. I love it here, and Lotus is glad to be home. Just imagine the specimens we'll find!'

'It's no holiday, Setau. Nubian warriors have earned their fierce reputation.'

'Why not let the poor devils have their gold, and things will quieten down?'

286

'They committed robbery and murder. No one can flout the rule of Ma'at with impunity.'

'Nothing can change your mind, I suppose.'

'No, nothing.'

'Have you considered your personal safety?'

'This mission isn't one I can delegate.'

'Tell your men to take special care. Snakes are especially venomous at this time of year. Use asafedita: the odour of the gum resin will repel some reptiles. If anyone is bitten, send for me at once. Lotus and I will be sleeping in our wagon.'

The expeditionary force marched along the rocky trail, led by a scout. Next came Serramanna and Ramses on sure-footed horses, then oxen pulling wagons, donkeys laden with weapons and water gourds, and finally the foot-soldiers.

The Nubian scout was convinced that the rebels were still close by the site of the attack. Nearby was an oasis, the perfect place to stash their booty until they attempted to trade it.

According to the map supplied by the Viceroy, the gold route was studded with wells, and reports from the Nubian mines had indicated no recent problem with the water supply. They could advance without fear through the heart of the desert.

The scout was surprised to encounter a decomposing donkey. Usually the convoy leaders selected only the healthiest animals for their long marches.

As they neared the first well, the men's spirits rose. To quench their thirst, refill their gourds, sleep in the shade of their cloth shelters . . . From the officers down, every soldier was looking forward to the same prospect. Since night would fall in three hours or less, the king would certainly make camp here.

When the scout reached the well, his blood ran cold despite the heat. He ran back to Ramses.

'Majesty! The well is dry.'

The troops did not have enough water to go back the way they had come. The only option was to march forward, in hope of making it to the next well. But since the provincial government's information had proved unreliable, the next well might be just as dry.

'We could leave the main road,' suggested the scout, 'and branch out to the right towards the rebels' oasis. Between here and there is a well they must use on their raids.'

'Rest until dusk,' ordered Ramses. 'Then we'll continue.'

'A night march is dangerous, Majesty! Snakes, the potential for ambush—'

'We have no choice.'

Ramses was reminded of an earlier expedition, with his father. Their soldiers had faced a similar situation – local insurgents had poisoned the wells. In his heart of hearts, he admitted that this time he'd underestimated the danger. He knew from experience that a simple mission to restore order could end in disaster.

The king addressed his men and told them the truth. They were worried, but the more experienced soldiers kept morale high. Pharaoh was their leader, and Pharaoh was a miracle-worker, they told their comrades.

Despite the risks, the foot-soldiers enjoyed the night march. The rearguard, more alert than ever, would counter surprise attacks. In front, the scout advanced cautiously. Thanks to the full moon, he could see far into the distance.

Ramses thought of Nefertari. If he failed to return, the burden of ruling Egypt would fall on her. Kha and Meritamon were too young to take the throne. Faction fighting would resume, more desperate than ever for having been temporarily quelled.

Suddenly Serramanna's horse reared, throwing him to the rocky ground. Half-stunned, he rolled down a sandy slope and came to rest in a crater not visible from the trail.

A curious sound, like heavy breathing, caught his attention.

Just in front of him, a viper rasped, threatening and ready to strike.

Serramanna had lost his sword in the fall. Unarmed, all he could do was back away, avoiding any sudden movements. But the hissing viper, slithering sideways, blocked his path.

He tried to stand, but an excruciating pain in his right ankle stopped him. Unable to run, he'd be easy prey.

'Get away from me, snake! I promised I'd die by the sword!'

The viper inched closer. Serramanna threw sand in its face, making it even more furious. Just as it was about to strike at him, a forked stick pinned it to the ground.

'Nice shot!' Setau said admiringly. 'Only one chance in ten I'd make it.' He grabbed the snake by the neck; its tail thrashed wildly.

'What a beauty. Light blue, dark blue and green – a lovely specimen, don't you agree? Luckily for you, the hissing carries and it's pretty easy to recognize.'

'I suppose I should thank you.'

'Its bite causes local swelling. Then the whole limb is affected and begins to haemorrhage. That's all. Only a small amount of venom, but very toxic. With a strong heart, you might survive it. Honestly, this snake isn't half as dangerous as it looks.'

51

Setau plastered Serramanna's sprained ankle with herbs, then applied linen dressings soaked in salve to reduce the swelling. In a few hours, it would be fine. Ever suspicious, the Sard wondered if the snake-charmer might not have masterminded the whole incident to make himself look like a hero, and to convince Serramanna that he was innocent of any wrongdoing and a true friend to Ramses. However, Setau had made no attempt to capitalize on the rescue, which was a point in his favour.

At dawn, they stopped to rest until mid-afternoon. Then the march resumed. There was still enough water for man and beast, but soon it would have to be rationed. Despite the men's fatigue and anxiety, Ramses stepped up the pace and exhorted the rearguard not to relax their vigilance. The insurgents would never attack head-on: they would try for the advantage of surprise.

In the ranks, there was no more joking or talk of home. In time, the men fell silent.

'There it is,' announced the scout, pointing.

Puny weeds, a circle of parched stones, a wooden frame to hold the weight of a large water-skin hanging from a frayed rope: the well. Their only hope of survival.

The scout and Serramanna ran forward. They peered down for a long moment, then slowly straightened.

The Sard shook his head. 'The place has been dry for ages. We're all going to die of thirst. No one's been able to find a permanent water source. We'll have to fill our skins in the great beyond.'

Ramses called the men together and told them that the situation was serious. By the next day, their water would be gone. They could neither advance nor retreat.

Several soldiers threw down their weapons.

'Pick those up,' ordered Ramses.

'What's the use,' asked an officer, 'if we're going to die of thirst?'

'We've come here to re-establish order, and we won't leave until we've done so.'

'How can our dead bodies fight the Nubians?'

'My father once found himself in a similar situation,' said Ramses, 'and he saved his men.'

'Then you save us, too.'

'Take shelter from the sun and water the animals.'

The king turned his back on his army and faced the desert.

Setau came to join him. 'What do you plan to do?'

'Walk until I find water.'

'That's crazy.'

'I have to do as my father taught me.'

'Stay here with us.'

'A pharaoh doesn't simply give up and wait for death.'

Serramanna approached them. 'Majesty . . .'

'Don't let the men panic, and keep up the watch, day and night. They must remember they're under threat of attack.'

'I can't let you go off alone into this desert. As your head of security—'

Ramses put his hand on the Sard's shoulder. 'Keep my army safe for me.'

'Hurry back. Your troops need a general.'

As the foot-soldiers looked on in horror, the king walked

away from the dried-up well and into the red desert towards a rocky promontory. He scaled it easily, and surveyed the desolate scene from the top.

Like his father, he needed to probe the earth's hidden secrets, find the veins of water that sprang from the ocean of energy, flowed through the rocks, and filled the heart of the mountains. Ramses' solar plexus ached, his vision was blurred, his body burned as if consumed with fever.

He took the divining-rod tied to the sash of his kilt, the same wand his father had used to see into the earth. Its magic, he knew, would still work, but where should he search in all this sand?

A voice spoke within the king's body, a voice from the beyond, a voice as ringing as Seti's. The pain in his solar plexus forced him to move, to climb down from the promontory. He no longer felt the heat that had killed many a traveller. His heartbeat slowed like an oryx's.

The sand and rocks changed shape and colour. Ramses' gaze gradually penetrated deep into the desert sand; his fingers gripped the two pliable acacia branches bound together at the tip with linen thread.

The rod quivered, paused, went dead. He walked on and the voice grew more distant. He retraced his steps, going left, the direction of death. The voice became louder again and the rod twitched. Ramses bumped into a huge pink granite boulder, lost in the sea of stone.

The force from the earth tore the rod out of his hands.

He had found water.

Parched, sunburned and with aching muscles, the soldiers rolled the boulder away and dug where the king told them. Thirty cubits down, they hit a huge pool of water. Their cheers reached the sky.

Ramses had them sink a series of wells, linked by an underground gallery, a technique he had picked up from

292

miners. In this way, he could not only save his army, but provide for future irrigation over a wide area.

'Are you imagining gardens already?' asked Setau.

'Fertility and prosperity are the best footprints we could leave,' answered the king.

'I thought we were here to put down an insurrection,' protested Serramanna.

'We are.'

'Then why are your soldiers digging ditches?'

'It's often part of their mission, according to our custom.'

'Pirates don't try to be fishermen,' he sniffed. 'If we're attacked, will we be able to defend ourselves?'

'I thought I put you in charge of our security.'

While the soldiers completed the wells and gallery, Setau and Lotus were busy trapping snakes, outstanding in both variety and size. They milked a quantity of priceless venom.

Serramanna uneasily stepped up the scheduled watches and also instituted barracks-style training. The men seemed to have forgotten about the stolen gold and the rebel threat. Their pharaoh worked wonders, and soon he'd be leading them home.

Amateurs, thought the ex-pirate. These Egyptian soldiers were temporary recruits who soon reverted to the labourers or peasants they really were. They had never experienced the heat, blood, and death of combat. There was no better training for war than being a pirate, always on the alert and ready to dispatch any enemy with any weapon. Discouraged, Serramanna hadn't even tried to teach the men about vicious attacks and surprise defences. These 'foot-soldiers' would never learn to fight.

Yet he had the feeling that the Nubian rebels were not far off and for the past two days or more had been sneaking up on the Egyptian camp, spying. Ramses's lion and dog also sensed a hostile presence. They grew agitated, slept less and prowled around sniffing the air.

If the Nubians were anything like some of the pirates Serramanna had known, the Egyptian forces were doomed.

The new capital of Egypt was going up at an astonishing rate, but Moses no longer saw it. To him, Pi-Ramses was now a foreign place, full of false gods and men deluded into meaningless beliefs.

Faithful to his promise, he kept the work moving along. Yet everyone noticed how short his temper was becoming, especially when he dealt with the Egyptian foremen; his complaints about their strictness were usually unfounded. He spent more and more time with his Hebrew brethren, discussing their people's future with small groups of men each evening. Many were satisfied with their life in Egypt and felt no urge to go in search of an independent homeland. The risk seemed too great.

Moses persisted, stressing their faith in a single god, their unique culture, the need to throw off the Egyptian yoke and reject false idols. He changed a few minds, but many more remained closed to him. Still, Moses was recognized as a leader who had done them a world of good. No one took his opinion lightly.

Ramses' old friend was sleeping less and less. His waking dream was of a fertile land where the god he cherished would reign supreme, a land the Hebrews would govern on their own, defending its borders as their most prized possession.

At last he understood the nature of the fire that had been consuming his soul for so many years. He could name this unquenchable desire; he could see the truth and lead his people towards it. He knew, and was filled with dread. Would Ramses accept such a defection, such a challenge to his power? Moses would have to convince him, make him see the light.

Memories flooded his mind. Ramses was far more than an old playmate. He was a true friend, who burned with a different version of the fire that consumed Moses. He would never betray Ramses by plotting against him. He would meet him face to face and win him over. No matter how impossible that might seem, Moses was confident.

For God was with him.

52

The Nubian rebels had half-shaved heads, hoop earrings, broad noses, ritual scars on their cheeks, beaded necklaces and panther-skin loincloths. They encircled the Egyptian encampment while most of Ramses' soldiers dozed in the afternoon heat. Their huge acacia bows launched a number of successful hits before the Egyptians could muster a response.

What kept the rebel chief from giving the order to attack was the sight of a small band of men, also armed with sturdy bows, behind a palisade of shields and palm fronds. In the lead was Serramanna, who had been expecting them. His hand-picked archers would have a clear shot into the Nubian ranks, as the Nubian chief could see. The advantage was his, but even so . . .

Time stood still. No one moved a muscle.

The rebel chief's main adviser urged him to start shooting and bring down as many of the enemy as possible, while a few fleet-footed warriors stormed the palisade. But the chief had been in a battle or two, and didn't like the look of Serramanna. The bewhiskered giant might well have a trick or two up his sleeve. He didn't look like the Egyptians they'd killed. The chief's hunter's instincts warned him to be careful.

When Ramses emerged from his tent, all eyes were

upon him. In a close-fitting blue crown which flared out at the back, a short-sleeved, pleated linen tunic and gold-trimmed kilt with a wild bull's tail dangling from the sash, the pharaoh held in his right hand the sceptre 'Magre', shaped like a shepherd's crook. He clutched the end of it to his chest.

Behind him came Setau, bearing the king's white sandals. He thought of Ahmeni, the king's official sandal-bearer, and almost smiled despite the tenseness of the situation. How amazed their friend would be to see Setau decked out in wig and white loincloth, clean-shaven, exactly like a seasoned courtier except for the odd-looking sack suspended from his waist and hanging down behind him.

As the Egyptian soldiers looked on nervously, Pharaoh and Setau walked to the edge of the camp, stopping less than a hundred paces from the Nubians.

'I am Ramses, Pharaoh of Egypt. Who is your chief?'

'I am,' said the Nubian, stepping forward.

Two feathers stuck in his red headband, muscles bulging, the rebel chief held a light spear trimmed with ostrich plumes.

'If you're not a coward, come here.'

The chief's adviser made a sign of disapproval. But neither Ramses nor his sandal-bearer was armed, while he had his spear and his adviser carried a double-edged dagger. The chief glanced over at Serramanna.

'Stay on my left,' he ordered his adviser. If the bewhiskered giant gave the order to shoot, the chief would be protected by a human shield.

'Are you afraid?' asked Ramses.

The two Nubians broke away from the war party and walked towards the king and his sandal-bearer, coming to a halt only ten paces in front of them.

'So you're the pharaoh who oppresses my people.'

'Nubians and Egyptians live in peace. You broke that

297

peace when you killed the members of the convoy and stole
the gold being shipped to our temples.'

'The gold is ours, not yours. You're the one who's
a thief.'

'Nubia is an Egyptian province, subject to the Rule of
Ma'at. Murder and robbery must be severely punished.'

'Your laws mean nothing to me, Pharaoh. I make my own.
Other tribes are prepared to join us. Killing you will make
me a hero! Every warrior in Nubia will be at my command,
and we'll rid our country of Egyptians once and for all!'

'Kneel down,' ordered the king.

The chief and his adviser looked at each other, bewildered.

'Lay down your arms, kneel, and submit to the Rule.'

The chief grimaced at him. 'If I bow to you, will you
grant me your pardon?'

'You've placed yourself outside the Rule. To pardon you
would also go against it.'

'You show me no mercy.'

'I know none.'

'Why should I bow to you?'

'Because it's the only freedom permitted you as a rebel.'

The adviser jumped in front of his chief, waving his
dagger. 'Let Pharaoh's death set us free, then!'

Setau, who hadn't taken his eyes off the two men, opened
the sack at his waist and released a sand viper. Slithering
across the sand with deadly speed, it bit the Nubian's foot
before he could spear it.

Crying out, he bent over to slash the bite with his dagger
and let out the poison.

'He's already colder than water and hotter than flame,'
intoned Setau, looking the chief straight in the eye. 'He's
sweating, his eyes are glazing over, he's starting to drool.
Now his eyes and eyelids are stiffening, his face is swelling, his throat is burning. He's about to die. He can't

get up, his skin is turning purple, his whole body is shaking.'

Setau held up his sack full of vipers. The Nubian war party backed away.

'Kneel,' Pharaoh ordered again, 'or prepare to die an awful death.'

'You're the one who's going to die!'

The chief lifted his spear over his head, then froze as a terrible roaring filled his ears. Turning, he barely caught a glimpse of the lion's mane and gaping jaws before it ripped his chest open with it's claws and its jaws closed on his head.

At a signal from Serramanna, the Egyptian bowmen fired at the scattering Nubians. The foot-soldiers advanced and disarmed the war party.

'Tie their hands behind their backs!' shouted the Sard.

As news of Ramses' victory spread, hundreds of Nubians left their hideouts and villages to pay him homage. The king gave a white-haired tribal chief the use of the newly created fertile zone around the water hole, and also put him in charge of the prisoners of war, who were to do farm work under the supervision of the Nubian police. Escapees and repeat offenders would get the death penalty.

Then the Egyptian forces marched to the oasis that had served as the rebel stronghold. They met with only feeble resistance, and took possession of the gold that would one day grace statues and temple doors in the motherland.

At nightfall, Setau found two lengths of well-dried palm rib, held them between his knees, set a piece of dead wood between them and rubbed them together faster and faster until sparks flew. The soldiers on watch would have a fire to keep away cobras, hyenas and other pests.

'Have you collected more snakes?' asked Ramses.

He nodded. 'Lotus is delighted. Tonight we'll rest.'

'It's a wonderful country.'

'You seem to like it as much as we do.'

'It tests me and makes me excel myself. Its power is mine.'

'Without my viper, the rebels would have killed you.'

'But they didn't, did they?'

'It was still a risky plan.'

'It prevented a great deal of bloodshed.'

'Do you ever consider being more cautious?'

'What for?'

'I'm only Setau the snake-charmer. It's all right if I fool around with reptiles. But you, Ramses, are Lord of the Two Lands. Your death would plunge Egypt into disarray.'

'Nefertari would reign wisely.'

'You're only twenty-five, Ramses, I know. But you no longer have the right to behave like a young man. You must consider your safety. You'll have to send others into battle.'

'Is Pharaoh to be a coward?'

'Don't exaggerate. I'm only telling you to be a bit more careful.'

'But I'm protected on all sides: Nefertari's magic, you and your snakes, Serramanna and his Royal Bodyguard, Wideawake and Invincible . . . I'm the luckiest man on earth.'

'Save your luck for when you need it.'

'It'll never run out.'

'Pig-headed as ever, I see. I might as well go to bed.'

Setau turned his back on the king and went and stretched out beside Lotus. Her contented sigh told Ramses that it was time to slip away. His friend might not be allowed to rest for long.

How could he make Setau realize his real place was high in the government? Ramses' failure to recruit him was his first major setback. Should Setau be free to go his own way or be forced into an official position?

Ramses spent the night gazing at the starry sky, the luminous home of his father's soul and the souls of all the pharaohs before him. He was proud of having found water in the desert and put down the rebellion, just as his father had done, but he was not content with his victory. The earlier campaign had not had lasting results. This time would be the same. He would have to get to the root of the problem, but how could he determine what it was?

In the first light of dawn, Ramses sensed a presence at his back and slowly, very slowly, turned round.

There stood an enormous elephant. It had come into the oasis as silently as the wind, avoiding the dried palm ribs strewn all around. The lion and watchdog had opened their eyes but sounded no warning, as if they knew their master was safe.

As Ramses looked, he fancied that there was something familiar about the beast. Of course: the big bull elephant with flapping ears and long tusks was his friend. Years earlier, Ramses had saved it, removing a spearhead from its trunk.

The King of Egypt stroked that trunk now, and the lord of the savannahs trumpeted in joy, waking the whole encampment.

The elephant moved away, then turned to look back at the king.

'We must follow him,' said Ramses.

53

Ramses, Serramanna, Setau and a handful of armed soldiers followed the elephant across a strip of arid plain, then up a thorny slope to a plateau topped with a venerable acacia.

The elephant waited for Ramses to catch up.

Following the huge beast's gaze, he discovered a splendid view. The huge spur of rock where they stood, a landmark for navigation, looked down on a vast bend in the Nile. Ramses, spouse of Egypt, contemplated the life-giving waters, the divine river in all its majesty. On the nearby rocks, hieroglyphic inscriptions dedicated the spot to the goddess Hathor, sovereign of the stars and of sailors, who often stopped here.

With its right front foot, the elephant sent a boulder tumbling down the cliff. It landed in a deep sandy ravine between two promontories. To the north, the cliffs were vertical, dropping almost straight down to the water. To the south, they sloped gradually into a vast open stretch, broadening westward.

On the shore below, a boat hollowed out of a palm trunk was moored, with a young boy sleeping inside.

'Go and get him,' the king ordered two of his soldiers.

The young Nubian saw them coming and took to his heels. He would have got away if he hadn't tripped on a rock and sprawled on the riverbank. The Egyptian soldiers twisted the young Nubian's arms behind his back and brought him before the king.

The runaway's eyes rolled in panic: he was afraid his nose would be cut off. 'I'm not a thief,' he cried. 'The boat belongs to me, I swear it, and—'

'Answer my question,' Ramses told him, 'and you'll go free. What do they call this place?'

'Abu Simbel.'

'You may go.'

The boy ran back to his boat and paddled away with all his might.

'We can't stay here long,' advised Serramanna. 'I don't think this spot is safe.'

'No sign of any snakes,' complained Setau. 'Bizarre. Could Hathor have driven them off ?'

'Don't follow me,' the king commanded.

Serramanna stepped forward. 'Majesty!'

'Must I say it again?'

Ramses began the descent towards the river.

Setau restrained the Sard. 'You'd better do as he says.'

Grumbling, Serramanna gave in. The king on his own, in the middle of nowhere, in hostile territory! If danger arose, despite his orders he would step in.

When he reached the riverbank, Ramses turned to face the sandstone cliff.

This was the heart of Nubia, though she didn't know it. He, Ramses, the Son of the Light, would reveal it, make of Abu Simbel a wonder that would outlast time and seal the pact between Egypt and Nubia.

The pharaoh meditated at Abu Simbel for several hours, steeping himself in the purity of the sky, the sparkling of the Nile and the strength of the rocks. The province's main temple would be built here, concentrating divine energy and radiating a protective force so strong that the clash of arms would be for ever stilled.

Ramses observed the sun. Its rays did not merely glance off the cliff, but penetrated to the heart of the rock, lighting it from within. When his architects worked on the site, they must capture this miracle.

By the time the king climbed back to the top of the cliff, Serramanna's nerves were stretched to the limit. He was tempted to quit for good, but the elephant's placid attitude changed his mind. He refused to appear less patient than an animal, even the most majestic of animals.

'We're going back to Egypt,' decreed the king.

After cleansing his mouth with natron, Shaanar surrendered his face to the barber, who was skilled in the painless removal of body hair. He was extremely fond of massage, and particularly liked having his scalp rubbed with perfumed oils before the hairdresser came to do his wig. These small pleasures lightened his days and helped him present his best face to the world. He might not be as handsome or athletic as Ramses, but he could be just as well groomed, if not better so.

His water-clock, a costly piece, told him that the hour of his meeting was near.

His litter, comfortable and roomy, was the finest in Memphis except for the pharaoh's, which he one day planned to occupy. Shaanar had the bearers drop him off at the canal that gave heavy barges passage to the main river landing.

Ofir was sitting in the shade of a willow tree. Shaanar leaned against the trunk and watched a fishing boat go by.

'Any progress, Ofir?'

'Moses is an exceptional man, with a mind of his own.'

'In other words, you can't persuade him.'

'I didn't say that.'

'I need facts, Ofir. Vague impressions won't do.'

304

'The road to success is often a long and winding one.'

'Spare me the philosophy. Have you succeeded, yes or no?'

'He didn't reject my proposal. That's quite something, isn't it?'

'Interesting, I admit. Did he admit that your plan is feasible?'

'Moses is familiar with Akhenaton's ideas. He knows they helped shape the Hebrew faith and that we could do great things together.'

'And the Hebrews will follow him?'

'He's more popular than ever. Moses is a born leader. Once Pi-Ramses is finished, he'll rally his people.'

'How long will that take?'

'A few more months. He has the brickmakers working at lightning speed.'

'That damned capital! Ramses' fame will spread beyond the northern border, I'm afraid.'

'Where is pharaoh now?'

'In Nubia.'

'A dangerous place.'

'Don't fool yourself, Ofir. The royal couriers have brought excellent news. More miracles for Ramses: he found an underground spring in the desert and opened up new farmland. He's bringing back the stolen gold for the temples. A successful expedition, a signal victory.'

'Moses knows that he'll have to confront the pharaoh.'

'His closest friend . . .'

'His belief in the One God will be stronger than their friendship: a clash is inevitable. When it comes, we must support Moses.'

'That's your role, Ofir. You understand why I have to remain in the background.'

'I'll need your help.'

'What do you need?'

'A place in Memphis, servants, a communication network.'

'Granted, on condition that you send me regular reports on your activities.'

'Confidential reports.'

'When are you going back to Pi-Ramses, Ofir?'

'Tomorrow. I plan to tell Moses how our numbers are growing.'

'I'll take care of your everyday routine; you concentrate on persuading Moses to fight for his faith, against Ramses' tyranny.'

Abner the brickmaker hummed to himself. In less than a month, the first Pi-Ramses barracks would be finished and the initial detachment of foot-soldiers transferred from Memphis. The premises were spacious and well ventilated, the fittings remarkable.

Thanks to Moses, who had recognized his talent, Abner now headed a small crew of his fellow craftsmen, as experienced and industrious as himself. Sary's extortion was only a bad memory. Abner would move his family to the new capital and work in public building maintenance. The future was looking bright.

Tonight he would enjoy a meal of Nile perch with his comrades. Then they would play a game of snake, advancing their pieces along the board and trying to avoid various traps marked on the reptile's body. Abner had a feeling it was his lucky night.

Pi-Ramses was coming to life. The construction site was gradually turning into a real city. It didn't seem long now until the time for the dedication, the moment when Pharaoh would bring his capital to life. It had been his special privilege, Abner reflected, to serve a great king's vision and work with Moses.

'How are you, Abner?'

Sary wore a Libyan tunic with wide vertical stripes of black and yellow, caught at the waist with a green leather belt. His face had grown even more emaciated.

'What do you want with me?'

'Asking after your health, that's all.'

'Move along.'

'Is that any way to talk to me?'

'I think you've forgotten I was promoted. I don't report to you any more.'

'Proud as a peacock, aren't we, Abner? Now, now, don't get worked up.'

'I'm busy.'

'Too busy to talk to your old friend Sary?'

The Hebrew was growing uneasy, to Sary's amusement.

'You're a reasonable fellow, Abner. You want a nice little life for yourself, but you know that everything has a price. And I'm the one who sets it.'

'Go to hell!'

'Hebrew, you're nothing more than an insect and bugs don't complain when you squash them. I demand half your wages and bonuses. When the work is done here, you'll volunteer to stay on as my servant. Mmm, I'd love to have a Hebrew houseboy. I'll keep you busy, don't worry. You're lucky, Abner. If I hadn't noticed you, you'd have ended up as vermin.'

'You can't make me, I tell you, I—'

'Stop babbling and do as I say,' the foreman snarled in parting.

Abner crouched in a corner, hanging his head. This time Sary had gone too far. This time he'd speak to Moses.

54

Peerless Nefertari, her beauty like the morning star at the dawn of a good year, her touch like a lotus flower. Luminous Nefertari, catching him in the dark loops of her fragrant hair.

To love her was to be reborn.

Ramses gently massaged her feet, then kissed her legs, letting his hands wander over her lithe, sun-gilded body. She was the garden where the rarest flowers grew, the pool of clear water, the distant country of frankincense trees. When they came together, their desire was strong as the surge of a wave cresting the inundation, tender as a flute tune in the twilight.

As soon as the expedition had returned from Nubia, the king had made straight for his wife, ignoring well-wishers and advisers. Nefertari and Ramses had celebrated their reunion beneath the verdant foliage of a sycamore. The refreshing shade of the great tree, its turquoise leaves and notched fruit red as jasper were one of the treasures of the palace at Thebes where they had managed to slip away.

'You were gone for so many, many months . . .'

'The baby?'

'Kha and Meritamon are both doing wonderfully. Your son thinks his little sister is very pretty but a little noisy. He's already trying to teach her to read. His tutor made him stop.'

Ramses took his wife in his arms. 'That's wrong. Why hold him back?'

Before Nefertari could answer, her husband's lips sought hers as the sycamore branches bent discreetly over them in the cool north wind.

Bakhen, carrying a long staff, marched in front of the royal pair. It was the tenth day of the fourth month of the inundation season, Year Three of Ramses' reign, and he was leading them to inspect the newly completed additions to the temple of Luxor. A long procession followed them down the avenue of sphinxes leading from the temple of Karnak.

The new façade of Karnak imposed silence. The two obelisks, the colossal royal statues and the massive yet elegant pylon gateway formed a perfect whole, worthy of the greatest builders of old.

The obelisks repelled negative energy and attracted divine power to the temple, where it would nourish the *ka* produced here. At their bases were carved dog-faced baboons, symbols of the mind of the god Thoth, uttering the sounds that helped bring forth each new dawn. Each element, from hieroglyph to colossal statue, contributed to the daily rebirth of the sun, which now sat in glory above the twin towers of the pylon and central gateway.

Ramses and Nefertari passed through it, entering a great open-air forecourt with huge columns lining the walls, a powerful expression of the *ka*. Between them stood colossal statues of the king, a testimony to his indomitable strength. Leaning lovingly against one of the giant's legs was Nefertari, at once frail and steadfast.

Nebu, the High Priest of Karnak, slowly made his way towards the royal pair, his golden staff tapping. The old man bowed. 'Majesty, here is the home of your *ka*, the endless source of energy for your reign.'

The feast of the dedication of Luxor involved the entire population of Thebes and its environs, from the humblest to the wealthiest. For ten days, there was singing and dancing in the streets; taverns and open-air drinking establishments were crammed. By the grace of Pharaoh, free beer would fill every belly.

The king and queen presided at a banquet recorded in the royal annals. Ramses proclaimed the temple to his *ka* completed, decreeing that no architectural feature would be added in the future. It remained only for him and the queen to choose the themes and symbolic figures that would adorn the façade of the pylon and the walls of the great forecourt. It was generally agreed that the young pharaoh was wise not to make his decision until he had conferred with the ritualists of the House of Life.

Ramses appreciated Bakhen's attitude. The Fourth Prophet of Amon made no mention of his own contributions, but praised the architects who had designed Luxor in accordance with the laws of harmony. When the feasting was over, the king presented the High Priest of Amon with the Nubian gold, which would henceforth be shipped with stringent security measures.

Before departing northward, the royal pair visited the site of the Temple of a Million Years. Bakhen's competence was in evidence there as well. Graders, unskilled labourers, and stone-cutters were hard at work. The temple was beginning to rise from the desert floor.

'Hurry, Bakhen. I want the foundations laid as quickly as possible.'

'The Luxor work gangs will start working here tomorrow. Then we'll have full crews and enough skilled workers.'

Ramses noted that his plan for the complex had been followed to the letter. He could already picture the shrines, the great Hall of Pillars, the offering tables, the laboratory, the library . . . Millions of years would flow through the building's stone veins.

The king toured the holy site with Nefertari, describing his

310

vision as if he were already touching the carved walls and columns covered with hieroglyphs.

'This temple will be your greatest monument.'

'Perhaps.'

'Why do you doubt it?'

'Because I hope to build temples all over the country, make hundreds of homes for the gods. I want my country drenched with their energy. I want the land of Egypt to be heaven on earth.'

'What could surpass your Temple of a Million Years?'

'In Nubia I met an old friend, an elephant. He led me to an extraordinary place.'

'Does it have a name?'

'Abu Simbel. A stopping place for sailors, protected by Hathor, where the Nile is at its most beautiful. The river blends with the rock, the sandstone cliffs seem ripe to give birth to a temple.'

'But so far south . . . Won't the technical difficulties be overwhelming?'

'We won't let them overwhelm us.'

'No pharaoh before you has attempted such a thing.'

'True, but I'll succeed. From the moment I first saw Abu Simbel, I haven't been able to get it out of my mind. The elephant was a messenger from the gods, I'm sure of it. Abu stands for elephant, and as you know its hieroglyph can also be read as 'start' or 'beginning'. A new start for Egypt, the beginning of her territory, must be there in the heart of Nubia, at Abu Simbel. It's the only way to assure a lasting peace.'

'It's a wild idea.'

'Of course it is! But it's also an expression of my *ka* – the fire within me captured for ever in stone. Luxor, Pi-Ramses and Abu Simbel are each my desire and my brainchild. If I spent my time on day-to-day matters, I wouldn't be acting like a pharaoh.'

'My head rests on your shoulder and I feel secure in your

love. But you can also rest on me, like a colossal statue on its pedestal.'

'Do you approve of my Abu Simbel project?'

'Think more about it. Let it grow inside you until your vision is dazzling and imperious. Then act upon it.'

Within the enclosure of the Temple of a Million Years, Ramses and Nefertari felt a strange force move within them, making them invulnerable.

Workshops, warehouses, barracks – all were ready to be occupied. The main streets led through residential neighbourhoods and ended at the major temples, still under construction but with each inner sanctum in usable condition.

The brickmakers' work was finished, and an army of landscapers and painters took their place, not to mention the decorative artists who would give Pi-Ramses its outward face. But would Ramses smile on it?

Moses climbed to the roof of the palace and contemplated the city. Like Pharaoh, he had worked miracles. The men's physical labour and his own careful organization had not been enough. The spark had come from enthusiasm, not human but divine in origin, the sign of God's love for his creation. And Moses longed to offer this city to God, not leave it to Amon, Set and the like. Such an outpouring of talent wasted on those mute idols . . .

His next city would be built to the glory of the One God, in his own country, on holy ground. If Ramses was truly his soulmate, he would understand.

Moses pounded his fist on the edge of the balcony.

The King of Egypt would never tolerate a minority revolt, never let a descendant of Akhenaton take over the throne. To believe otherwise was, at best, an impossible dream.

Below, near one of the side entries to the palace, stood Ofir. 'May I speak to you?' he called.

'Come up.'

Ofir had learned to blend in wherever he went. At Pi-Ramses he could pass for an architect coming to offer Moses valuable advice.

'I'm giving up,' declared Moses. 'It's no use arguing any more.'

The sorcerer eyed him coolly. 'Has something happened to change your mind?'

'I've thought it over, that's all. Our plans are crazy.'

'I came to tell you that our ranks have been growing steadily. There are influential people who believe Lita will take the throne with the blessing of the One God. In that case, the Hebrews will be free.'

'You mean to overthrow Ramses? Are you mad?'

'Our convictions are firm.'

'Do you think your sermons will sway the king?'

'Who said we'll stop at sermons?'

Moses stared at Ofir as if he were meeting a stranger. 'You can't mean—'

'Of course I can, Moses. You've reached the same conclusion I have, and that's what alarms you. Akhenaton was defeated and persecuted only because he refused to use force against his enemies. No fight can be won without bloodshed. Ramses will never give up a single morsel of his power. We'll have to fight him from within. And you will lead the Hebrews in their revolt.'

'The dead will number in the hundreds, even thousands. Is carnage what you want?'

'If you prepare your people, they'll win. God is with us.'

'I won't listen to another word. Get out of here, Ofir.'

'I can see you in Memphis as well as here.'

'Don't count on it.'

'There's no other way, and you know it. Don't try to ignore the voice inside you. We'll fight the good fight together, and God will triumph.'

55

Raia, the Syrian merchant, fingered his beard. Business was booming. The quality of his preserved meats and Asian vases attracted an ever-growing clientele among the upper classes of Memphis and Thebes. The creation of the new capital, Pi-Ramses, meant yet another market would open up. Raia had already secured a permit to open a large shop in the heart of the commercial district and was training the sales force to deal with demanding customers.

In preparation, he had ordered a hundred precious vases, all new designs, from his Syrian sources. Each piece was unique and would be priced accordingly. Raia's personal opinion was that Egyptian craftsmen did better work, but the buying public's taste for the exotic (not to mention its rampant snobbery) was lining his pockets.

Although the Hittites had ordered their spy to back Shaanar and oppose Ramses, after a single unsuccessful attempt on the king Raia had given up trying. Pharaoh was too well protected and a second unsuccessful attempt might lead the investigators to him.

Over the last three years, Ramses had proved as strong a ruler as his father, with the added energy of youth. He was like a raging torrent, sweeping all obstacles out of his way. No one had the authority to oppose him, even if the number of building projects he had undertaken was sheer madness. The court and the people were at once enthralled and subjugated.

Raia checked his shipment. Among the new pieces were two alabaster vases.

He shut the storeroom door, then put his ear to it for several moments. Satisfied that he was alone, he stuck his hand inside the vase with the small, distinctive red mark under the rim and pulled out a pine tablet inscribed with the vase's dimensions and origin.

Raia knew the code by heart and easily worked out the message his contact in southern Syria had forwarded from the Hittites.

Stunned, the secret agent destroyed the message and went running out of the shop.

'Superb,' said Shaanar, admiring the blue swan-necked vase Raia had just unpacked for him. 'The price?'

'Rather high, I'm afraid, Your Highness. But it's a unique piece.'

'Let's discuss it, shall we?'

Clutching the vase to his chest, Raia followed Shanaar to one of his villa's roofed terraces, where they could speak without fear of being overheard.

'If I'm not mistaken, Raia, you're following emergency procedure.'

'Correct.'

'Why?'

'The Hittites have decided to take action.'

It was the news Shaanar had hoped for, but also dreaded. If he were Pharaoh, he would put Egyptian troops on high alert and reinforce the border defences. But Egypt's most dangerous enemy was offering him a way to win the throne. He would have to use this vital secret to his sole advantage.

'Could you be more specific, Raia?'

'You look disturbed.'

'Who wouldn't be?'

'It's true, Your Highness. I'm still in shock myself. This decision will shatter the existing state of affairs.'

'More than that, Raia, much more. The fate of the whole world hangs on it. You and I will be major players in the drama that unfolds.'

'But I'm only a humble information-gatherer.'

'You'll be my contact with the Hittites. A good part of my strategy depends on the accuracy of the information you provide.'

'You make it sound so important.'

'Do you hope to stay in Egypt, once we win?'

'I'm at home here.'

'You'll be rich, Raia, very rich. I shan't be ungrateful to the people who help me to power.'

The merchant bowed. 'Your humble servant, Prince.'

'Do you have any details?'

'Not yet.'

Shaanar took a few steps, leaned over the balustrade, and looked towards the north.

'This is a great day, Raia. One day we'll tell ourselves it marked the beginning of the end of Ramses.'

Ahsha's Egyptian mistress was a marvel. Playful, inventive and insatiable, she had elicited from him new and subtle responses. She was a definite improvement over her pretty but boring predecessors, two Libyan girls and three Syrians. Ahsha demanded imagination in his lovemaking. That alone could release the unexpected melodies straining within the body. He was just getting round to sucking his lady love's sweet little toes when he heard his steward hammering at the door, despite strict orders.

Outraged, Ahsha flung the door open without thinking to cover himself.

316

'Forgive me, sir. An urgent message from your office.'

Ahsha consulted the wooden tablet. Just two words: 'Report immediately.'

At two in the morning, the streets of Memphis were deserted. Ahsha's horse quickly covered the distance between his house and the secretariat. Not stopping to make the customary offering to Thoth, Ahsha took the stairs four at a time and sped to his office. He found his secretary waiting.

'I thought I should let you know immediately.'

'About what?'

'A dispatch from one of our agents in northern Syria.'

'If it's another false alarm, I'll deal with him.'

The bottom of the papyrus scroll looked blank, but when heated over the flame of an oil lamp, hieratic characters appeared. This shorthand method of writing hieroglyphs sometimes made them almost illegible. The hand of the Egyptian spy on their payroll in northern Syria was unmistakable.

Ahsha read and reread the message.

'Glad I sent for you?' asked the secretary.

'Please leave.'

Ahsha spread out a map and checked the information against it. If his calculations were correct, the worst was in store.

'The sun hasn't even risen,' grunted Shaanar, yawning.

'Read this,' advised Ahsha, handing his minister the secret message.

Shaanar's eyes opened wide. 'What? The Hittites have taken control of several villages in central Syria, well outside the zone of influence acceptable to Egypt . . .'

'He's categorical.'

'No one killed or wounded. They could just be testing the waters.'

'It wouldn't be the first time. But the Hittites have never gone so far south.'

'What do you make of it?'

'They're preparing a fully fledged campaign in southern Syria.'

'Is that a statement or a guess?'

'A guess.'

'How can we find out for sure?'

'In the light of the situation, I assume more messages will soon follow.'

'Whatever the case, let's keep this quiet as long as possible.'

'We're taking quite a risk.'

'I know we are, Ahsha. But that's what we have to do. We were trying to coax Ramses into making mistakes that would cost him dearly, but it seems the Hittites are restless. We'll have to delay the mobilization of the Egyptian army as long as we can.'

'I'm not so sure,' objected Ahsha.

'Why?'

'On one hand, that would only buy us a few more days, hardly enough time to stop a counteroffensive. On the other, my secretary knows I received an urgent message. Any delay in informing the king will look suspicious.'

'Then having advance information does us no good at all!'

'Wrong, Shaanar. Ramses appointed me head of the Secret Service. He trusts me. In other words, he'll believe what I tell him.'

Shaanar smiled. 'A very dangerous tactic. They say Ramses is a mind-reader.'

'A diplomat's thoughts are unreadable. What I want you to do is tell him your concerns, once I've alerted him. That will make you look honest and credible.'

Shaanar settled into an armchair. 'Damnably intelligent, Ahsha.'

'I know Ramses. Underestimating his insight would be a fatal error.'

'I agree. We'll follow your plan.'

'Just one more problem: being sure of the Hittites' real intentions.'

Shaanar knew what those intentions were. But he judged it wiser not to reveal his sources to Ahsha, whom he might be forced to sacrifice to his Hittite friends as the situation evolved.

56

Moses raced from building to building, checking the walls and windows. He drove his chariot all the way across town, urging the painters to hurry and finish their work. It was only a matter of days until the king and queen arrived for the official dedication of Pi-Ramses.

A thousand flaws jumped out at him, but how could they be fixed in so short a time? The brickmakers had agreed to lend a hand to the frantic workmen finishing the site. In the final rush, Moses' popularity remained intact. His enthusiasm was catching, even more so as the dream was transformed into reality.

Despite his exhaustion, Moses had spent long evenings with his Hebrew brethren, listening to their grievances and hopes. He had grown comfortable in his role as leader of a people in search of its identity. His ideas frightened most of the men, yet they were drawn to him. When the grand adventure of Pi-Ramses was finished, would Moses be taking his fellow Hebrews in a new direction?

Overtired, the young supervisor slept only fitfully. In his dreams, Ofir's gaunt face loomed. The worshipper of Aton had spoken the truth: in a crisis sermons and speeches were not enough. They would have to act, and action often meant violence.

Moses had fulfilled the mission Ramses had entrusted

to him, thus discharging any obligation to the King of Egypt. Yet he still owed loyalty to his oldest friend and vowed to warn him of the dangers facing him. Once his conscience was eased on that score, Moses would be free – completely free.

According to the royal courier, the pharaoh and his wife would arrive around noon the following day. The population of the surrounding towns and villages had flocked to the outskirts of the new capital so as not to miss the event. Overwhelmed, the security forces could not stop the curious from spilling in.

Moses was hoping to spend his last few hours as construction supervisor outside the city, strolling in the countryside. Just as he reached the edge of town, however, an architect ran up to him.

'The statue is breaking loose! The giant statue!'

'At the Temple of Amon?'

'We can't stop it.'

'I told you not to touch it!'

'We thought—'

Moses' chariot sped like the wind through the city. The scene in front of the Temple of Amon was chaotic. A two-hundred-ton statue of the king seated on his throne was slowly slipping towards the façade. It could either collide with the building, causing enormous damage, or fall from its sledge and shatter. What a sight to greet Ramses at the dedication!

Fifty or more men strained desperately, holding the ropes that secured the giant sculpture to a wooden sledge. Where rope touched stone, several leather pads had already split.

'What happened?' asked Moses.

'The foreman climbed up on the statue to help guide it into place. He fell, and to avoid crushing him the men pulled the wooden brakes to stop the sledge. It jumped the track and kept going. There was dew on the ground, the runners were already wet . . .'

'You should have had at least a hundred and fifty men!'

'There isn't a hand to spare.'

'Bring me jugs of milk.'

'How many?'

'Thousands! And get more men here as fast as you can.'

Heartened by Moses' arrival, the struggling workers quieted. When he climbed along the right side of the statue, perched on its granite apron and poured milk in front of the sledge to lay a new track, they took hope. A chain formed to pass jugs to Moses. Following his directives, the first spare hands to arrive on the scene tied long ropes to the sides and back of the sledge, slowing the statue's momentum.

Little by little, the colossus moved back on track.

'The braking beam!' shouted Moses.

Thirty men sprang into action, hauling the notched log into place. It would halt the sledge at the spot where Ramses' statue would sit, in front of the Temple of Amon.

The colossus, righted and slowed, slid easily into place.

Dripping with sweat, Moses hopped down, glowering. The men feared the punishment that was sure to come.

'Bring me the man responsible for this fiasco, the man who fell off the statue.'

'Here he is.'

Two workmen pushed Abner forward. He fell to his knees in front of Moses.

'Forgive me,' he groaned, 'I had a dizzy spell, I—'

'Aren't you one of my brickmakers?'

'Yes. My name is Abner.'

'Why were you working here?'

'I . . . I'm in hiding,' he gulped.

'Have you lost your mind?'

'I can explain.'

Abner was a Hebrew: he deserved a hearing before being punished. Moses could see that the man was distraught and would talk to him only if they were alone.

'Come with me, Abner.'

An Egyptian architect stepped forward. 'This man is responsible for a serious incident. Letting him off would be an insult to his co-workers.'

'I'll question him and then decide what to do.'

The architect bowed to the project supervisor. If Abner had been an Egyptian, Moses would surely have shown less consideration. Lately he had shown a favouritism towards his fellow Hebrews that was bound to rebound on him.

Moses helped Abner into his chariot and fastened a leather strap round him.

'Enough falls for one day, don't you think?'

'Please, Moses, forgive me!'

'Stop whining, man, and tell me what happened.'

In front of Moses' house, there was a small courtyard sheltered from the wind. The two men got down from the chariot and went inside. Moses took off his wig and kilt, and gestured towards a large jug.

'Get up on the ledge,' he ordered Abner, 'and pour that water slowly over my shoulders.'

As Moses briskly rubbed his skin with herbs, the brick-maker emptied the heavy jug.

'Cat got your tongue, Abner?'

'I'm afraid.'

'Why?'

'Someone's after me.'

'Who?'

'I can't say.'

'If you won't tell me, I'll turn you over to the tribunal for disciplinary action.'

'No! I'll never work again.'

'Wouldn't that be fair?'

'No! I swear it.'

'Then talk.'

'I've been the victim of extortion,' Abner sighed.

'Who's doing this to you?'

'An Egyptian.'

'What's his name?'

'I can't tell you! He has connections.'

'Then I can't help you.'

'If I tell you, he'll kill me!'

'Don't you trust me?'

'I wanted to tell you, but I was too scared.'

'Stop shaking and give me a name. I'll take care of him for you.'

Abner trembled so violently that the jug slipped from his hands and shattered.

'Sary,' he said. 'It's Sary.'

The royal fleet entered the grand canal leading to Pi-Ramses. Every member of the court, it seemed, was accompanying Pharaoh and the Great Royal Wife. No one could wait to see the new capital, which would be the place to live if you sought the king's favour. There was a great deal of negative speculation, bordering on criticism: how could a city built so quickly be any match for Memphis? It would be a major setback for Ramses, and sooner or later he'd be forced to abandon his new capital.

In the prow, the pharaoh was watching the Nile fan into its Delta when the boat tacked towards the canal.

Shaanar sidled up to his brother. 'I know this is hardly the time, but I have a serious matter to discuss with you.'

'Can't it wait?'

'I'm afraid not. If I'd been able to speak to you sooner, I wouldn't have intruded on this happy occasion. But you were out of reach.'

'I'm listening, Shaanar.'

'You did me a favour appointing me minister for foreign affairs, and I wish I could repay you with nothing but the best of news.'

'And that's not the case?'

'If reports reaching me are to be believed, the international situation leaves something to be desired.'

'Get to the point.'

'The Hittites seem to have gone beyond the limits our late father established and invaded central Syria.'

'Is that fact or hearsay?'

'It's too early to tell, but I wanted to be the first to warn you. In the recent past, the Hittites have tended to engage in provocation, then back away. We can hope that this is simply another bluff. Still, it would be wise to take certain precautions.'

'I'll consider it.'

'Are you sceptical?'

'You said yourself that the reports haven't been verified. Once you have solid information, let me know.'

'At your service, Majesty.'

The current was strong, there was a good following wind, and the boat sailed briskly. Shaanar's announcement left Ramses thoughtful. Did his elder brother really take his new position seriously? He was capable of inventing reports of a Hittite invasion, just to show how well he was running his secretariat.

Central Syria was a neutral zone where neither nation maintained a military presence, relying on a patchy intelligence network. Since Seti had refrained from taking the Hittite stronghold of Kadesh, the fighting had been small-scale and intermittent.

Perhaps the creation of Pi-Ramses, which occupied a strategic position, had roused the Hittites to action. They might have decided the young pharaoh was looking toward Asia and their empire. Only one man could sort out the truth for him: his friend Ahsha, head of the Secret Service. The official reports that reached Shaanar would be fragmentary, while Ahsha's sources would reveal the enemy's real intentions.

A sailor who had climbed to the top of the mast began to cheer.

'Ahoy! There it is, the port, the town – Pi-Ramses!'

57

Alone in a golden chariot, the Son of the Light rode down the main thoroughfare of Pi-Ramses, towards the Temple of Amon. At high noon, he shone like the sun that had given life to the city. Alongside his two plumed horses marched his lion, head high, mane blowing in the wind.

Stunned by the power their monarch radiated, and by the magic that permitted him to have the king of beasts as a bodyguard, at first the crowd was silent. Then a voice shouted, 'Long live Ramses!' Then another, ten more, a hundred, a thousand took up the chant . . . The jubilation was passionate and clamorous as the king made his slow and majestic way down the avenue.

Nobles, tradesmen and country folk were all dressed for a feast day. Their hair shone with moringa oil, the women wore their best wigs, children and servants threw armfuls of flowers and greenery in the royal chariot's path.

An open-air banquet was being prepared. The steward of the new palace had ordered a thousand loaves of the whitest bread, two thousand rolls, ten thousand pastries, mounds of dried meat, milk, bowls of carob, grapes, figs, pomegranates. Roast goose, game, fish, cucumbers and leeks would also be on the menu, not to mention thousands of jars of wine from the royal cellars and vats of beer brewed for the noble occasion.

The king had invited all his people to celebrate his capital's birthday.

No little girl was without a colourful new dress, no horse without bright bands of cloth and copper rosettes, no donkey without a garland of flowers around its neck. Pet dogs, cats, and monkeys would have an extra feed. Elders, no matter what their station in life, would be served first, seated in comfort beneath sycamore and persea trees. Petitions would be collected – for a house, a job, a plot of land, a cow – and carefully examined by Ahmeni. Generosity and indulgence were the order of the day.

The Hebrews joined in the festivities. Their labours had earned them a long well-paid rest, as well as the satisfaction of having built the new capital of the Kingdom of Egypt with their own hands. Their accomplishments would go down in history.

A hush fell over the assembled crowd as the chariot drew to a halt before the colossal statue of the pharaoh that had come so close to causing a disaster the day before.

Ramses looked up, meeting the giant's stony stare. On its forehead the statue wore the uraeus, the figure of a spitting-cobra, whose venom would blind the king's enemies. On its head were the 'Two Powers', the White Crown of Upper Egypt and the Red Crown of Lower Egypt. Seated on his throne, his hands placed flat on his kilt, the granite pharaoh gazed out over his city.

Ramses stepped down from his chariot. He, too, wore the double crown, and was dressed in a billowing full-sleeved robe of gauzy linen; beneath it shone a gilded linen kilt held in place by a belt of silver. A broad gold collar covered his chest.

He addressed the statue. 'You are my *ka* incarnate, the spirit of my reign and my city. I open your mouth, your eyes, your ears. I pronounce you a living being. Anyone who dares attack you will be punished by death.'

The sun was at its zenith, directly above the pharaoh. He turned to his people.

'Pi-Ramses is born, Pi-Ramses is our capital!'

Thousands of enthusiastic voices took up the chorus.

All day long, Ramses and Nefertari had travelled broad avenues, streets and alleys, visiting each section of Pi-Ramses. Dazzled, the Great Royal Wife dubbed it 'the Turquoise City', a phrase that was instantly on everyone's lips. That was Moses' final surprise for the king: the façades of villas, houses and modest dwellings had been covered with blue-glazed tiles of exceptional luminosity. The faience workshop had been Ramses' idea, but he had never imagined that so many tiles could be produced in so short a time, providing the city with a visual unity.

A dashing Moses served as master of ceremonies. There was no doubt now that Ramses would name his old friend vizier and first minister of the country. It was obvious how well they understood each other and how perfectly Moses had realized the pharaoh's plans and wishes for his new capital.

Shaanar was furious. Ofir had either lied about his influence over the Hebrew, or grossly miscalculated. Moses was poised to become a rich man, a devoted courtier. Confronting Ramses over religious differences would be suicide. Besides, his people were so well assimilated that they had no desire to change things. Shaanar's only true allies remained the Hittites. Dangerous as vipers, but allies.

A reception was held in the royal palace, its great columned hall adorned with peaceful, ordered scenes from nature. In this enchanted setting, Nefertari appeared lovelier and more charming than ever. The king's consort, magical protectress of the royal residence, found the right thing to say to each courtier.

Everyone admired the painted-tile flooring, in delightful patterns evoking garden ponds, flowers in bloom, ducks flying in a veritable forest of papyrus, lotuses in full bloom, darting fish. Pale green, light blue, off-white, golden yellow and deep purple blended in a song of colour, praising the perfection of creation.

Scoffers and nay-sayers were reduced to silence. Pi-Ramses' temples were still far from completion, but in terms of luxury and refinement the palace was in every way the equal of Memphis and Thebes. The court could feel quite at home. The aristocracy and government officials were already planning their villas in Pi-Ramses.

Another miracle for Ramses – an incredible string of miracles.

'Nothing you see would exist without this man,' declared Pharaoh, laying a hand on Moses' shoulder. Conversations broke off.

'Protocol dictates that I should sit upon my throne, Moses should prostrate himself before me and I should reward him for his faithful service with collars of gold. But he is my friend, my friend since childhood, and we have worked side by side. I conceived the idea for this capital; he carried out my plans.'

Ramses took Moses in a solemn embrace, the highest accolade a pharaoh could bestow.

'Moses will remain a few more months as head of construction, until his replacement is trained. Then he will come to work at my side for the greater glory of Egypt.'

Shaanar's worst fears were realized. The two of them combined would be harder to deal with than an entire army.

Ahmeni and Setau congratulated Moses and were surprised to note his nervousness. They put it down to the emotion of the moment.

'Ramses is mistaken,' said the Hebrew. 'He's crediting me with qualities I don't possess.'

'You'll make an excellent vizier,' Ahmeni said firmly.

'But you'll have to answer to this wretched little scribe,' teased Setau. 'He's the one who really gives the orders.'

'Watch it, snake man!'

'The food is wonderful. If Lotus and I can unearth some lovely new snakes, we may find a place nearby. Has anyone seen Ahsha? Why isn't he here?'

'No idea,' said Ahmeni.

'You'd think he'd be more diplomatic.'

The three friends saw Ramses walk up to his mother, Tuya, and kiss her on the forehead. Despite the hint of sadness that would never leave her grave and lovely face, Seti's widow shone with pride. When she had announced she was moving her household to the palace for an extended stay at Pi-Ramses, her son's triumph had been complete.

The palace aviary was finished but not yet stocked with the exotic birds that would delight both the ear and the eye. Leaning against a pillar, arms crossed, features drawn and tense, Moses avoided looking Ramses in the eye. He had to forget the man and address an adversary, the Pharaoh of Egypt.

'Everyone is sleeping, except you and me.'

'You look exhausted, Moses. Can't this talk wait until tomorrow?'

'No. I have to stop pretending.'

'Pretending what?'

'I'm a Hebrew. I believe in the One True God. You're an Egyptian and you worship idols.'

'Not this childish nonsense again.'

'It disturbs you because it's the truth.'

'You've been instructed in the wisdom of the Egyptians, Moses. Your One God, shapeless and unknowable, is the hidden power within each speck of life.'

'He isn't incarnated in a sheep!'

331

'Amon is the secret of life, revealing himself in the gust of invisible wind that fills the sails of the barque, in the ram's horns whose spiral traces the harmonious development of all creation, in the stone that gives shape to our temples. He is all that and none of that. You know these ancient teachings as well as I do.'

'It's all an illusion. There's only one God.'

'Does that prevent him from taking the form of his many creatures, while remaining One?'

'He doesn't need your temples and your statues.'

'I'm telling you again, Moses, you've been under too much strain.'

'I know what I believe. Even you can't change that.'

'If your god makes you intolerant, be careful. He'll turn you into a fanatic.'

'You're the one who ought to be careful, Ramses! A movement is gathering strength in this country, still tentative, but a force for the truth.'

'What do you mean?'

'Do you remember Akhenaton and his belief in One God. He blazed the trail. Listen to his voice, Ramses. Listen to me. Or else your empire will crumble.'

58

For Moses, the situation was clear. He hadn't betrayed Ramses' trust and had even warned him of the peril that lay ahead. He could proceed with an easy conscience, following his destiny and unleashing the fire in his heart.

The One God, Yahweh, lived on a mountain. He would go in search of it, no matter how difficult the journey might prove. A few other Hebrews had decided to risk losing everything and leave Egypt with him. As he finished packing, Moses remembered the one pressing matter he should resolve before he said goodbye to his native land.

It was only a short distance to Sary's estate on the west of the city. The house was set in an old and thriving palm grove. He found his old teacher drinking cool beer by a fish pond.

'Moses! What a pleasure to see the real power behind Pi-Ramses! To what do I owe this honour?'

'The pleasure is all yours, and it certainly isn't an honour.'

Sary rose, insulted. 'You may be the man of the hour, but you have no right to be rude. Remember who you're talking to.'

'To a scoundrel.'

Sary struck out at Moses, but the Hebrew caught his wrist. He crumpled and fell to his knees.

'You've been hounding a fellow by the name of Abner.'

'Never heard of him.'

'You're lying, Sary. You stole from him and blackmailed him.'

'He's only a Hebrew brickmaker.'

Moses tightened his grip. Sary groaned.

'I'm only a Hebrew, too,' said Moses, 'but I could break your arm and cripple you.'

'You wouldn't dare.'

'My patience is wearing thin, I warn you. Stop bothering Abner or I'll drag you into court by the scruff of your neck. Now swear it!'

'I . . . I swear not to bother him again.'

'In the name of Pharaoh?'

'The name of Pharaoh.'

'Break your oath and a curse will fall on you.' Moses released him. 'You're getting off easy, old man.'

If he hadn't been in such a hurry to leave the country, he'd have initiated formal proceedings. He hoped a warning would be sufficient, but as he left the house, his mind was not at ease. He had read hatred, not submission, in Sary's eyes.

Moses hid behind a palm tree. He didn't have to wait long.

Carrying a cudgel, Sary slipped out of the house and headed south towards the brickmakers' quarters.

Moses kept a good distance between them until he saw him go through the open door of Abner's house. Almost at once, he heard cries of pain.

He ran into the house and in the semi-darkness saw Sary clubbing Abner, who crouched on the dirt floor, shielding his face with his hands. Moses grabbed the cudgel from Sary and whacked him on the back of the skull. The Egyptian collapsed, blood streaming down his neck.

'Get up, Sary, and get out!'

But Sary lay still.

Abner crept closer. 'Moses . . . it looks like . . . he's dead!'

'He can't be. I didn't hit him that hard!'

'He isn't breathing.'

Moses bent over and touched the body – the corpse?

He had just killed a man.

In the street outside it was quiet.

'Run for it,' said Abner. 'If they arrest you . . .'

'You'll defend me, Abner. You'll explain I was saving your life!'

'Who'd believe me? They'd say it was a cover-up. Go, Moses, go quickly!'

'Have you got a big sack?'

'Yes, for my tools.'

'Let me have it.'

Moses stuffed Sary's body inside and hoisted the sack over his shoulder. He'd find some sandy spot where he could dig a shallow grave, then hide in an unoccupied villa until he could gather his wits.

The police dog let out a high-pitched whine and strained on his leash, which was most unusual for him. When the patrolling guard released him, the hound bolted towards a piece of sand-strewn vacant land.

The dog was digging fast. By the time the patrol caught up, they saw him unearth an arm, then a shoulder, then the face of a dead man.

'I know him,' said one of the policemen. 'It's Sary.'

'The king's brother-in-law?'

'That's the one. Look, there's dried blood on his neck!'

They uncovered the body. There could be no doubt: Sary had been killed by a blow to the back of the head.

All night long, Moses paced like a Syrian bear in its cage. What he'd done was wrong, trying to hide the body of a villain like Sary, fleeing justice when it would have absolved him. But there had been Abner, his fear, his hesitation – and they were both Hebrews. Moses' enemies would be sure to use the incident to bring about his downfall. Even Ramses would side with them and punish him harshly.

Someone had just entered the half-finished villa. The police, so soon? He would put up a fight. He would never surrender.

'Moses, Moses, it's me, Abner! Come out if you're hiding here!'

He stepped from the shadows. 'Will you testify in my favour, Abner?'

'The police have discovered Sary's body. You're accused of murder.'

'But who—'

'My neighbours. They saw you.'

'But they're Hebrews, like us!'

Abner hung his head. 'They don't want trouble with the law. I know how they feel. Run, Moses. You have no future here in Egypt.'

Moses was appalled. The king's construction supervisor and potential first minister reduced to being a fugitive from justice! In the space of a few hours, to fall from the pinnacle into the abyss . . . God must have sent him this suffering to try his faith. Instead of a comfortable but empty life in a heathen country, God was offering him freedom.

'I'll leave at dark. Farewell, Abner.'

Moses passed through the brickmakers' quarters. He hoped to persuade a handful of followers to leave with him and form a sect that would eventually attract other Hebrews, even if their first homeland was only an isolated desert region. He had to set an example, no matter what the cost.

A few lamps shone. Children slept, housewives chatted on doorsteps. Beneath the awnings, their husbands drank herb tea before going off to bed.

In the street where his closest followers lived, two men

were fighting. As he drew near, he could see that it was his two most vocal supporters, quarrelling over a stepladder one had supposedly stolen from the other.

Moses broke up the fight.

'You!' they exclaimed, almost in unison.

'Stop fighting over a trifle and come with me. Let's leave Egypt and go in search of our true homeland.'

The older man eyed Moses with disdain. 'Who made you our prince and our guide? If we don't obey you, will you kill us, as you murdered the Egyptian?'

Stricken, Moses found no answer. A grandiose dream shattered inside him. He was no better than a criminal on the run, utterly abandoned.

59

Ramses insisted on viewing Sary's body. This was the first death in Pi-Ramses since its dedication.

'It was murder, Majesty,' confirmed Serramanna. 'A violent blow to the back of the head with some kind of club.'

'Does my sister know yet?'

'Ahmeni saw to it.'

'Is the suspect in custody?'

'Majesty . . .'

'What aren't you telling me? No matter who it is, he'll be tried and sentenced.'

'Majesty . . . there's a warrant out for Moses.'

'That's absurd.'

'The police have witnesses.'

'Reliable witnesses?'

'All Hebrews. The main accuser is a brickmaker named Abner. He saw it happen.'

'What does he say?'

'That they scuffled and it got out of hand. Moses and Sary were not on the best of terms. My sources tell me they'd already quarrelled in Thebes.'

'What if all the witnesses are wrong? Moses can't be a murderer.'

'Police scribes have recorded sworn statements from all the brickmakers.'

'Moses will explain.'

'No, Majesty. He's fled.'

The pharaoh ordered a search of every house and building in Pi-Ramses, but nothing came of it. Mounted policemen combed the Delta, questioning villagers, but found no trace of Moses. The north-eastern border patrol received strict orders, but they were probably too late.

Ramses was frustrated to find that his daily updates gave no clue as to which route Moses had taken. Was he hiding in a fishing village along the Mediterranean? Had he stowed away in a boat heading south, or taken refuge in some remote temple?

'You must eat something,' urged Nefertari. 'Since Moses disappeared, you really haven't had a good meal.'

Ramses gave his wife's hands a tender squeeze. 'Moses was exhausted. Sary must have provoked him. If he were here in front of me, he could explain. The fact that he ran away tells me he was at his wits' end.'

'Will he be able to live with himself ?'

'I'm afraid he won't.'

'Your dog is sad. It thinks you're neglecting it.'

Ramses let Wideawake jump on his lap. Wriggling with joy, the dog licked its master's face, then rested its head on his shoulder.

Ramses' three years on the throne had been wonderful. The additions to Luxor completed, the Temple of a Million Years under way, the new capital dedicated, Nubia under control and now this calamity! Without Moses, the world Ramses had begun to build would begin to crumble.

'You've been neglecting me, too,' said Nefertari in a hushed voice. 'Can't I help you rise above this suffering?'

'Yes. Only you can do it.'

Shaanar and Ofir met by the docks at Pi-Ramses, now bustling with activity. Foodstuffs, furnishings, household goods and countless other supplies needed in the new capital were being unloaded every day. Boats brought in donkeys, horses and cattle. The grain silos filled, cellars were stocked with fine wines. Discussions as heated as any in Memphis or Thebes were heard among the merchants vying to establish trade in the new capital.

'Now Moses is only a wanted killer, Ofir.'

'It doesn't seem to upset you much.'

'You were wrong about him. He would never have changed sides. His rash action has cost Ramses a valued associate.'

'Moses is an honest man. His faith in the One God is no mere whim,' said the sorcerer.

'Let's stick to the facts. Either he'll turn himself in or he'll be arrested and sentenced. We no longer have any hope of using the Hebrews.'

'Those who believe in Amon are no strangers to adversity. We've struggled on for years. This won't stop us. I hope we can count on your help.'

'Don't press me. I need to know about your concrete plans,' said Shaanar.

'Every night I work to undermine the health of the royal couple.'

'He's at the height of his power! Then there's the Temple of a Million Years too.'

'Pi-Ramses is the only one of his projects that Ramses has completed. We'll have to capitalize on the slightest sign of weakness, be ready to rush in when the first breach opens.'

The sorcerer's manner, calm yet firm, impressed Shaanar. If the Hittites succeeded with their plan, Ramses' *ka* would certainly be weakened. Ofir's magical attacks would further sap the king's strength. Resilient as he was, eventually Ramses would falter.

'Keep it up, Ofir. Perhaps you've heard that I never forget a favour.'

Setau and Lotus had decided to set up a new laboratory at Pi-Ramses. Ahmeni, in his smart new offices, worked day and night. Tuya kept the court running smoothly. Nefertari performed her religious and queenly duties. Iset the Fair and Nedjem were busy bringing up Kha. Meritamon was blooming. Remet the steward puffed from palace kitchens to wine cellar, wine cellar to state dining-room. Serramanna tinkered with his security procedures. Life in Pi-Ramses was orderly and peaceful, but for Ramses nothing was the same without Moses.

Despite their differences, his old friend's strength had been a gift that helped Ramses achieve his vision. Moses had put his soul into the city he left behind, and it showed. Their final conversation proved that his friend had fallen victim to evil influences, was caught in invisible bonds.

A spell – someone had cast a spell on him.

Ahmeni, juggling an armload of scrolls, hurried towards the king as he paced his audience chamber.

'Ahsha has just arrived. He wants to see you.'

'Show him in.'

Although suave in his elegant pale-green robe with red trim, the young diplomat looked less stylish than usual.

'It distressed me that you missed the dedication,' Ramses told him.

'The head of the secretariat represented me, Majesty.'

'But where were you?'

'In Memphis, collecting the dispatches from my information network.'

'Shaanar mentioned Hittite troop movements in central Syria.'

'It's more than troop movements, and it goes much farther than Syria,' Ahsha said with uncharacteristic gruffness.

'I thought my dear brother might be exaggerating. He likes to make himself look important.'

'If anything, he minimized the danger. Now that I've checked my own sources, I'm convinced that the Hittites have launched a full-scale campaign in Caanan and Syria – all of Syria. Even the ports of Lebanon are under threat.'

'Have there been direct attacks on our garrisons?'

'Not yet, but they've moved into areas we considered neutral and taken villages. Before this it's only been political manoeuvring in our territories, apparently non-violent, but in practice the Hittites have taken control of Egyptian territory – provinces under our jurisdiction and supposedly sending us tributes.'

Ramses bent over the map of the Near East spread out on a low table.

'The Hittites are working their way down a corridor to our north-east. They plan to invade,' the king predicted.

'It's too early to be sure, Majesty.'

'Why else would they be heading in this direction?'

'To extend their territory, cut us off, sow panic in our protectorates, hurt Egypt's reputation, demoralize our army . . . Take your pick.'

'What does it look like to you?'

'Like war.'

Ramses drew a quick slash of red ink across the Anatolian peninsula, home of the Hittites.

'These people love only savagery, blood and violence. Unless we stop them, they will endanger civilization as we know it.'

'Diplomacy . . .'

'Too late for that.'

'Your father negotiated—'

'A buffer zone around Kadesh, I know. But the Hittites won't honour it. They honour nothing. I demand a daily report on their movements.'

Ahsha bowed. Ramses no longer spoke as a friend, but as a commanding pharaoh.

'Have you heard that Moses is a fugitive from justice, wanted for murder?'

'Moses? It's unbelievable.'

'I think he's the victim of a plot. Put out a message through your network, Ahsha, and find him for me.'

Nefertari was playing the lute in the palace garden. To her right lay the cradle where her plump and rosy-cheeked daughter napped; on her left sat Kha, cross-legged, reading a tale full of wizards and demons. Just in front of her was Wideawake, trying to dig up a tamarisk sapling Ramses had planted the day before. Nose in the dirt, front paws flying, he worked so hard that the queen didn't have the heart to scold him.

Suddenly he stopped and ran to the garden gate. His joyful barking and jumping could only mean a visit from his master.

The sound of her husband's footsteps told Nefertari that his heart was heavy. She rose to meet him.

'Is it Moses?'

'No, I'm sure he's all right.'

'Not . . . not Tuya.'

'My mother is fine.'

'Tell me what's wrong.'

'It's Egypt, Nefertari. The dream is over – the dream of a country where peace and prosperity rule, where each day is a blessing.'

The queen shut her eyes. 'War?'

He nodded. 'It's unavoidable.'

'You're leaving, then.'

'Who else should command the army? If we don't stop the Hittites, it's death to Egypt.'

Little Kha glanced up at the embracing couple, then

went back to his story. Meritamon napped. Wideawake kept digging.

In the tranquil garden, Nefertari clung to Ramses. In the distance, a white ibis took flight above the wheat fields.

'War will separate us, Ramses. Where will we find the courage to go on?'

'In the love that unites us and always will, no matter what happens. While I'm gone, you, my Great Royal Wife, will reign in my Turquoise City.'

Nefertari gazed into the distance.

'You're right to go,' she told him. 'Never negotiate with evil.'

The white ibis soared majestically above the royal pair, bathed in the glow of sunset.